Food Toxicology
A Perspective on the
Relative Risks

ift Basic Symposium Series

Edited by
INSTITUTE OF FOOD TECHNOLOGISTS
221 N. LaSalle St.
Chicago, Illinois

Foodborne Microorganisms and Their Toxins:
Developing Methodology *edited by Merle D.
Pierson and Norman J. Stern*

Water Activity: Theory and Applications to
Food *edited by Louis B. Rockland and
Larry R. Beuchat*

Nutrient Interactions *edited by C. E. Bodwell
and John W. Erdman, Jr.*

Food Toxicology: A Perspective on the Relative
Risks *edited by Steven L. Taylor and Richard
A. Scanlan*

Food Toxicology
A Perspective on the Relative Risks

edited by

Steven L. Taylor
University of Nebraska—Lincoln
Lincoln, Nebraska

Richard A. Scanlan
Oregon State University
Corvallis, Oregon

Marcel Dekker, Inc.   New York and Basel

Library of Congress Cataloging-in-Publication Data

Food toxicology : a perspective on the relative risks / edited by
  Steven L. Taylor, Richard A. Scanlan.
      p.   cm. -- (IFT basic symposium series)
    Proceedings of a symposium sponsored by the Institute of Food
  Technologists (IFT) and the International Union of Food Science and
  Technology, held June 17-18, 1988 in New Orleans.
    Includes bibliographies and index.
    ISBN 0-8247-8141-4 (alk. paper)
    1. Food contamination--Health aspects--Congresses.
  2. Carcinogens--Congresses. 3. Food poisoning--Congresses.
  I. Taylor, Steven L. II. Scanlan, Richard A.
  III. Institute of Food Technologists. IV. International Union of
  Food Science and Technology. V. Series.
    [DNLM: 1. Carcinogens--toxicity--congresses. 2. Food Additives-
    -toxicity--congresses. 3. Food Contamination--congresses. 4. Risk
  Factors--congresses. WA 712 F686 1988]
  RA1258.F65   1989
  615.9'54--dc20
  DNLM/DLC
                                                          89-12081
                                                              CIP

This book is printed on acid-free paper.

MARCEL DEKKER, INC.
270 Madison Avenue, New York, New York 10016

Current printing (last digit);
10 9 8 7 6 5 4 3 2 1

PRINTED IN THE UNITED STATES OF AMERICA

Preface

The Institute of Food Technologists (IFT) and the International Union of Food Science and Technology each year sponsor a two-day basic symposium, held in conjunction with the annual IFT meeting. The contents of this book are the proceedings of the 12th Basic Symposium, "Food Toxicology: A Perspective on the Relative Risks," which was held June 17–18, 1988, immediately prior to the 48th Annual IFT Meeting in New Orleans.

During the past 20 years we have witnessed a dramatic increase in public awareness of the safety and wholesomeness of the food supply. A very specific example of the public's concern and anxiety regarding protection from exogenous carcinogens was the passage of Proposition 65 in California several years ago. During the past 20 years there have been significant changes in the way in which food is processed and distributed on a worldwide basis. These changes present formidable challenges to people in the food industry and in regulatory agencies who are responsible for the safety and wholesomeness of our food.

During this same period of time, and particularly over the past decade, there has been a great deal of activity on the part of academicians, people in the food industry, and people in regulatory agencies to improve our knowledge base and to improve our ability to define and control risks associated with deleterious substances in food. Some of the people from academia, from the food industry, and from governmental agencies who have been involved in these activities were speakers at the symposium and are authors of the chapters in this book.

Much of the attention has been focused on the carcinogens that find their way into our food. Accordingly, several chapters are devoted to selected groups of carcinogens such as mycotoxins and N-nitroso compounds. Not all food toxicology problems relate to risks for cancer, so we included several chapters that deal with risk factors other than carcinogens. Finally, there are several chapters in which authors from various backgrounds provide overall perspectives on how risk assessment has progressed and how it is being used in making difficult regulatory decisions.

This symposium was the result of discussions by the symposium organizers when they were members of the Committee on Food Protection, National Research Council/National Academy of Sciences several years ago. The purpose of the symposium was to provide an update and a discussion of the many issues involved in defining and dealing with risk from deleterious substances in our food.

The symposium organizers want to thank the members of the IFT Basic Symposium Committee for approval and support of the program. The committee members included Drs. Merle D. Pierson (Chairman), R. V. Josephson (Past Chairman), J. A. Maga, R. A. Scanlan, C. Akin, B. Klein, V. N. Mohan Rao, L. Wicker, and N. Fogg-Johnson. We are grateful for enthusiastic support and help from R. E. Morse, 1987–1988 IFT President, H. W. Mattson, IFT Executive Director, J. B. Klis, IFT Director of Publications, Anna May Schenck, JFS Associate, Scientific Editor, and other IFT staff members who provided support and coordination for the symposium.

Most especially, the speakers and contributing authors are gratefully acknowledged for their contributions to the symposium and this book. It is their expertise and hard work that resulted in a successful symposium and publication of this volume.

Steven L. Taylor
Richard A. Scanlan

Contributors

Paul B. Addis, Ph.D. Professor, Department of Food Science and Nutrition, University of Minnesota, St. Paul, Minnesota

George S. Bailey, Ph.D. Professor, Department of Food Science and Technology, Oregon State University, Corvallis, Oregon

Wayne R. Bidlack, Ph.D. Associate Professor, Department of Pharmacology and Nutrition, University of Southern California School of Medicine, Los Angeles, California

R. H. Dashwood, Ph.D. Research Associate, Department of Food Science and Technology, Oregon State University, Corvallis, Oregon

Bob J. Dull, Ph.D. Senior Research Biochemist, Technical Resource Center/Corporate Research and Development, McCormick & Company, Inc., Hunt Valley, Maryland

Andrew G. Ebert, Ph.D. Senior Vice President, The Robert H. Kellen Company, Atlanta, Georgia

Clausen Ely, Jr. Partner, Covington & Burling, Washington, D.C.

W. Gary Flamm, Ph.D.* Director, Office of Toxicological Sciences,

---

Present affiliation: Health Science Solutions, Rockville, Maryland, and Reston, Virginia

Department of Health and Human Services, Food and Drug Administration, Reston, Virginia

Dian A. Gans, Ph.D. Assistant Scientist, Department of Nutritional Sciences, University of Wisconsin–Madison, Madison, Wisconsin

Richard L. Hall, Ph.D. Vice President, Science and Technology, McCormick & Company, Inc., Hunt Valley, Maryland

Jerry D. Hendricks, Ph.D. Professor, Department of Food Science and Technology, Oregon State University, Corvallis, Oregon

Sara Hale Henry, Ph.D. Toxicologist, Division of Toxicology, Food and Drug Administration, Washington, D.C.

Joseph H. Hotchkiss, Ph.D. Associate Professor, Institute of Food Science, Cornell University, Ithaca, New York

Dennis P. H. Hsieh Department of Environmental Toxicology, University of California at Davis, Davis, California

Ian C, Munro, Ph.D., FRCPATH Director, Canadian Center for Toxicology, Guelph, Ontario, Canada

Minako Nagao National Cancer Center, Tokyo, Japan

Julie A. Nordlee Department of Food Science and Technology and Food Processing Center, Institute of Agriculture and Natural Resources, University of Nebraska-Lincoln, Lincoln, Nebraska

Hiroko Ohgaki National Cancer Center, Tokyo, Japan

Michael W. Pariza, Ph.D. Director, Chairman, Professor, Department of Food Microbiology and Toxicology, Food Research Institute, University of Wisconsin–Madison, Madison, Wisconsin

Seok-Won Park, Ph.D.* Assistant Research Chemist, Food Protein Research and Development Center, Texas A&M University, College Station, Texas

Donald J. Reed, Ph.D. Professor, Department of Biochemistry and Biophysics, Oregon State University, Corvallis, Oregon

John F. Riebow, M. S. Graduate Student, Department of Pharmacology and Nutrition, University of Southern California School of Medicine, Los Angeles, California

Alan M. Rulis, Ph.D. Chief, Regulatory Food Chemistry Branch, Center for Food Safety and Applied Nutrition, Food and Drug Administration,

---

*Present affiliation: Food and Nutrition Research, Bristol-Meyers U.S. Pharmaceutical and Nutritional Group, Evansville, Indiana

Washington, D.C.

John H. Rupnow Department of Food Science and Technology and Food Processing Center, Institute of Agriculture and Natural Resources, University of Nebraska—Lincoln, Lincoln, Nebraska

Robert J. Schleuplein, Ph.D. Acting Director, Office of Toxicological Sciences, Center for Food Safety and Applied Nutrition, Food and Drug Administration, Washington, D.C.

Takashi Sugimura National Cancer Center, Tokyo, Japan

Steven L. Taylor, Ph.D. Professor and Head, Department of Food Science and Technology and Food Processing Center, Institute of Agriculture and Natural Resources, University of Nebraska—Lincoln, Lincoln, Nebraska

Keiji Wakabayashi National Cancer Center, Tokyo, Japan

David E. Williams, Ph.D. Assistant Professor, Department of Food Science and Technology, Oregon State University, Corvallis, Oregon

Contents

Preface   iii

Contributors   v

1 A Perspective on Diet and Cancer   1
Michael W. Pariza

Introduction   1
Trends in Cancer Mortality   2
Carcinogens in Food   3
Anticarcinogens in Food   3
Enhancement of Carcinogenesis by Diet   6
Conclusion   8
References   8

2 Carcinogenic Potential of Mycotoxins in Foods   11
Dennis P. H. Hsieh

Mycotoxins in Foods   11
Evidence of Carcinogenicity   14
Carcinogenicity Bioassays in Animals   14
Human Susceptibility to Aflatoxin Carcinogenicity   16
Epidemiological Evidence   17

Evidence Against Aflatoxin as a Human Carcinogen   20
Role of Hepatitis B Virus   21
Joint Effect of Aflatoxin and HBV in LCC Development   22
Control of Mycotoxins in the Prevention of Human   23
    Liver Cancer
Perspective of Relative Risks   24
References   25

3 **Heterocyclic Amines in Cooked Food**   31
   Takashi Sugimura, Keiji Wakabayashi,
   Minako Nagao, and Hiroko Ohgaki

Introduction   31
History of Studies on Heterocyclic Amines in   32
    Cooked Foods
Chemistry of Heterocyclic Amines   33
Carcinogenicity of Heterocyclic Amines   36
Metabolism and Mutagenicity of Heterocyclic Amines   38
Relation Between Carcinogenicity and Mutagenicity   40
    of Heterocyclic Amines
Relevancy of Heterocyclic Amines to Carcinogenicity   43
    in Humans and Primates
Enhancement and Suppression of Biological Activity   43
    of Heterocyclic Amines
Quantitation of Heterocyclic Amines in Foods   44
Other Effects of Heterocyclic Amines   46
Future Prospects and Implications   46
References   47

4 **Relative Exposure to Nitrite, Nitrate, and N-Nitroso**   57
   Compounds from Endogenous and Exogenous Sources
   Joseph H. Hotchkiss

Introduction   57
Exposure to Exogenously Formed Nitrate and Nitrite   64
Exposure to Endogenously Formed Nitrate and Nitrite   67
Exposure to Exogenously Formed N-Nitroso Compounds   70
Endogenous Formation of Nitroso Compounds   76
Factors Affecting Endogenous Nitrosation   82
Relative Exposure/Risks from Endogenous Versus   85
    Exogenous Nitroso Compounds
Conclusions   90
References   92

5 **Anticarcinogens and Tumor Promoters in Foods**   101
   David E. Williams, R.H. Dashwood, Jerry D. Hendricks,
   and George S. Bailey

   Introduction   101
   Anticarcinogenesis by Food Components   103
     and Additives
   Tumor Promoters in Foods   117
   Protocol-Dependent Tumor Enhancement by   119
     Some Anticarcinogens
   Mechanisms of Anticarcinogenesis   123
   Summary   135
   References   135

6 **A Case Study: The Safety Evaluation of Artificial**   151
   Sweeteners
   Ian C. Munro

   Introduction   151
   Toxicological Studies on Cyclamate   152
   Toxicological Studies on Saccharin   153
   Promotion Studies with Sweeteners   154
   Mouse Studies with Cyclamate   155
   Conclusions   161
   References   162

7 **Glutathione and Vitamin E in Protection Against**   169
   Mutagens and Carcinogens
   Donald J. Reed

   Introduction   169
   General Concepts of Protection   170
   Types of Protection   173
   Cellular Aspects of Protection   184
   References   192

8 **Comparison of the Carcinogenic Risks of**   205
   Naturally Occurring and Adventitious Substances in Food
   Richard L. Hall, Bob J. Dull, Sara Hale Henry, Robert J.
   Schleuplein, and Alan M. Rulis

   Introduction   205
   Risk Comparisons   208
   Risk Assessment   209

Pesticides   211
Naturally Occurring Compounds   214
Discussion   219
References   221

9   Behavioral Disorders Associated with Food Components   225
Dian A. Gans

Introduction   225
Influence of Nutritional Status on Behavior   226
Nutritive Sweeteners and Behavior   230
Towards a More Objective Methodology   241
References   245

10   Food Allergies and Sensitivities   255
Steven L. Taylor, Julie A. Nordlee, and John H. Rupnow

Introduction   255
True Food Allergies   258
Food Sensitivities   271
References   283

11   Role of Lipid Oxidation Products in Atherosclerosis   297
Paul B. Addis and Seok-Won Park

Introduction   297
Atherosclerosis   300
Role of Oxidized Lipids   310
Lipoproteins and Diet   317
Thrombosis and Spasm   320
Conclusions   321
References   324

12   Toxicological and Pharmacological Interactions as   331
Influenced by Diet and Nutrition
Wayne R. Bidlack and John F. Riebow

Introduction   331
Physiological Parameters   333
Conclusions   376
References   378

13 Regulatory Distinctions Between Naturally   397
Occurring and Added Substances in Food
Clausen Ely, Jr.

Regulation of Naturally Occurring Substances   398
  in Food
Regulation of Added Substances in Food   400
Regulation Under California Proposition 65   402
Conclusion   405
Notes   405

14 Strengths and Limitations of Toxicological   407
Testing Procedures
Andrew G. Ebert

Introduction   407
Systems in Toxicology Testing—The Decision Tree   408
Limitations in Toxicological Testing   416
Limitations in Toxicology Studies—The Decreasing Zero   418
IARC/NTP and Expert Committees   421
Lists from Lists   422
References   427

15 Pros and Cons of Quantitative Risk Analysis   429
W. Gary Flamm

Introduction and Background   429
Basic Assumptions of QRA   433
Alternatives to QRA   437
The Pros   440
The Cons   442
Hope for the Future   444
References   445

Index   447

Food Toxicology
A Perspective on the
Relative Risks

1
A Perspective on Diet and Cancer

Michael W. Pariza

University of Wisconsin–Madison
Madison, Wisconsin

INTRODUCTION

Food safety is a complex and multifaceted subject. It is a matter that the public is intensely interested in, and for this reason hardly a day goes by without some mention of food safety in the popular press. Unfortunately, but perhaps understandably, the public's perception of this issue is somewhat different from that of many scientists conducting research in the area or charged with maintaining the safety of the food supply.

Popular articles written for the public often focus on diet/health issues. Examples include numerous articles on diet and cancer, which tend to conclude that the risk of developing some major cancers may be reduced by selecting the "right foods." Invariably such articles include a list of foods to eat and foods to avoid.

By contrast, the U.S. Food and Drug Administration (FDA), the federal agency that is charged with protecting the nation's food supply, has expressed a somewhat different view of food safety risks (Schmidt, 1975). The FDA has concluded that of the potential sources of harm associated with foods, the largest by far is microbiological contamination, followed closely by nutritional imbalance including the excessive consumption of food as well as nutritional deficiencies. By contrast, the emotionally

1

charged issues of pesticide residues and the use of food additives are of much less public health significance.

Microbiological issues are usually straightforward: dangerous microorganisms and microbial toxins should not be in food, and foods that contain them at levels that can cause illness should not be consumed. Anyone who is familiar with the evidence is bound to agree with the FDA's conviction that microbial contamination is the most serious of the known hazards to health that are associated with food.

By contrast, issues like diet and cancer are considerably more uncertain. Cancer is a very complex disease, the origins of which are only dimly understood. Diet and nutrition may affect it, but we don't yet know how.

TRENDS IN CANCER MORTALITY

The American Cancer Society (ACS) publishes annual summaries of changes in cancer mortality in the U.S. (ACS, 1987). Cancer is basically a disease of old age, meaning that your chance of contracting it goes up with each birthday, so the ACS adjusts their data to compensate for the fact that the average age of Americans is higher today than it was in years past.

The ACS data reveal some surprising trends. Death from stomach cancer used to be very common but today is rare. Since the 1930s it has steadily declined. On the other hand, death from lung cancer used to be very rare but today is common. Since the 1930s it has steadily increased. Death from virtually all other forms of cancer has remained relatively constant for the past 50 years. In fact, were it not for lung cancer we would be experiencing a significant overall decline in age-adjusted cancer mortality.

These trends have developed in the face of the revolutionary changes in food production, processing, and preservation methods that have occurred during the past 50 years, including the now widespread use of pesticides, food additives, and processed fats and oils. There is nothing in the U.S. cancer death statistics to indicate that any of these changes has been harmful.

There's another side to this coin, however. (Did I hear someone say that there always is—just ask any professor?) Since cancer risk increases with age, and because the U.S. population is aging, it follows that the overall cancer death rate (not adjusted for age) must also be on the rise. This in fact is true, all the more given that deaths from other killer diseases, such as heart disease and stroke, are declining (CAST, 1987). More of us will die of cancer because we will live longer, and our risk of dying from another chronic affliction is declining. Whether this represents good or bad news is, of course, a subject for debate.

CARCINOGENS IN FOOD

It does not take an expert to note that there is widespread public concern about carcinogens in food. This too is a bad news/good news issue, but the former is often emphasized to the neglect of the latter.

The bad news is that exposure to dietary carcinogens is an unavoidable fact of life. Given the large number of naturally occurring carcinogens in the environment, it is now (and undoubtedly always will be) impossible to eat a meal devoid of traces of these substances (Ames, 1983; CAST, 1987). Further, as analytical methods are refined and more chemicals studied for carcinogenic activity, this bad news will seemingly mount.

On the other hand, the concentration of carcinogens in the diet is amenable to management through technology. Improvements in detection and control continuously move the dietary carcinogen exposure level downward. More importantly, based on growing scientific evidence (Boutwell, 1985), it is virtually certain that today in the U.S. the levels of dietary carcinogens are not the limiting factor in determining cancer risk. There is no reason whatever to believe that further reduction in the already very low levels of carcinogens in our diet will perceptibly reduce the incidence of cancer. This view may seem extraordinary, perhaps even revolutionary, but it is one that I share with many colleagues in the diet/cancer research field (Boutwell, 1985).

ANTICARCINOGENS IN FOOD

Another bit of good news about our food supply is that it contains numerous anticarcinogens, substances that inhibit carcinogenesis in animal models (Wattenberg, 1983). Personally I find anticarcinogens to be particularly interesting. They belong to a larger class of substances that modulate carcinogenesis and hence may appropriately be referred to as modulators.

Modulators include tumor promoters and enhancers as well as inhibitors. Paradoxically, many modulators both inhibit and enhance carcinogenesis in animals, depending on conditions of test. Some modulators, like the phenolic antioxidant butylated hydroxyanisole (BHA), may actually appear to cause (initiate) cancer in some rodent strains when fed at relatively high levels for prolonged periods (Lam, 1988). However, when fed at lower levels for limited periods of time, the same substance affords protection against the deleterious effects of concurrent exposure to a carcinogen such as benzo[a]pyrene (Wattenberg, 1983).

There is limited epidemiological evidence that anticarcinogens in food may provide humans with some protection against cancer. It has been suggested that ensuring adequate intake of such substances may prove to be the most practical way to reduce cancer risk via dietary means (Doll and Peto, 1981). Of course, implementation of this proposal depends on identifying the most important dietary anticarcinogens and establishing a safe and effective level of intake. Unfortunately studies to date of specific potential anticarcinogens, such as *beta*-carotene, have been disappointing (Pariza, 1988).

Perhaps we expect too much. The process of carcinogenesis is multidimensional and its modulation complex and paradoxical. It is naive to hope for a single dietary "magic bullet." We must even consider the possibility that a factor that inhibits cancer in me may have no effect upon, or may even enhance, cancer in you.

However, there is reason for guarded hope. In an ongoing prospective epidemiological investigation in Japan, Hirayama (1985) has found that the risk of dying from colon cancer is much lower among subjects who report consuming both meat and green and yellow vegetables on a daily basis (Table 1.1). By contrast, colon cancer mortality was 3 to 4 times greater for those eating on a daily basis meat but not vegetables, but not meat, or neither meat nor vegetables. One interpretation of these findings is that anticarcinogens in foods of both plant and animal origin may act in concert to reduce cancer risk.

TABLE 1.1 Relationship Between Daily Meat or Vegetable Consumption and Colon Cancer Risk

Dietary pattern	Colon cancer risk (rate per 100,000)
Neither meat nor vegetables on a daily basis	14.9
Meat but not vegetables on a daily basis	18.43
Vegetables but not meat on a daily basis	13.67
Meat and vegetables on a daily basis	3.87

Source: Hirayama (1985).

Much has been written about potential cancer inhibitors from foods of plant origins (Wattenberg, 1983), but what of inhibitors from foods of animal origin? There's calcium, of course (Lipkin and Newmark, 1985), but what else? Recently, in my laboratory, we isolated and identified a new anticarcinogen from fried ground beef (Ha et al., 1987). The material, which we call CLA, is composed of four isomeric derivatives of linoleic acid each and containing a conjugated double bond system. Figure 1.1 depicts a model for CLA formation from linoleic acid during heating. Synthetically prepared CLA, containing all four isomers, provides partial protection to mice from the initiation of epidermal and forestomach carcinogenesis by chemical carcinogens. The individual isomers have not yet been separated in sufficient quantity for individual testing. We are finding CLA in many heat-processed foods (Ha et al., 1988). Obviously the significance of these observations in terms of the potential for reducing the risk for certain cancers in humans in not yet known, but we are struck

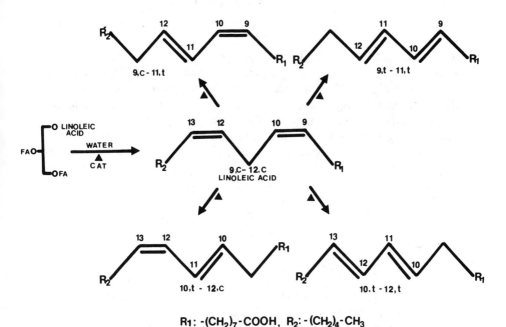

R_1: -$(CH_2)_7$-COOH, R_2: - $(CH_2)_4$-CH_3

FIG. 1.1 Model for the formation of CLA (isomeric derivatives of linoleic acid containing a conjugated double bond system) in ground beef during frying. (*From Ha et al., 1987.*)

by the fact that a derivative of a fatty acid, a constituent of fats and oils, is also an anticarcinogen.

ENHANCEMENT OF CARCINOGENESIS BY DIET

The prevalent scientific view is that diet influences cancer risk by modulating (either inhibiting or enhancing) the process of carcinogenesis. We have some hints as to what dietary factors might be involved, but there are still numerous, serious gaps in our knowledge base (Pariza, 1984;1988). In my opinion a good deal of the difficulty is conceptual. Diet and nutrition are all too often thought of in an isolated sense, as though they can be cleanly separated from other lifestyle factors. An individual's cancer risk is better thought of as the result of several interacting factors, specifically genetic, physiological, and lifestyle factors. Diet should be considered a part of lifestyle, but certainly not the whole of lifestyle.

We have considered inhibition of cancer by dietary factors. What about enhancement? The factor most closely linked to enhancement of carcinogenesis is dietary fat (NRC, 1982). In fact, it is commonly asserted that dietary fat has been conclusively shown to increase one's risk of developing certain cancers, particularly breast and colon cancer. However, two recently published prospective epidemiological studies (Willett et al., 1987; Jones et al, 1987) have failed to confirm a relationship between dietary fat consumption and breast cancer risk. Mormons, a religious group residing predominately in the Western United States, exhibit a relatively low death rate from breast (and colon) cancer, yet they are not vegetarians and in fact consume at least as much dietary fat as non-Mormon Americans (Doll and Peto, 1981). The relatively low death rate from breast cancer among U.S. Seventh-Day Adventist women has been attributed in part to the result of better survival due to earlier diagnosis and treatment rather than to dietary practice (Zollinger et al., 1984). (Seventh-Day Adventists are a religious group that practice lacto-ovo vegetarianism.)

Based on these and other epidemiological studies as well as new data from experiments with animals, there is now a notable shift in thinking among scientists away from concentrating on dietary fat per se in favor of more encompassing lifestyle issues like total energy intake vs. expenditure (Pariza and Simopoulos, 1987). This change in thinking is the result of a recognition of complications that involve various factors such as ad libitum feeding and differences in efficiency of utilization of calories from different sources. In particular, total caloric intake appears to be more important than the amount of dietary fat per se.

For example, in the study (Boissonneault et al., 1986) summarized in Table 1.2, female F344 rats were treated with a carcinogen to initiate mammary carcinogenesis and then divided into three groups. Two groups were fed a diet containing 30% fat by weight, referred to as "high-fat" because 60% of the calories came from fat (this is considerably higher than the typical U.S., diet where 35–40% of the calories come from fat).The third group was fed a diet containing 5% fat by weight, referred to as "low-fat" because only about 10% of the calories came from fat. The low-fat group and one of the high-fat groups were fed ad libitum. The other high-fat group was fed under conditions of very modest calorie restriction of about 15%.

Rats in both the high-fat and low-fat ad libitum fed groups consumed similar numbers of calories, but the animals on the high-fat diet ate more fat. This group was also heavier because the calories in the high-fat diet were utilized more efficiently, a conclusion supported by body composition analyses. During the experimental period 73% of the high-fat ad libitum fed rats developed mammary cancer compared with 43% for the low-fat ad libitum fed animals.

For the rats fed the high-fat diet under modest conditions of restriction the calorie consumption was reduced, but the animals weighed the same

TABLE 1.2 Effect of Dietary Regimen on Carcinogen-induced Mammary Carcinoma Incidence in Rats

	Dietary regimen		
	High-fat ad lib.	Low-fat ad lib.	High-fat restricted
Kcal consumption per day	41 Kcal	42 Kcal	34 Kcal
Fat consumption per day	2.7 g	0.6 g	2.2 g
Linoleic acid intake per day	1.5 g	0.3 g	1.2 g
Body weight	217 g	190 g	182 g
Body composition			
% body fat	24%	16%	25%
% body protein	20%	23%	20%
Retained energy	752 Kcal	532 Kcal	634 Kcal
Tumor incidence	73%	43%	7%

Source: Boissonneault et al. (1986).

as those fed the low-fat diet ad libitum. Their body compositions were more like the rats fed the high-fat diet ad libitum. They had simply matured at a smaller body size. For this group the tumor incidence was only 7%, even though these animals ate three times as much fat as the low-fat ad libitum fed group and almost as much as the high-fat ad libitum fed group. Hence, total caloric intake was much more important than total fat intake.

There is now a considerable and growing body of evidence indicating that excessive caloric intake may be a risk factor for cancer in man, whereas physical activity may be protective (Pariza and Simopoulos, 1987). Animal studies indicate that moderate levels of calorie restriction and physical activity induce favorable changes in hormonal balance. Hormones thought to be important are prolactin, excessive levels of which may promote mammary cancer, and the glucocorticoids, which have been shown to retard the development of several tumor types, including mammary cancer. Moderate calorie restriction appears to decrease the levels of prolactin while also increasing the levels of the glucocorticoids (Pariza, 1987).

CONCLUSION

We urgently need comprehensive and thorough studies on the biochemical mechanisms whereby dietary and related lifestyle factors affect (enhance or inhibit) carcinogenesis in animal models. A thorough understanding of mechanisms will permit us to determine how humans might respond. With such information it may be possible to formulate an anticancer strategy involving diet and lifestyle considerations that is both effective and safe.

REFERENCES

ACS. 1987. *Cancer Facts and Figures.* American Cancer Society, New York

Ames, B. N. 1983. Dietary carcinogens and anticarcinogens. *Science* 221: 1256

Boissonneault, G. A., Elson, C. E., and Pariza, M. W. 1986. Net energy effects of dietary fat on chemically induced mammary carcinogenesis in F344 rats. *J. Natl. Cancer Inst.* 76: 335.

Boutwell, R. K. 1985. Tumor promoters in human carcinogenesis. Ch. 2. In *Important Advances in Oncology,* (Ed.) DeVita, V. T., Hellman, S., and Rosenberg, S. A., p. 16. J.B. Lippincott, Philadelphia.

CAST. 1987. *Diet and Health,* Report No. 111. Council for Agricultural Science and Technology, Ames, IA.

Doll, R. and Peto, R. 1981. The causes of cancer: Quantitative estimates of avoidable risks of cancer in the United States today. *J. Natl. Cancer Inst.* 66: 1191

Hirayama, T. 1985. Diet and cancer: feasibility and importance of prospective cohort study. In *Diet and Human Carcinogenesis,* (Ed.) Joossens, J.V., Hill, M.J., and Geboers, J. Elsevier, Amsterdam/New York.

Ha, Y. L., Grimm, N. K., and Pariza, M. W. 1987. Anticarcinogens from fried ground beef: heat-altered derivatives of linoleic acid. *Carcinogenesis* 8: 1881.

Ha, Y. L., Grimm, N. K., and Pariza, M. W. 1988. Anticarcinogenic fatty acids from fried ground beef. *FASEB J.* 2: A1192 (Abs. 5208).

Jones, D. Y., Shatzkin, A., Green, S. B., Block, G., Brinton, L. A., Ziegler, R. G., Hoover, R., and Taylor, P. R. 1987. Dietary fat and breast cancer in the National Health and Nutrition Examination Survey I epidemiologic follow-up study. *J. Natl. Cancer Inst.* 79: 465.

Lam, L. 1988. Carcinogenesis. In press.

Lipkin, M. and Newmark, H. 1985. Effect of added dietary calcium on colon epithelial-cell proliferation in subjects at high risk for familial colonic cancer. *New England J. Med.* 313: 1381

NRC. 1982 *Diet, Nutrition, and Cancer.* National Academy Press, Washington, DC.

Pariza, M. W. 1984. A perspective on diet, nutrition, and cancer *JAMA* 251: 1455

Pariza, M. W. 1987. Dietary fat, calorie restriction, ad libitum feeding, and cancer risk. *Nutr. Rev.* 45: 1.

Pariza, M. W. 1988. Dietary fat and cancer risk: Evidence and research need. *Ann. Rev. Nutr.* 8: 167

Pariza, M. W. and Simopoulos, A.P. (Guest Ed.). 1987. Calories and energy expenditure in carcinogenesis. *Amer. J. Clin. Nutr.* 45(Supp.): 149.

Schmidt, A. M. 1975. Address given at the symposium, *Food Safety—A Century of Progress,* celebrating the hundredth anniversary of the Food and Drugs Act at London, Oct. 20–21, 1975 [cited in *Fd. Cosmetics Toxicol.* 16 (Supp. 2): 15, 1978].

Wattenberg, L. W. 1983. Inhibition of neoplasia by minor dietary constituents. *Cancer Res.* (Supp.) 43: 2448s.

Willett, W. C., Stampfer, M. J., Colditz, G. A., Rosner, B. A., Hennekens, C. H., et al. 1987. Dietary fat and the risk of breast cancer. *New England J. Med.* 316: 22.

Zollinger, T. W., Phillips, R. L., and Kuzma, J. W. 1984. Breast cancer survival rates among Seventh-day Adventists and non-Seventh-day Adventists. *Amer. J. Epidemiol.* 119: 503.

2

Carcinogenic Potential of Mycotoxins in Foods

Dennis P. H. Hsieh
University of California at Davis
Davis, California

MYCOTOXINS IN FOODS

Mycotoxins are highly toxic, small molecular weight compounds produced by fungi. Under laboratory conditions, hundreds of such compounds have been produced and characterized chemically and toxicologically (Cole and Cox, 1981). Only those mycotoxins that occur in food commodities under natural conditions are of food safety significance. As reviewed by Stoloff (1982), the following 13 mycotoxins have been detected in food commodities in recent years with some degree of frequency: aflatoxin, zearalenone, zearalenol, trichothecene, ochratoxin, citrinin, penicillic acid, patulin, sterigmatocystin, alternariol methyl ether, mycophenolic acid, penitrem A, and PR toxin.

Both aflatoxin and trichothecene are a family of structurally related compounds. Of all these mycotoxins, nine individual compounds stand out as especially significant based on the frequency of their occurrence (Stoloff, 1982, 1976; Pohland and Wood, 1987). They are aflatoxin B_1, aflatoxin G_1, aflatoxin M_1, zearalenone, ochratoxin A, patulin, penicillic acid, nivalenol, and deoxynivalenol.

The chemical structures of these major foodborne mycotoxins are shown in Fig. 2.1. The occurrence of each is highly commodity and region

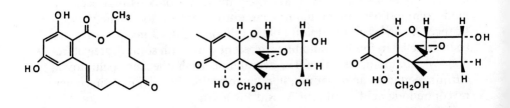

Aflatoxin B₁   Aflatoxin G₁   Aflatoxin M₁

Patulin   Penicillic acid   Ochratoxin A

(S)-Zearalenone   Nivalenol   Deoxynivalenol

FIG. 2.1 Chemical structures of nine major foodborne mycotoxins.

specific. These mycotoxins are mostly produced by three genera of fungi: *Aspergillus, Penicillium, and Fusarium.* Undoubtedly, as new monitoring analytical methods become available and curiosity impels the search, more foodborne mycotoxins will be added to this list.

Mycotoxins have been recognized as an important class of potentially hazardous substances in the human food chain for the following reasons:

1. These compounds can sustain heat treatment and are persistent in processed foods. They possess a spectrum of biological activities due to the diversity of their chemical structures (Hsieh, 1987).
2. Many toxigenic fungi are able to invade and subsequently develop in foodstuffs before or during harvest, resulting in widespread occurrence of mycotoxins in foods (Pohland and Wood, 1987).
3. Human diseases caused by mycotoxins in foods, or mycotoxicoses, have been documented in different parts of the world (Pohland and Wood, 1987), indicating that exposure to acutely toxic levels of mycotoxins in foods can occur in certain populations under certain conditions. Long-term, low-level exposure is certainly more common.
4. Some mycotoxins are highly carcinogenic to laboratory animals, making the long-term, low-level exposure to these toxins a potential health problem (Stoloff, 1982).

The strong interest in mycotoxins shown by the scientific community and regulatory agencies in the last 25 years is largely due to the discovery in the 1960s of the potent carcinogenicity of aflatoxins, especially aflatoxin B_1, the principal member of this family of mycotoxins (Wogan and Newberne, 1967). There has been concern that mycotoxins in general may be a significant class of naturally occurring carcinogens in foods (Ames et al., 1987). This concern is legitimate in view of the extremely high carcinogenic potency of aflatoxin B_1 to some species of laboratory animals (Wogan, 1973) and its widespread occurrence in some food commodities (Stoloff, 1976).

Based on the current practice of toxicological risk assessment (NRC, 1983), in order to assess the human cancer risk posed by mycotoxins, the following four questions need to be addressed for each toxin:

1. Is there sufficient evidence of carcinogenicity of the mycotoxin in experimental animals?
2. To what extent are humans exposed to carcinogenic mycotoxins?

3. Is it valid to extrapolate the animal data to humans?
4. Is there epidemiological evidence to support or contradict the animal evidence?

The following discussion of the carcinogenic potential of mycotoxins in foods is guided by these questions.

EVIDENCE OF CARCINOGENICITY

Evidence that a substance may be a carcinogen to humans comes from the following four sources of information, in order of decreasing significance (U.S. EPA, 1986):

1. Epidemiological studies in human populations.
2. Bioassays in experimental animals.
3. Short-term in vitro tests for DNA modification.
4. Similarity in chemical structures to known carcinogens.

Chemical structure analysis is not likely to yield much useful information regarding the carcinogenicity of mycotoxins because the chemical structure of each class of mycotoxins is unique and a minor change in chemical structure may represent a great difference in biological activity.

It has been generally accepted that initiation of the development of cancer involves DNA modification, and therefore a number of short-term in vitro tests for DNA modification have been used to predict the cancer-initiating activity of many fungal metabolites (Stark, 1980; Hsieh, 1986). Of the nine major foodborne mycotoxins mentioned earlier, eight have been found to possess such activity in one test or another, leaving deoxynivalenol as the only one that has not been proven genotoxic. The results of these short-term tests are not directly useful in determining the carcinogenicity of mycotoxins, because there is a high degree of uncertainty in the predictability of the results, and also these tests are not able to detect cancer promoters, whose crucial role in the development of cancer has become increasingly evident. We shall therefore focus attention on the information from animal carcinogenic bioassays and epidemiologic studies.

CARCINOGENICITY BIOASSAYS IN ANIMALS

The ability of a chemical to induce tumors in experimental animals has been generally used, in the absence of other evidence, as an indication of the carcinogenic potential of the chemical in humans. This assumption is supported by recent biochemical and genetic studies on the mechanism of carcinogenesis, which give increasing evidence that the molecular basis for carcinogenesis in humans is remarkably similar to that in experimental animals (Harris, 1985). Based on established animal assay procedures, at present only aflatoxin, as represented by aflatoxin B_1, and sterigmatocystin are considered by the International Agency for Research on Cancer (IARC) as having sufficient evidence of carcinogenicity in experimental animals (IARC, 1986). Both compounds have induced liver

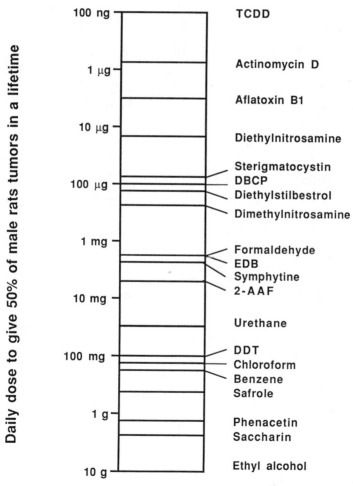

FIG. 2.2 TD_{50} values of a number of selected chemicals.

tumors in more than two species of experimental animals. Ochratoxin A
may be added to the list as more evidence of its animal carcinogenicity
becomes available (Kanisawa and Suzuki, 1978; Kanisawa 1984).

Based on the response of the most sensitive animal species, Ames and
coworkers estimated the 50% toxic doses (TD_{50}), or the tumorigenic dose
rate for 50% of the test animals, as a measure of potency for a large number
of chemical carcinogens (Peto et al., 1984; Gold et al., 1984, 1986). The
TD_{50} values of a number of selected chemicals are shown in Fig. 2.2. The
lower the value, the more potent the carcinogen.

Despite the extremely high potency of aflatoxin B_1 in Fischer rats, it was
not classified as a "human carcinogen" by IARC until 1987. Prior to that,
the evidence for the carcinogenicity of aflatoxin in humans was considered "limited," that is, "a causal interpretation is credible, but alternate
explanations such as chance, bias or confounding, could not adequately
be excluded" (IARC, 1986). It is now generally accepted that chronic
hepatitis B virus infection is a predominating confounding factor of the
carcinogenicity of aflatoxin in humans (Beasley, et al., 1981; Blumberg
and London, 1982).

It is noteworthy that, after more than two decades of active research,
there are only two (aflatoxin and sterigmatocystin) or three (if ochratoxin
A is included) mycotoxins that have sufficient evidence of carcinogenicity
in experimental animals. Their human carcinogenicity, however, is yet to
be established by IARC.

HUMAN SUSCEPTIBILITY TO AFLATOXIN CARCINOGENICITY

The potency of aflatoxin in different species of animals differs considerably because of species differences in metabolism and disposition of
aflatoxin (Hsieh and Wong, 1982). Aflatoxin is a promutagen and pro-
toxin that requires metabolic activation for its mutagenicity and toxicity.
Whereas the rat is highly sensitive to the hepatocarcinogenic effect of
aflatoxin, the mouse is highly resistant (Wogan, 1973). The rhesus monkey
is also considerably more resistant than the rat to aflatoxin carcinogenicity (Seiber et al., 1979).

Humans appear more resistant than the rat to the hepatocarcinogenicity of aflatoxin based on differences in metabolism. Post-
mitochondrial preparations of human liver metabolize aflatoxin in a
manner very similar to preparations of rhesus monkey liver, but in a manner very different from preparations of rat liver (Buchi et al., 1974; Hsieh et
al., 1977a). The ability to activate aflatoxin is greater in enzyme prep-

arations of rat liver than in enzyme preparations of human liver, whereas the opposite is true with respect to ability to detoxify aflatoxin (Hsieh, et al., 1977a, b).

Therefore, the aflatoxin carcinogenicity data obtained from the rat should not be directly extrapolated to humans. The results of epidemiological studies should be closely examined for evidence of the carcinogenicity of aflatoxin in humans.

EPIDEMIOLOGICAL EVIDENCE

To date, aflatoxin is the only class of mycotoxins that has been a subject of extensive epidemiological studies, necessitating that our assessment of the carcinogenic potential of mycotoxins in foods is focused on aflatoxin. Nonetheless, aflatoxin is a good representative carcinogenic mycotoxin because its potency in animals is at least an order of magnitude greater than that of other mycotoxins, and its occurrence in foods is more widespread and frequent than many other mycotoxins.

Animal studies have indicated that aflatoxins are capable of inducing cancer in liver, kidney, intestine, colon, and lung, with the liver being the principal and the most sensitive target organ (Newberne and Rogers, 1981).Therefore, all the epidemiological studies of aflatoxin have been directed toward liver-cell carcinoma (LCC).

Most of the evidence that implicates aflatoxin in the etiology of LCC comes from epidemiological studies conducted in African and Asian countries where LCC is a major form of cancer (Van Rensberg, 1986). Of special interest are the following findings.

Dose-Response Relationship

Quantitative population studies in Thailand and four African countries (Table 2.1), involving a total of 17 regions, have shown a strong correlation, both regionally and within a single country, between unadjusted combined crude LCC rates for both sexes and estimated dietary aflatoxin intake based on current levels of aflatoxin contamination of prepared food (Van Rensberg et al., 1985). Analysis of part of the data for African males also indicates a dose-response relationship between estimated dietary aflatoxin intakes and calculated lifetime risks of liver cancer (Carlborg, 1979). In general, the data from similar studies conducted in China as well as a case-control study conducted in the Philippines sup-

TABLE 2.1 Countries and Regions Involved in the Epidemiologic Studies Used to Demonstrate the Dose-Response Relationship between Liver Cancer and Exposure to Aflatoxin

Country	Region	Reference
Thailand	Songkhla	Shank et al. (1972)
	Ratburi	
Kenya	High altitude	Peers and Linsell (1973)
	Middle altitude	
	Low altitude	
Swaziland	Highveld	Peers et al. (1976)
	Middleveld	
	Lebombo	
	Lowveld	
Mozambique	Manhica-Magude	Van Rensberg et al. (1974)
	Massinga	
	Inharrime	
	Inhambane	
	Morrumbene	
	Homoine-Maxixe	
	Zavala	
Transkei		Van Rensberg et al. (1985)

port this correlation (Sun and Wang, 1983; Sun et al., 1986; Bulatayo-Jayme et al., 1982).

Seasonal Variation

There was a marked seasonal variation found in the level of aflatoxin contamination of foods and the clinical presentation of LCC in four different African populations (Van Rensberg, 1986). LCC frequency peaked in two regions in Mozambique during May to August (Van Rensberg, 1977), but peaked exactly 6 months later north of the equator in Senegal (Diop et al., 1981) and Nigeria (Okonkwo and Obionu, 1981), an indication that the peak for all four populations was mid-winter. Correspondingly, aflatoxin contamination of foodstuffs peaked in mid-summer, 6 months prior to the peak season of LCC incidence.

The seasonal variation of the aflatoxin contamination and the clinical presentation of LCC in Africa suggests that aflatoxin may act at a stage of the disease process, possibly as a promotor or by precipitating final malignant transformation of hepatocytes. The 6-month period between the peak season of aflatoxin exposure and the peak season of LCC presentation does not necessarily imply a malignancy within 6 months of exposure. The latency period could well be 18 months (6 months plus one year), during which a single fully malignant hepatocyte may be able to grow to a large, clinically apparent tumor (Purves, 1973, Van Rensberg, 1986).

Effectiveness of Intervention

Withdrawal of exposure to aflatoxin effectively reduces LCC risk. Urbanization and the consequent reduction in exposure to aflatoxin-contaminated foods led to a decline in the LCC incidence in Johannesburg blacks (Robertson et al., 1971). Similarly, the LCC rates for black goldminers from Mozambique declined steadily over a 17-year period from 1964 to 1981; the miners were given commercial food supplies subject to statutory control of aflatoxin contamination (Harington et al., 1983). This decline was detectable after only 6 months to a year, if employment turnover was considered (Purves, 1973).

The decline in LCC incidence among Mozambican Africans during the last three decades can be plausibly explained in terms of the effects of intervention (Bijisma, 1981; Van Rensberg et al., 1985). The dissemination of information to the public regarding the association of moldy food and liver cancer probably has alerted people to exercise more selectivity in the preparation and storage of foodstuffs. Also, the increasing replacement of peanuts with less costly maize as the main staple has probably helped to reduce dietary aflatoxin intake. In Mozambique, maize does not seem as susceptible to aflatoxin contamination as peanuts or cassava (Van Rensberg et al., 1975).

These epidemiological findings indicate not only that aflatoxin is involved in the etiology of human liver cancer, but also that aflatoxin has an effect at the late stage of the development of LCC. In the high-risk regions in Africa, such as Zavala of Mozambique where aflatoxin contamination of food is frequent, it is conceivable that long-term human exposure to subacute levels of aflatoxin would result in the late stage effect in the development of LCC. Aflatoxin has been found at levels of 1 ppm or higher in meals consisting mainly of ground nuts (Van Rensberg et al., 1985). At these levels of contamination, daily food intake may become subacutely toxic. Human exposure to acute levels of aflatoxin in foods has been reported in different parts of the world (Tung and Ling, 1968; Krishnamachari et al., 1975; Ngindu et al., 1982).

EVIDENCE AGAINST AFLATOXIN AS A HUMAN CARCINOGEN

A geographical association between LCC incidence and dietary aflatoxin intake was not found in the United States. In a retrospective study, rural white males from the southeast, north, and west regions were selected for the comparison of lifetime risk of death from liver cancer and past dietary exposure to aflatoxin (Stoloff, 1983). For an approximately 100-fold interregional difference in aflatoxin intake, there was only a 6 to 10% increase in excess LCC death risk in the expected direction of comparison, indicating a very low probability that aflatoxin is the cause of liver cancer in U.S. rural white males. No dose-response association was evident in a case-control study conducted in Hong Kong (Lam et al, 1982). In regions in Mozambique where heavy aflatoxin contamination of foodstuffs occurred, only a subset of the population had a high risk of LCC (Van Rensberg, 1977; Van Rensberg et al., 1985). In Taiwan, illness and mortality have been associated with acute levels of aflatoxin intake (Tung and Ling, 1968), yet in a large prospective study of LCC conducted by Beasley et al. (1981), there was no evidence of aflatoxin involvement. Also, aflatoxin was not found in food samples from villages of Alaska although the resident Eskimos had a high LCC incidence (Lanier et al., 1976). Presumably, the dietary aflatoxin intake of this population is very low due to the cold environment, which is unfavorable for the growth of aflatoxin-producing fungi.

In addition, the date base, methodology, and interpretation of the studies that provide positive evidence as presented in the preceding section were questioned and criticized by several investigators. For example, Wagstaff (1985) and Stoloff (1986) pointed out that none of the cancer incidence data used in those studies was adjusted for differences in the age distribution of the separate populations; the time intervals and population sizes studied were rather small in relation to the amount and scatter of both aflatoxin intake and cancer incidence data; there was no control for other possible hepatocarcinogenic agents; no validation was done of retrospective projection of the aflatoxin ingestion data; and in all regions, the great majority of meal samples contained no measurable aflatoxin, and therefore interregional differences in exposure were based on a limited number of positive samples that showed large annual, daily, and person-to-person variations in the aflatoxin level within each region. Wagstaff (1985) expressed concern about the validity of the dose-response correlation shown by these studies because of the difficulty of performing exposure assessment at an individual level and the lack of complete LCC incidence records in developing nations. Another concern is the possible biased selection of studies to fit a preset hypothesis.

ROLE OF HEPATITIS B VIRUS

The most important argument against aflatoxin being a causal agent in the development of LCC stems from the observation by a number of investigators that liver cancer in African and Asian populations is strongly associated with chronic hepatitis B virus (HBV) infection (Hadziyannis, 1980; Blumberg and London, 1982). As pointed out by Stoloff (1987), the odds ratio of 223 for liver cancer in HBV carriers (Beasley et al., 1981) is more than 20 times greater than the odds ratio for lung cancer in cigarette smokers (Doll and Peto, 1981). It has been estimated that HBV infection is responsible for 80% of the LCC cases in high incidence countries and about 50% in other countries (WHO, 1983; Nishioka, 1985). Some investigators believe that HBV infection is a prerequisite for the development of LCC (Blumberg and London, 1985). Moreover, it has been found that multiplication of HBV may occur even in the absence of any conventional serological marker for HBV (Brechot et al., 1985). Evidence of an HBV-LCC link also comes from natural and experimental incidences of LCC in woodchucks and ducks infected with viruses similar to human HBV (Summers et al., 1978; Mason et al., 1984; Abe et al., 1988).

The reason HBV infection is so effective is probably due to the ability of the virus to proliferate and develop in the host liver tissues causing continuous cytotoxic damage to the tissues through chronic active hepatitis. This type of continuous subacute damage, or "microhepatectomy," constitutes a most effective promotional treatment. Rarely does exposure to any hepatotoxic chemical reach a subacute dose level for a duration long enough to be as effective as chronic HBV infection in the promotion of carcinogenicity.

The effective promoting activity of HBV infection and the possible late stage effect of aflatoxin in the development of LCC offer some plausible explanations for the observed low LCC risk in those regions of the United States where exposure to aflatoxins is as high as in high-risk regions of Africa. Any one or more of the following possible reasons would result in a reduction of the carcinogenic effect of aflatoxin.

1. The incidence of HBV infection is low among U.S. rural white males.

2. The dietary variety available to these populations would render continuous exposure to subacute levels of aflatoxin rather unlikely.
3. The resistance to chronic active hepatitis and aflatoxin toxicity is better developed in U.S. populations due to better nutritional conditions (Newberne, 1987).

HBV infection, though very strongly associated with LCC, does not constitute the sole, essential, and sufficient cause of the disease. The fact that aflatoxin and other hepatocarcinogens, such as nitrosamines, can induce LCC in the rat, which is not susceptible to HBV infection, would indicate that viral infection is not essential for LCC development. The great variation in the LCC risk of hepatitis B surface antigen (HBsAg) carriers among different regions in the world, as reviewed by Van Rensberg (1986), indicates that HBV infection is not the sole etiological factor. Among populations that have a high HBsAg carrier rate, there is an excellent positive association between LCC risk and climatic conditions suitable for the growth of aflatoxin-producing fungi, suggesting that aflatoxin is a strong confounding factor for the carcinogenic effect of HBV infection (Bagshawe et al., 1975; Peers and Linsell, 1973; Ziegler et al., 1977; Girgis et al., 1977; Skinhoj, et al., 1978). The striking difference in LCC rate between whites and blacks in Africa (Van Rensberg, 1977) and between whites and Asians in the United States (Stoloff, 1983) may be more easily explained as due to differences in dietary pattern than due to differences in the rate of HBV infection.

JOINT EFFECT OF AFLATOXIN AND HBV IN LCC DEVELOPMENT

Recently, a study was carried out in Swaziland to specifically assess the relationship between aflatoxin exposure, HBV infection, and the risk of LCC. Hepatocellular carcinoma is the most commonly occurring malignancy among males in this country (Peers et al., 1987). A nationwide cancer registration system was established, samples of prepared foods and crops were assayed for aflatoxin, and HBV exposure was assessed from blood donor samples. The results indicated that the prevalence of the HBsAg carrier status was high with little variation throughout Swaziland and that, on a regional basis, estimated aflatoxin exposure was more strongly correlated with LCC rate. Thus, in Swaziland, aflatoxin appears to act as an independent risk factor for LCC, rather than simply as a cofactor to HBV.

Mechanistically, an interesting multifactorial etiological explanation for LCC involving HBV and aflatoxin has been advanced by Harris and Sun (1984). In the multistep process of hepatocarcinogenesis, which consists of initiation and promotion steps, aflatoxin is undoubtedly a potent initiator able to damage DNA and cause genetic alterations or mutagenesis in liver cells. Following initiation, a "programmed" cellular response is triggered, producing a phenotype that has a survival-growth advantage, including resistance to both the cytotoxicity of environmental chemicals and the cytopathology related to the development of HBV in host cells. During the promotion process, clones of these resistant cells expand into groups of preneoplastic cells or foci, in response to an endogenous proliferative factor. This proliferative factor is released either following partial hepatectomy or after injury of nonresistant, normal cells by either chemicals (e.g., aflatoxin) or viral agents (e.g., hepatitis B virus).

Based on this "selective clonal cell expansion" theory, it is apparent that HBV can promote LCC in people already exposed to aflatoxin and other genotoxic hepatocarcinogens. It also offers an explanation as to why hepatotoxic agents such as alcohol and aflatoxin can also promote the development of liver cancer. Aflatoxin can be a promoter as well as an initiator. The mechanism of a possible synergistic effect between aflatoxin and HBV, however, is yet to be elucidated.

The requirement of both the initiating and the promoting activities of a chemical for inducing liver carcinogenesis has been experimentally demonstrated by a relatively short-term animal assay established by Ito and coworkers using Fischer 344 male rats as the animal model (Ito et al., 1980). Using this assay system, they analyzed five mycotoxins: citrinin, ochratoxin A, sterigmatocystin, rugulosin, and patulin (Imaida et al., 1982). They reported that ochratoxin A, sterigmatocystin, and rugulosin possess both initiating and promoting activities, whereas citrinin and patulin possess only initiating activity. They concluded that the first three mycotoxins are liver carcinogens, whereas the last two are not. Data from animal bioassays reported so far are consistent with this conclusion.

CONTROL OF MYCOTOXINS IN THE PREVENTION OF HUMAN LIVER CANCER

Based on the preceding elaborations, it seems clear that the carcinogenic potential of mycotoxins in humans comes from their promoting as well as their genotoxic or initiating activity. Exposure to genotoxic mycotoxins at low dose levels may increase the mutagen load or the density of initiated liver cells, but until sufficient promotion takes place, either by active HBV infection or by continuous exposure to subacute levels of mycotoxins, there seems to be little risk of cancer progression.

In view of the potent mutagenicity of aflatoxin, its possible late stage effect in LCC development, and its widespread occurrence in foodstuffs, government-imposed intervention into aflatoxin exposure may be a more rapid and cost-effective approach to the reduction of LCC risk in humans than vaccination against HBV infection. The steady decline in the LCC rate in certain Mozambican populations has been credited to such an approach (Van Rensberg, 1986). However, any benefit from aflatoxin control procedures will only be seen in countries where the HBV infection rate is high. In advanced socioeconomic groups, aflatoxins may seem irrelevant as a cause of cancer.

The only other form of cancer possibly associated with mycotoxins is esophageal cancer, which has been shown to be associated with exposure to moldy foods in Africa (Van Rensberg, 1986). In light of the controversy about the role of aflatoxins in LCC, the cause-effect relationship will not be certain until sufficient supporting epidemiological data become available.

PERSPECTIVE OF RELATIVE RISKS

Recent public awareness and intense interest in chemical safety has prompted governmental regulatory agencies to make a massive investment in an attempt to control the presence of certain carcinogenic chemicals in the environment (Denney, 1986). Very few of these chemicals are designated by IARC as human carcinogens, and the regulatory actions are justified totally based on their animal carcinogenicity (U.S. EPA, 1986). For example, ethylene dibromide (EDB) was recently banned as a pesticide by the U.S. Environmental Protection Agency because of the discovery of both its ability to induce tumors in experimental animals and the presence of residues in EDB-treated commodities (U.S. EPA, 1983). If the carcinogenic potency in the most sensitive animal species is to be used as a basis of concern (Ames et al., 1987), then mycotoxins, especially aflatoxin, should be considered an important class of potential human carcinogens, in view of their high carcinogenic potency and their widespread natural occurrence in foodstuffs.

In keeping with the conservative approach taken by the U.S. governmental agencies to control hazardous substances in the environment, for the greatest margin of safety, mycotoxins should continue to warrant rigorous regulatory action as a significant class of potential human carcinogens.

ACKNOWLEDGMENTS

The author gratefully acknowledges the substantial input from Mr. Leonard Stoloff for the preparation of this paper. His advice and critique were most helpful. Ms. Linda Beltran edited the manuscript. Ms. Lucy Hsieh helped compile the references.

REFERENCES

Abe, K., Kurata, T., Shikata, T., and Tennant, B. C. 1988. Enzyme-altered liver cell foci in woodchucks infected with woodchuck hepatitis virus. *Jap. J. Cancer Res.* (Gann) 79: 466–472.

Ames, B. N., Magaw, R., and Gold, L. S. 1987. Ranking possible carcinogenic hazards. *Science* 236: 271–280

Bagshawe, A. F., Gacengi, D. M., Cameron, C. H., Dorman, J., and Dane, D. S. 1975. Hepatitis B surface antigen and liver cancer. A population based study in Kenya. *Brit. J. Cancer* 31: 581–584.

Beasley, R. P., Hwang, L. Y., Lin, C. C., and Chien, C. S. 1981.Hepatocellular carcinoma and hepatitis B virus. *Lancet* 2: 1129–1132.

Bijlsma, F. 1981. Malignant tumours in Mozambican Africans with special reference to primary liver carcinoma. *Trans. Soc. Trop. Med. Hyg.* 75: 451–454.

Blumberg, B. S. and London, W. T. 1985. Hepatitis B virus and prevention of primary cancer of the liver. *J. Nat. Cancer Inst.* 74: 267–273.

Blumberg, B. S. and London W. T. 1982. Primary hepatocellular carcinoma and hepatitis B virus. *Curr. Probl. Cancer* 6: 1–23.

Brechot, C., Degos, F., Lugassy, C., Thiers, V., Zafrani, S., Franco, D., Bismuth, H., Trepo, C., Benhamou, J-P., Wands, J., Isselbacher, K., Tiolias, P., and Berthelot, P. 1985. Hepatitis B virus DNA in patients with chronic liver disease and negative tests for hepatitis B surface antigen. *New England J. Med.* 312: 270–276.

Buchi, G. H., Muller, P. M., Roebuck, B. D., and Wogan, G. N. 1974. Aflatoxin Q1: A major metabolite of aflatoxin B1 produced by human liver. *Res. Commun. Chem. Pathol. Pharmacol.* 8: 585–591.

Bulatao-Jayme, J., Almero, E. M., Castro, M. C. A., Jardeleza, M. T. R., and Salamat, L. A. 1982. A case-control dietary study of primary liver cancer risk from aflatoxin exposure. *Int. J. Epidemiol.* 11: 112–119.

Carlborg, F. W. 1979. Cancer, mathematical models and aflatoxin. *Fd. Cosmet. Toxicol.* 17: 159–166.

Cole, R. J. and Cox, R. H. 1981. *Handbook of Toxic Fungal Metabolites,* Academic Press, New York.

Denney, R. J. 1986. California's Proposition 65: Coming soon to your neighborhood. *Toxics Law Reporter* 12: 789–793.

Diop, B., Denis, F., Barin, F., Perrin, J., Chiron, J. P., Goudeau, A., Coursaget, P., and Maupas, P. 1981. Epidemiology of primary hepatocellular carcinoma in Senegal. *Prog. Med. Virol.* 27: 35–40.

Doll, R. and Peto, R. 1981. the causes of cancer: Quantitative estimates of avoidable risks of cancer in the United States Today. *J. Natl. Cancer Inst.* 66: 1191.

Girgis, A. N., El-Sherif, S., Rofael, N., and Nesheim, S. 1977. Aflatoxins in Egyptian foodstuffs. *J. Assoc. Off. Anal. Chem.* 60: 746.

Gold, L. S., de Veciana, M., Backman, G. M., Magaw, R., Lopipero, P., Smith, M., Blumenthal, M., Levinson, R., Bernstein, L., and Ames, B. N. 1986. Chronological supplement to the carcinogenic potency database: Standardized results of animal bioassays published through December 1982. *Env. Health Persp.* 67: 161–200.

Gold, L. S., Sawyer, C. B., Magaw, R., Backman, G. M., deVeciana, M., Levenson, R., Hooper, N. K., Havender, W. R., Bernstein, L., Peto, R., Pike, M. C., and Ames, B. N. 1984. A carcinogenic potency database of the standardized results of animal bioassays. *Env. Health Persp.* 58: 9–319.

Hadziyannis, S. J. 1980. Hepatocellular carcinoma and type B hepatitis. *Clin. Gastroenterol.* 9: 117–134.

Harlington, J. S., Bradshaw, E. M., and McGlashan, N. D. 1983. Changes in primary liver and oesophageal cancer rates among black goldminers, 1964–1981. *S. Afr. Med. J.* 64: 185–191.

Harris, C. C. 1985. Future directions in the use of DNA adducts as internal dosimeters for monitoring human exposure to environmental mutagens and carcinogens. *Env. Health Persp.* 62: 185–191.

Harris, C. C. and Sun, T. 1984. Multifactoral etiology of human liver cancer. *Carcinogenesis* 5: 697–701.

Hsieh, D. P. H. 1987. Mode of action of mycotoxins. In *Mycotoxins in Food.* (Ed.) Krogh, P., pp. 149–176. Academic Press. London.

Hsieh, D. P. H. 1986. Gentoxicity of mycotoxins. In *New Concepts and Developments in Toxicology.* (Ed.) Chambers, P. L., Gehring, P. and Sakai, F., pp. 251–260. Elsevier, Amsterdam.

Hsieh, D. P. H. and Wong, J. J. 1982. Metabolism and toxicity of aflatoxins. In *Biological Reactive Intermediates II: Chemical Mechanisms and Biological Effects.* (Ed.) Snyder, R., Parke, D. V., Kocsis, J. J., Jollow, D. J., Gibson, G. G., and Whitmer, C. M., pp. 847–863. Plenum Publ. Corp., New York.

Hsieh, D. P. H., Wong, Z. A., Wong, J. J., Michas, C., and Ruebner, B. H. 1977a. Comparative metabolism of aflatoxin. In *Mycotoxins in Human and Animal Health.* (Ed.) Rodricks, J. V., Hesseltine, C. W., and Mehlman, M. A., pp. 37–50. Pathotox Publishers, Park Forest South, IL.

Hsieh, D. P. H., Wong, Z. A., Wong, J. J., Michas, C., and Ruebner, B. H., 1977b. Hepatic transformation of aflatoxin and its carcinogenicity. In *Origins of Human Cancer.* (Ed.) Hiatt, H. H., Watson, J. D., and Winsten, J. D., pp. 697–707. Cold Spring Harbor Lab., Cold Spring Harbor, NY.

IARC. 1986. Some halogenated hydrocarbons and pesticide exposures. In *Evaluation of the Carcinogenic Risk of Chemicals to Humans* 41: 22. World Health Organization, Lyon.

Imaida, K., Hirose, M., Ogiso, T., Kurata, Y., and Ito, N. 1982. Quantitative analysis of initiating and promoting activities of five mycotoxins in liver carcinogenesis in rats, *Cancer Letters* 16: 137–143.

Ito, N., Tatematsu, M., Imaida, K., Hasegawa, R., and Murasaki, G. 1980. Effects of various promoters on the induction of hyperplastic nodules in rat liver. *Gann* 71: 415–416.

Kanisawa, M. 1984. Synergistic effect of citrinin on hepatorenal carcinogenesis of Ochratoxin A in mice. In *Toxigenic Fungi—Their Toxins and Health Hazard.* (Ed.) Kurata, H. and Ueno, Y., pp. 245–254. Elsevier, Amsterdam.

Kanisawa, M. and Suzuki, S. 1978. Induction of renal and hepatic tumors in mice by ochratoxin A, a mycotoxin. *Gann* 69: 599–600.

Krishnamachari, K. A. V. R., Bhat, R. V., Nagarajan, V., and Tilak, T. B. G. 1975. Hepatitis due to aflatoxicosis: An outbreak in western India. *Lancet* 1: 1061–1063.

Lam, K. C., Yu, M. C., Leung, J. W. C., and Henderson, B. E. 1982. Hepatitis B virus and cigarette smoking: Risk factors for hepatocellular carcinoma in Hong Kong. *Cancer Res.* 42: 5246–5248.

Lanier, A. P., Bender, T. R., Blot, W. J., Fraumeni, J. F., and Hurlburt, W. B. 1976. Cancer incidence in Alaska natives. *Int. J. Cancer* 18: 409–412.

Mason, W. S., Halpern, M. S., and London, W. T. 1984. Hepatitis B viruses, liver disease, and hepatocellular carcinoma. *Cancer Surv.* 3: 25–49.

National Research Council. 1983. *Risk Assessment in the Federal Government: Managing the Process.* National Academy Press, Washington, DC.

Newberne, P. M. 1987. Interaction of nutrients and other factors with mycotoxins. In *Mycotoxins in Food.* (Ed.) Krogh, P., pp. 177–216. Academic Press, London.

Newberne, P.M. and Rogers, A. E. 1981. Animal toxicity of major environmental mycotoxins. In *Mycotoxing and N-Nitroso Compounds: Environmental Risks.* (Ed.) Shank, R. C., pp. 51–106. CRC Press, Inc., Boca Raton,FL.

Ngindu, A., Johnson, B. K., Kenya, P. R., Ngira, J. A., Ocheng D. M., Nandwa, H., Omonde, T.N., Jansen, A. J., Ngare, W., Kaviti, J. N., Gatei, D., and Siongok, T. A. 1982. Outbreak of acute hepatitis caused by aflatoxin poisoning in Kenya. *Lancet* 1: 1346–1348.

Nishioka, K. 1985. Hepatitis B virus and hepatocellular carcinoma: Postulates for an etiological relationship. *Adv. Viral Oncol.* 5: 173–199.

Okonkwo, P. O. and Obionu, C. N. 1981. Implications of seasonal variations in aflatoxin B1 levels in Nigerian market food. *Nutr. Cancer* 3: 35–39.

Peers, F., Bosch, X., Kaldor, J., Linsell, A., and Pluijmen, M. 1987. Aflatoxin exposure, hepatitis B virus infection and liver cancer in Swaziland. *Int. J. Cancer* 39: 545–553.

Peers, F. G., Gilman, G. A., and Linsell, C. A. 1976. Dietary aflatoxins and human cancer. A study in Swaziland. *Int. J. Cancer* 17: 167–176.

Peers, F. G. and Linsell, C. A. 1973. Dietary aflatoxins and liver cancer—a population-based study in Kenya. *Brit. J. Cancer* 27: 473–484.

Peto, R., Pike, M. C., Bernstein, L., Gold, L. S., and Ames, B. N. 1984. The TD50: A proposed general convention for the numerical description of the carcinogenic potency of chemicals in chronic-exposure animal experiments. *Env. Health Persp.* 58: 1–8.

Pohland, A. E. and Wood, G. E. 1987. Occurrence of mycotoxins in food. In *Mycotoxins in Food.* (Ed.) Krogh, P., pp. 35–64. Academic Press, London.

Purves, L. R. 1973. Primary liver cancer in man as a possible short duration seasonal cancer. *S. Afr. J. Sci.* 69: 173–178.

Robertson, M. A., Harington, J. S., and Bradshaw, E. 1971. The Cancer pattern in Africans at Baragwanath Hospital, Johannesburg, *Br. J. Cancer* 25: 377–384.

Seiber, S. M., Correa, P., Dalgard, D. W., and Adamson, R. H. 1979. Induction of osteogenic sarcomas and tumors of the hepatobillary system in non-human primates with aflatoxin B1. *Cancer Res.* 39: 4545–4554.

Shank, R. C., Bhamarapravati, N., Gordon, J. E., and Wogan, G. N. 1972. Dietary aflatoxins and human liver cancer. IV. Incidence of primary liver cancer in two municipal populations in Thailand. *Food Cosmet. Toxicol.* 10: 171–179.

Skinhol, P., Hansen, J. P., Nielson, N. H., and Mikkelsen, F. 1978. Occurrence of cirrhosis and primary liver cancer in an Eskimo population hyperendemically infected with hepatitis B virus. A. *J. Epidemiol.* 108: 121

Stark, A. A. 1980. Mutagenicity and carcinogenicity of mycotoxins: DNA binding as a possible mode of action. *Ann. Rev. Microbiol.* 34: 235–262

Stoloff, L. 1987. Carcinogenicity of aflatoxins. *Science* 237(4820): 1283.

Stoloff, L. 1986. A rationale for the control of aflatoxin in human foods. In *Mycotoxins and Phycotoxins,* (Ed.) Steyn, P. S. and Vleggaar, R., pp. 457–472. Elsevier, Amsterdam.

Stoloff, L. 1983. Aflatoxin as a cause of primary liver-cell cancer in the United States: A probability study. *Nutr. Cancer* 5: 165–168.

Stoloff, L. 1982. Mycotoxins as potential environmental carcinogens. In *Carcinogens and Mutagens in the Environment-1.* (Ed.) Stitch, H. F., pp. 97–119. CRC Press, Boca Raton, Fl.

Stoloff, L. 1976. Occurrence of mycotoxins in foods and feeds. In *Mycotoxins and Other Fungal Related Food Problems.* (Ed.), Rodricks, J. V., pp. 23–50. Adv. Chem. Ser. 149. American Chemical Society, Washington, DC.

Summers, J., Smolec, J. M., and Snyder, R. 1978. A virus similar to human hepatitis B virus associated with hepatitis and hepatoma in woodchucks. *Proc. Natl. Acad. Sci. USA* 75: 4533–4537.

Sun, T. and Wang, N. 1983. Studies on human liver carcinogenesis. In *Human Carcinogenesis.* (Ed.) Harris, C. C. and Autrup, H. N., pp. 757–780. Academic Press, New York.

Sun, T., Wu, S., Wu, Y., and Chu, U. 1986. Measurement of individual aflatoxin exposure among people having different risk to primary hepatocellular carcinoma. In *Diet, Nutrition and Cancer.* (Ed.) Hayashi, Y., Nagao, M., Sugimura, T., Takayama, S., Tomatis, L., Wattenberg, L. W., and Wogan, G. N. Japan Scientific Societies Press, Tokyo.

Tung, T. C. and Ling, K. H. 1968. Study on aflatoxin of foodstuffs in Taiwan. *J. Niutr. Sci. Vitaminol.* 14: 48–52.

U.S. EPA. 1986. Guidelines for carcinogen risk assessment. *Fed. Regist.* 51:

33992-34003.

U.S. EPA. 1983. Ethylene dibromide: intent to cancel registrations of pesticide products containing ethylene dibromide; Determination concluding the rebuttable presumption against registration; Availability of position document. *Fed. Regist.* 48: 46234-46248.

Van Rensburg, S. J. 1986. Role of mycotoxins in endemic liver and aesophageal cancer. In *Mycotoxins and Phycotoxins.* (Ed.) Steyn, P. S. and Vleggaar, R., pp. 483-494. Elsevier, Amsterdam.

Van Rensburg, S. J. 1977. Role of epidemiology in the elucidation of mycotoxin health risks. In *Mycotoxins in Human and Animal Health.* (Ed.) Rodericks, J. V., Hesseltine, C. W., and Mehlman, M. A., pp. 699-712. Pathotox Publishers, Park Forest South, FL.

Van Rensburg, S. J., Cook-Mozaffari, P., Van Schalkwyk, D. J., Van Der Watt, J. J., Vicent, T. J., and Purchase, I. F. 1985. Hepatocellular carcinoma and dietary aflatoxin in Mozambique and Transkei. *Br. J. Cancer* 51: 713-726

Van Rensburg, S. J., Kirsipuu, A., Coutinho, L. P., and Van der Watt, J. J. 1975. Circumstances associated with the contamination of food by aflatoxin in a high primary liver cancer area. *S. Afr. Med. J.* 49: 877.

Van Rensburg, S. J., Van Der Watt, J. J., Purchase, I. F. H., Pereira Coutinho, L., and Markham, R. 1974. Primary liver cancer rate and aflatoxin intake in a high cancer area. *S. Afr. Med. J.* 48: 2508a-d.

Wagstaff, D. J. 1985. The use of epidemiology, scientific data, and regulatory authority to determine risk factors in cancers of some organs of the digestive system. *Reg. Toxicol. Pharmacol.* 5: 384-404.

Wogan, G. N. 1973. Aflatoxin carcinogenesis. In *Methods in Cancer Research.* 7. (Ed.) Busch, J., pp. 309-344. Academic Press, New York.

Wogan, G. N. and Newberne, P.M. 1967. Dose response characteristics of aflatoxin B1 carcinogenesis in the rat. *Cancer Res.* 27: 2370-2376.

World Health Organization. 1983. Prevention of liver cancer. WHO Technical Report Series, Vol. 691. WHO, Geneva.

Ziegler, J. L., Adamson, R. H., Barker, L. F., Fraumeni, J. F., Gerin, J., and Purcell, R. H. 1977. National Institute of Health International Workshop on hepatitis B and liver cancer. *Cancer Res.* 37: 4672.

3
Heterocyclic Amines in Cooked Food

**Takashi Sugimura, Keiji Wakabayashi,
Minako Nagao, and Hiroko Ohgaki**
National Cancer Center
Tokyo, Japan

INTRODUCTION

The idea that lifestyle has an important influence on the development of cancer in humans is generally accepted by scientists, regulatory agencies, and the general public. Among the factors in lifestyle now recognized to influence cancer development are cigarette smoking, diet and nutrition, alcoholic beverages, and infectious diseases. Improvement of the lifestyle should be based as far as possible on scientific evidence. Cancers are caused by multiple factors, and carcinogenesis involves many complicated processes, so no single mutagen/carcinogen detected in food can be pinpointed as the direct cause of, or the only factor responsible for a certain type of cancer. But it is clearly important that exposure of humans to compounds that have been shown to be carcinogens in animal experiments should be reduced as far as possible. If this could be achieved simply without serious disturbance of our comfortable lifestyle, then, based on scientific evidence, recommendations for improvements should be made (Sugimura, 1982; 1986). The final goal of studies on mutagens/carcinogens in food should be prevention of cancer. With this aim in view, this article reports studies on the presence of mutagens/carcinogens in foods cooked in the usual way.

HISTORY OF STUDIES ON HETEROCYCLIC
AMINES IN COOKED FOODS

During studies on the mutagenicity of cigarette smoke tar, we wondered whether the smoke produced by broiling fish and meat in kitchens might also contain mutagens. To examine this possibility, we broiled fish over a gas flame and collected the smoke particles on a glass-fiber filter by suction with a motor pump. Then we dissolved the material on the filter in dimethyl sulfoxide and tested it for mutagenicity by Ames' Salmonella assay. As expected from our results on cigarette smoke tar, we found that the smoke condensate from broiling fish was in fact highly mutagenic (Nagao et al., 1977a; Sugimura et al., 1977a). We also found that charred surfaces of broiled fish and meat were mutagenic (Nagao et al., 1977a; Sugimura et al., 1977a). Calculations showed that the amounts of polycyclic aromatic hydrocarbons in the samples of smoke condensate and charred material could not account for all the mutagenic activity, and in fact most of the mutagenic activity was recovered in the basic fractions of the samples.

Further studies showed that charred amino acids, proteins, and proteinous foods all contained mutagenic substances (Nagao et al., 1977b; Matsumoto et al., 1977; Commoner et al., 1978; Kosuge et al., 1978; Pariza et al., 1979). Two potent mutagens, named Trp-P-1 and Trp-P-2, were isolated in pure states from a pyrolysate of D,L-tryptophan by monitoring mutagenic activity toward *Salmonella typhimurium* TA98 during their purification (Sugimura et al., 1977b). These compounds were the first of a series of heterocyclic amines discovered in pyrolysates of amino acids, proteins, and proteinous foods by scientists in this and other laboratories (Sugimura 1982, 1986; Felton et al., 1986; Becher et al., 1988).

IQ and MeIQ were isolated from broiled sardines (Kasai, et al, 1980a,b), and MeIQx was isolated from fried beef (Kasai et al., 1981). Creatinine in fish and meat may be important in the production of aminoimidazoquinoline and aminoimidazoquinoxaline compounds, because these compounds were formed on heating a mixture of creatinine, amino acids, and sugars (Jägerstad et al., 1984; Negishi et al., 1984, 1985; Grivas et al., 1985, 1986; Shioya et al., 1987).

Most aminoimidazoquinoline and aminoimidazoquinoxaline compounds were originally isolated from foods cooked under ordinary conditions, and some heterocyclic amines were originally isolated from pyrolysates of proteins and amino acids. Much of the work on the organic chemistry, analytical chemistry, mutagenicity, carcinogenicity, metabolism, and biological effects of these compounds, including their effects on the salivary gland, has been done by scientists from many countries.

CHEMISTRY OF HETEROCYCLIC AMINES

The chemical structures of the heterocyclic amines discovered at the National Cancer Center and in other laboratories are illustrated in Figs. 3.1 and 3.2. The chemical names and abbreviations of these compounds and references to their first reports are given in Table 3.1.

Heterocyclic amines are classified into two types: the IQ-type (Fig. 3.1) and the non-IQ-type (Fig. 3.2). Treatment with 2 mM nitrite does not affect the amino groups of IQ-type heterocyclic amines, but converts those

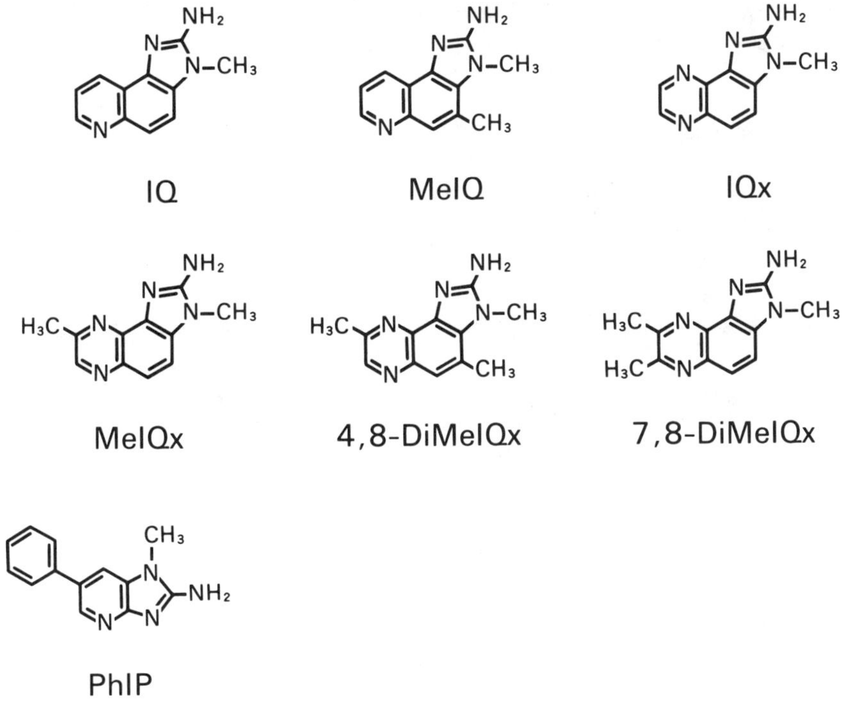

FIG. 3.1 Structures of IQ-type heterocyclic amines.

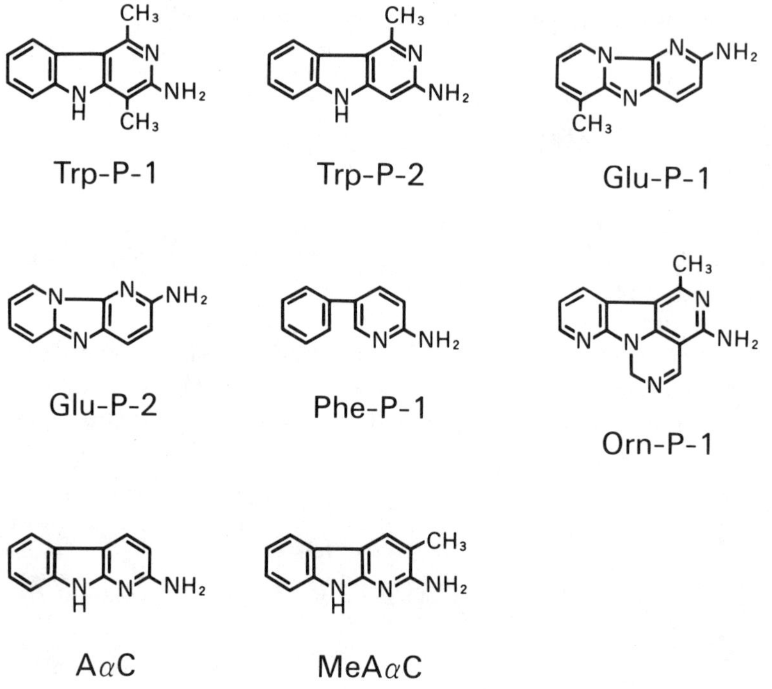

FIG. 3.2 Structures of non-IQ-type heterocyclic amines.

of non-IQ-type heterocyclic amines to hydroxy groups, and this conversion is associated with loss of mutagenicity (Tsuda et al., 1980; 1981; 1985). On the other hand, treatment with hypochlorite results in loss of mutagenicity of both IQ- and non-IQ-type heterocyclic amines(Tsuda et al., 1983; 1985). On the basis of the differential effects of nitrite on the two types of heterocyclic amines and the action of hypochlorite on both types, the contributions of IQ-type and non-IQ-type mutagens to the total mutagenicity of the basic fractions from various materials were determined, and results are given in Table 3.2 (Tsuda et al., 1985).

Treatment of IQ-type heterocyclic amines with a much higher concentration of nitrite (50 mM) resulted in conversion of amino groups to nitro groups (Matsushima, personal communication, 1988). The nitro derivatives of imidazoquinoline and imidazoquinoxaline showed almost the same mutagenicity in the absence and presence of S9 mix as parent amino derivatives.

TABLE 3.1 Chemical Names and Abbreviations of Heterocyclic Amines

Chemical name	Abbreviation	Reference
2-Amino-3-methylimidazo-[4,5-*f*]quinoline	IQ	Kasai et al. (1980a)
2-Amino-3,4-dimethyl-imidazo[4,5-*f*]quinoline	MeIQ	Kasai et al. (1980b)
2-Amino-3-methylimidazo-[4,5-*f*]quinoxaline	IQx	Becher et al. (1988)
2-Amino-3,8-dimethyl-imidazo[4,5-*f*]quinoxaline	MeIQx	Kasai et al. (1981)
2-Amino-3,4,8-trimethyl-imidazo[4,5-*f*]quinoxaline	4,8-DiMeIQx	Negishi et al. (1985)
2-Amino-3,7,8-trimethyl-imidazo[4,5-*f*]quinoxaline	7,8-DiMeIQx	Negishi et al. (1984)
2-Amino-1-methyl-6-phenyl-imidazo[4,5-*b*]pyridine	PhIP	Felton et al. (1986)
3-Amino-1,4-dimethyl-5*H*-pyrido[4,3-*b*]indole	Trp-P-1	Sugimura et al. (1977b)
3-Amino-1-methyl-5*H*-pyrido[4,3-*b*]indole	Trp-P-2	Sugimura et al. (1977b)
2-Amino-6-methyldipyrido[1,2-*a*:3′,2′-*d*]imidazole	Glu-P-1	Yamamoto et al. (1978)
2-Aminodipyrido[1,2-*a*:3′,2′-*d*]imidazole	Glu-P-2	Yamamoto et al. (1978)
2-Amino-5-phenylpyridine	Phe-P-1	Sugimura et al. (1977b)
4-Amino-6-methyl-1*H*-2,5,10,10b-tetraaza-fluoranthene	Orn-P-1	Yokota et al. (1981)
2-Amino-9*H*-pyrido[2,3-*b*]indole	AαC	Yoshida et al. (1978)
2-Amino-3-methyl-9*H*-pyrido[2,3-*b*]indole	MeAαC	Yoshida et al. (1978)

TABLE 3.2 Proportions of Mutagenicity Due to IQ and Non-IQ Types of Heterocyclic Amines in the Basic Fractions of Various Pyrolyzed Materials

Sample	IQ-type (%)	Non-IQ-type (%)
Cigarette smoke condensate	6	85
Broiled sardine	88	3
Fried beef	75	24
Broiled horse mackerel	48	42

These heterocyclic amines are readily soluble in many organic solvents and are also soluble in acidic aqueous solution. Details of the chemical properties and organic syntheses of these compounds are reviewed elsewhere (Sugimura et al., 1988). From the practical view point, these compounds are quite stable, and remain unchanged for at least 6 months when mixed with pellet diet and kept in dry conditions in a refrigerator. Thus, they are sufficiently stable for long-term animal experiments. In aqueous solution they are also stable in a refrigerator for 2 to 3 weeks when kept in the dark.

CARCINOGENICITY OF HETEROCYCLIC AMINES

Nine of the newly discovered heterocyclic amines have been subjected to long-term carcinogenesis tests in rats and mice. In these experiments one or two doses only were tested, namely, the maximal tolerated dose (MTD) and a lower dose than the MTD. Groups of 20 to 50 F344 strain rats and CDF_1 strain mice of both sexes were given a pellet diet containing 0.01 to 0.08% of the heterocyclic amines and water ad libitum continuously for up to 2 years (Sugimura, 1985). The results of these experiments are summarized in Table 3.3.

In rats, hepatocellular carcinomas, adenocarcinomas of the small and large intestines, and squamous cell carcinomas of the Zymbal glands, clitoral glands, oral cavity, and skin developed the most frequently (Takayama et al., 1984a,b; 1985a; Kato et al., 1988a,b). Male rats were more susceptible than females to induction of hepatocarcinomas by IQ, MeIQx, Glu-P-1, and Glu-P-2 (Takayama et al., 1984a,b; Kato et al., 1988a). Adenocarcinomas of the intestines were also more frequent in males fed on IQ, Glu-P-1, and Glu-P-2 (Takayama et al., 1984a,b). Squamous cell carcinoma originating from the oral cavity developed at high incidence in rats given a diet containing MeIQ (Kato et al., 1988b).

In mice, hepatocellular carcinomas, hemoangioendothelial sarcomas of the brown adipose tissue, and squamous cell carcinomas of the forestomach were frequently observed (Matsukura et al., 1981; Ohgaki et al., 1984a,b; 1986; 1987). Hepatocellular carcinomas were found at higher incidence in female mice than in males. Squamous cell carcinomas induced in the forestomach of mice given a diet containing MeIQ showed a high capacity for metastasis to the liver (Ohgaki et al., 1986). All the hetero-

TABLE 3.3 Carcinogenicity of Heterocyclic Amines

Chemical	Species	Concentration (%)	Target organs
IQ	Rats	0.03	Liver, small and large intestine, Zymbal gland, clitoral gland, skin
	Mice	0.03	Liver, forestomach, lung
MeIQ	Rats	0.03	Large intestine, Zymbal gland, skin, oral cavity, mammary gland
	Mice	0.04, 0.01	Liver, forestomach
MeIQx	Rats	0.04	Liver, Zymbal gland, clitoral gland, skin
	Mice	0.06	Liver, lung, hematopoietic system
Trp-P-1	Rats	0.015	Liver
	Mice	0.02	Liver
Trp-P-2	Mice	0.02	Liver
Glu-P-1	Rats	0.05	Liver, small and large intestines, Zymbal gland, clitoral gland
	Mice	0.05	Liver, blood vessels
Glu-P-2	Rats	0.05	Liver, small and large intestines, Zymbal gland, clitoral gland
	Mice	0.05	Liver, blood vessels
AαC	Mice	0.08	Liver, blood vessels
MeAαC	Mice	0.08	Liver, blood vessels

cyclic amines tested so far were found to be carcinogenic to rats and/or mice.

Some data are available on the effects of administration of these compounds by other routes. Administration of IQ by gavage induced mammary carcinomas in SD strain rats (Tanaka et al., 1985). Painting the skin of the back of mice with Trp-P-1, Trp-P-2, MeAαC, or Phe-P-1 and then phorbol ester resulted in the development of many papillomas and squamous cell carcinomas of the skin (Takahashi et al., 1986; Sato et al., 1987). Addition of Trp-P-1, Trp-P-2, or Glu-P-1 to cultured Syrian golden hamster embryo cells induced transformed foci (Takayama et al., 1977; 1979).

METABOLISM AND MUTAGENICITY OF
HETEROCYCLIC AMINES

Heterocyclic amines are not themselves mutagenic to *Salmonella typhimurium* strains. But they exert mutagenic activity in the presence of a metabolic activation system, namely S9 mix, prepared from the liver of rats treated with polychlorinated biphenyls or other inducers. Cytochrome P-450s in S9 mix convert the heterocyclic amines to their hydroxyamino derivatives (Kato and Yamazoe, 1987). Cytochrome P-448, which is induced in rat liver by 3-methylcholanthrene, is the most effective cytochrome for catalyzing this oxidation (Kato and Yamazoe, 1987). Synthetic hydroxyamino derivatives of the heterocyclic amines showed mutagenicity in the absence of a metabolic activation system. Like other aromatic amino compounds such as 2-acetylaminofluorene, the ultimate forms that react readily with DNA bases are reported to be esters of acetic acid and sulfuric acid, and the enzymes catalyzing these esterifications are present in bacterial cells (Kato and Yamazoe, 1987). This explains why the hydroxyamino derivatives themselves are mutagenic to bacteria. It is also noteworthy that heterocyclic amines themselves can induce hepatic P-450s (Degawa et al., 1988).

The optimum amount of S9 mix in the assay mixture varies depending on the chemical. The specific mutagenic activity of the compounds toward *Salmonella typhimurium* TA 98 and TA100 determined under optimal conditions are listed in Table 3.4 with those of other typical carcinogens (Sugimura, 1982; 1985). TA98 is more susceptible than TA100 to these heterocyclic amines. The planar structures of heterocyclic amines and their metabolites are favorable for their intercalation between bases of double stranded DNA and for efficiently causing a frameshift type mutation in TA98. The structures of adducts of some heterocyclic amines with guanine base were determined to be as shown in Fig. 3.3 (Hashimoto et al., 1980a,b; Snyderwine et al., 1988a). The adducts of Trp-P-2 and Glu-P-1 were purified from DNA extracted from the liver of rats treated with Trp-P-2 and Glu-P-1, respectively, and identified (Hashimoto et al., 1982). The adduct of IQ with guanine was obtained by treating DNA with the acetoxyamino derivative of IQ (Snyderwine et al. 1988a).

Incubation of a plasmid bearing the c-Ha-*ras*-1 proto-oncogene sequence with the acetoxyamino derivative of Glu-P-1 resulted in activation of c-Ha-*ras*-1, and this activated c-Ha-*ras*-1 transformed NIH3T3 cells in vitro. Of 14 transformants, six possessed a mutation in the sequence of

TABLE 3.4   Mutagenicities of Heterocyclic Amines and Typical Carcinogens in *Salmonella typhimurium*

Compound	Revertants/μg	
	TA98	TA100
IQ	433,000	7,000
MeIQ	661,000	30,000
IQx	75,000	1,500
MeIQx	145,000	14,000
4,8-DiMeIQx	183,000	8,000
7,8-DiMeIQx	163,000	9,900
PhIP	1,800	120
Trp-P-1	39,000	1,700
Trp-P-2	104,200	1,800
Glu-P-1	49,000	3,200
Glu-P-2	1,900	1,200
Phe-P-1	41	23
Orn-P-1	56,800	—
AαC	300	20
MeAαC	200	120
Aflatoxin B_1	6,000	28,000
AF-2	6,500	42,000
4-Nitroquinoline 1-oxide	970	9,900
Benzo[a]pyrene	320	660
MNNG[a]	0.00	870
N-Nitrosodiethylamine	0.02	0.15
N-Nitrosodimethylamine	0.00	0.23

[a]MNNG = *N*-Methyl-*N'*-nitro-*N*-nitrosoguanidine.

CCGG covering two bases each of the 11th and 12th amino acid codons of the c-Ha-*ras*-1 protein (Hashimoto et al., 1987). However, an activated *ras* family oncogene was found at only low frequency in hepatocellular carcinomas and intestinal adenocarcinomas induced by IQ and Glu-P-2, respectively, and thus this may not be the main mechanism of activation by heterocyclic amines (Ishizaka et al., 1987; Nagao et al., 1987). Trp-P-1, Trp-P-2, Glu-P-1, and AαC also induce sister chromatid exchanges in cultured mammalian cells (Tohda et al., 1980), and a hyroxyamino derivaive of Trp-P-2 induces single strand scission of DNA (Wakata et al., 1985).

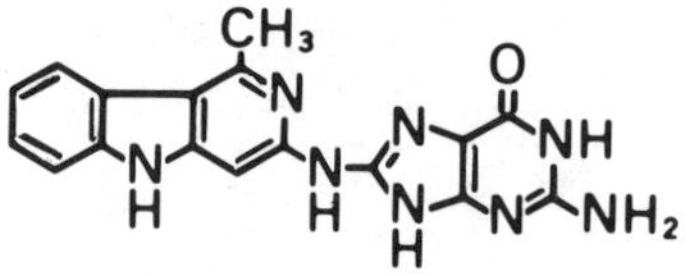

3-(C⁸-guanyl)amino-1-methyl-
5H-pyrido[4,3-b]indole

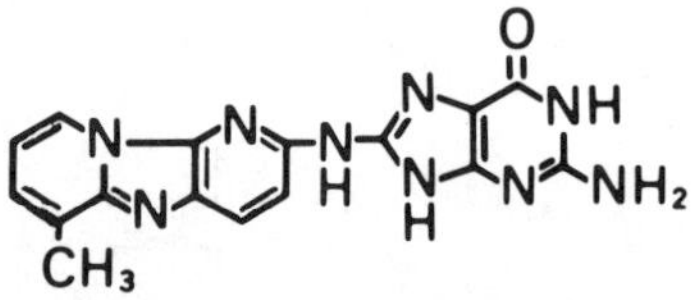

2-(C⁸-guanyl)amino-6-methyldipyrido-
[1,2-a:3',2'-d]imidazole

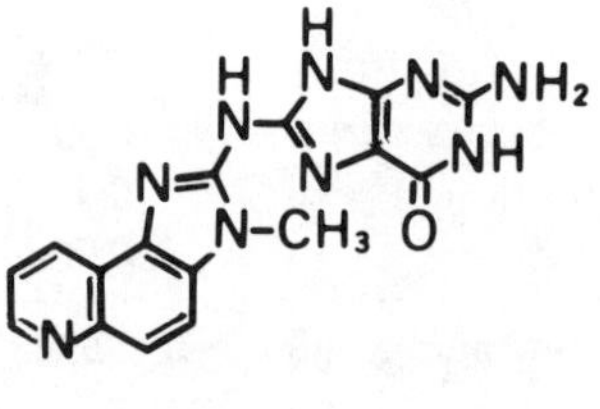

2-(C⁸-guanyl)amino-3-methylimidazo-
[4,5-f]quinoline

FIG. 3.3   Structures of adducts of Trp-P-2, Glu-P-1, and IQ with guanine.

RELATION BETWEEN CARCINOGENICITY AND MUTAGENICITY OF HETEROCYCLIC AMINES

Many heterocyclic amines are mutagenic to cultured Chinese hamster lung cells, producing diphtheria toxin resistant cells (Nakayasu et al., 1983). Their mutagenicities are given in Table 3.5. Their mutagenicities

TABLE 3.5 Mutagenicities of Heterocyclic Amines in Chinese Hamster Lung Cells

Compound	DT^r mutants/10^6 survivors induced by 1 μg/mL
IQ	40
MeIQ	38
MeIQx	5.7
Trp-P-1	33
Trp-P-2	160
Glu-P-1	1.2
Glu-P-2	0.3
AαC	20

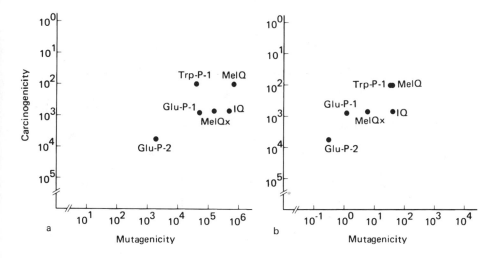

FIG. 3.4 Relation between carcinogenic potentials in rats and mutagenicities to *S. typhimurium* TA98 (a) and Chinese hamster lung cells (b) of heterocyclic amines. Carcinogenicity is expressed as the dose (μg/kg body weight/day) that causes cancers in 50% of the animals tested in ad libitum feeding experiments for life. Mutagenicity in Salmonella and Chinese hamster lung cells is shown as the number of revertants induced by 1 μg of compound and diphtheria toxin-resistant cells induced by 1 μg of compound, respectively.

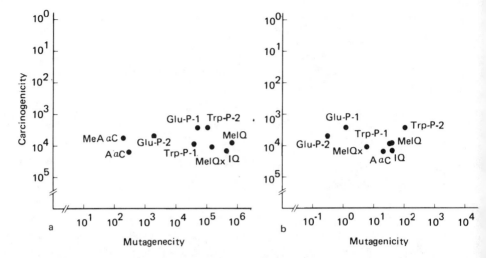

FIG. 3.5 Relation between carcinogenic potentials in mice and mutagenicities to *S. typhimurium* TA98 (a) and Chinese hamster lung cells (b) of heterocyclic amines. Carcinogenicity and mutagenicity are expressed as in Fig. 3.4.

toward Salmonella varied from 1 to 3000, whereas their mutagenicities to mammalian cells varied from 1 to 500. Their carcinogenic potentials, tentatively represented as TD_{50} values, which have been calculated as the doses causing cancers in 50% of the mice and rats tested in life-long feeding experiments, are plotted against their mutagenic potentials to *Salmonella typhimurium* TA98 and Chinese hamster lung cells. As shown in Fig. 3.4, correlation between the TD_{50} values calculated from the experiments in rats and their mutagenicities in *Salmonella typhimurium* TA98 was observed. In addition, a weak correlation between the TD_{50} values in rats and their mutagenicities in Chinese hamster lung cells was seen. On the other hand, no correlation between the TD_{50} values in mice and the mutagenic potentials in either Salmonella or Chinese hamster lung cells was observed (Fig. 3.5). Even in rodents, there are species differences in susceptibility to heterocyclic amines. Thus, it is, at present, still difficult to estimate the risk of heterocyclic amines to humans from their mutagenicities and carcinogenicities.

RELEVANCY OF HETEROCYCLIC AMINES TO CARCINOGENICITY IN HUMANS AND PRIMATES

An epidemiological survey indicated a higher risk of stomack cancer in people who frequently ate broiled fish (Ikeda et al., 1983).

Several studies have indicated that the metabolism of heterocyclic amines is similar in rodents and primates including humans. S9 mix from human liver was found to activate Trp-P-1 and Trp-P-2 (Sugimura, 1979). S9 mix prepared from the liver of a monkey without any previous treatment with an inducer also activated 11 heterocyclic amines including Trp-P-2, Glu-P-1, AαC, IQ, and MeIQx (Ishida et al., 1987). Consistent with these findings, possible metabolites of MeIQx were found in the urine and feces of persons who had eaten fried ground beef (Hayatsu et al., 1985a,b).

The ^{32}P-postlabeling method was used to demonstrate adduct formation with DNA in the liver of rats given IQ (Yamashita et al., 1988). DNA from the liver of a monkey given IQ by gavage showed exactly the same spots as those of DNA from rat liver (Snyderwine et al., 1988b). Moreover, hepatomas were found in a monkey given IQ (Adamson, personal communication, 1988). Thus some heterocyclic amines may well be carcinogenic in primates, including humans.

ENHANCEMENT AND SUPPRESSION OF BIOLOGICAL ACTIVITY OF HETEROCYCLIC AMINES

Tumors developed in the skin of the back of mice painted with a limited amount of Trp-P-2 and then phorbol ester, but they did not develop in skin painted with Trp-P-2 only (Takahashi et al., 1986). This indicates that the carcinogenicity of heterocyclic amines could be markedly enhanced by tumor promoter. On the contrary, the inclusion of quercetin in diet containing IQ suppressed the induction of hepatocellullar carcinomas in rats by IQ (Wakabayashi, unpublished data). Many substances inhibit the in vitro mutagenicity of heterocyclic amines toward *Salmonella typhimurium*. Typical examples are heme, hemin, unsaturated fatty acids, and fiber (Arimoto et al., 1980; Hayatsu et al., 1981; Kada et al., 1984). Porphyrins with planar structure form complexes with heterocyclic amines. Hydroxyamino derivatives of heterocyclic amines also form complexes with porphyrins (Arimoto et al., 1980). The mechanism of inhibition by fatty acids has not been clarified yet. A significant finding was that fried ground meat contains substances that inhibit the initiation of epidermal carcinogenesis by 7, 12-dimethylbenz[a]anthracene, and these substances were identified as derivatives of linoleic acid (Ha et al., 1987). The derivatives of linoleic acid might also inhibit initiating activities of heterocyclic amines.

QUANTITATION OF HETEROCYCLIC AMINES IN FOODS

The principle that heterocyclic amines form complexes with heme is now being used for partial purification of heterocyclic amines from crude extracts, such as extracts of cooked foods, feces, and urine. Heterocyclic amines also form complexes with trisulfocopper phthalocyanine, which has a planar structure. Trisulfocopper phthalocyanine can be covalently bound to cotton or rayon. The resulting materials are called blue cotton (Hayatsu et al., 1983) and blue rayon (Hayatsu et al., 1988), because trisulfocopper phthalocyanine is blue. Most heterocyclic amines are adsorbed to blue cotton or blue rayon and can then be eluted with methanol-ammonia solution. Partially purified samples obtained in this way were analyzed by HPLC with an electrochemical or fluorescence detector (Takahashi et al., 1985; Sugimura et al., 1988), and representative data are given in Table 3.6. MeIQx was found at highest concentration, and AαC was also frequently found at relatively high concentration. The specific mutagenicity of MeIQx is so high that MeIQx often accounts for 20 to 30% of the total mutagenicity in cooked foods. The mutagenic potential of AαC is only one-thousandth that of IQ, but the TD_{50} value of AαC in mice is about the same as that of IQ. Therefore, the risk of AαC to humans would be higher than that of IQ, because the amounts of AαC in foods are often higher than those of IQ.

PhIP was first isolated as a mutagen in fried beef by Felton et al. (1986). It has low mutagenic activity, but information on its carcinogenic potential is urgently required, because its concentration in cooked foods is often higher than that of other heterocyclic amines. Recently IQx, aminodimethylimidazopyridine (DMIP) and aminotrimethylimidazopyridine (TMIP) were found as mutagens in cooked foods (Becher et al., 1988). The exact positions of their methyl groups in DMIP and TMIP have not yet been determined, and the contributions of these three compounds to human cancer development also remain to be clarified.

TABLE 3.6 Amounts of Heterocyclic Amines in Cooked Foods

Sample	Amount (ng/g cooked food)							
	IQ	MeIQx	4,8-DiMeIQx	Trp-P-1	Trp-P-2	AαC	MeAαC
Broiled beef	0.19	2.11		0.21	0.25	1.20	
Fried ground beef		0.64	0.12	0.19	0.21		
Broiled chicken		2.33	0.81	0.12	0.18	0.21	
Broiled mutton		1.01	0.67		0.15	2.50	0.19
Food-grade beef extract		3.10					

OTHER EFFECTS OF HETEROCYCLIC AMINES

As described above, cooked foods contain mutagenic/carcinogenic heterocyclic amines. Some of these have other effects besides carcinogenicity.
Diets containing MeAαC caused atrophy of the salivary glands and pancreas in rats (Takayama et al., 1985b), but diets containing AαC did not
have this effect, and the salivary glands and pancreas of mice were not affected by MeAαC or AαC (Ohgaki et al., 1984a). With a preliminary experiment of 25 intramuscular injections of IQ at 10 mg/kg, chickens showed
atherosclerotic change of the aorta (Wakabayashi, unpublished data).
Trp-P-1 and Trp-P-2 inhibited both type A and type B monoamine oxidases in vitro (Ichinose et al.,1988) These findings suggest that heterocyclic amines may be related to development of degenerative changes, including those of the cardiovascular system, brain, and pancreas.

FUTURE PROSPECTS AND IMPLICATIONS

It is difficult but extremely important to estimate the risks to humans of
carcinogens, including polycyclic aromatic hydrocarbons, mycotoxins, N-
nitrosamines, and oxygen radicals. Heterocyclic amines are no exception.
At present, it is almost impossible to obtain precise quantitative information about them, but on the basis of the limited information available, we
recommend that exposure to smoke produced by broiling fish and meat
and a high intake of food containing significant amounts of hetercyclic
amines should be avoided. A fan should be used in the kitchen while
broiling meat and other foods to reduce inhalation of smoke containing
heterocyclic amines. Charring fish and meat by heating it directly over a
naked gas flame should also be avoided and, if possible, a microwave
oven range should be used to cook food. Of course, the way of cooking of
food and the taste should be chosen personally.

An experiment, in which Syrian golden hamsters were given a diet containing 5 to 40% fish meat pyrolysates, has been reported. In this experiment, the incidence of cancer in the test group was not significantly different from that in the control group (Takahashi et al., 1983). But in
another experiment, the presence of hyperplastic change was noticed in
the glandular stomach of rats given a diet containing 25% or 50% charred
fish meat (Fujii et al., 1987). The noncarcinogenic potential of crude
broiled fish can be explained reasonably by its low content of heterocyclic amines.

Even though the amounts of heterocyclic amines are so minute in comparison with their TD_{50} values, less exposure of humans to these chemicals is desirable. Humans are continuously being exposed to vast numbers of mutagens/carcinogens at very minute levels, but integration of these would result in the production of cancer in humans, especially under the condition of the presence of a tumor promoter. Experiments on the effects of various dose levels of heterocyclic amines are in progress in our laboratory. Preliminary results of experiments on the effects of combinations of five heterocyclic amines indicated that their effects were additive (Takayama et al., 1987). Experiments with appropriate tumor promoters are necessary. The recent finding of Trp-P-1, Trp-P-2, and MeIQx in dialysates from patients with uremia suggests the wide distribution of heterocyclic amines in our environment (Yanagisawa et al., 1986; Manabe et al., 1987). Thus, these compounds clearly require further collaborative studies by workers in various fields of science.

ACKNOWLEDGMENTS

The authors express their gratitudes to their many colleagues who have helped in this work. This series of research studies was supported by grants from the Ministry of Health and Welfare, the Ministry of Education, Science and Culture, the Agency for Science and Technology, the Foundation for Promotion of Cancer Research, Princess Takamatsu Cancer Research Fund, and Special Grants for a Comprehensive 10-Year Strategy for Cancer Control.

REFERENCES

Arimoto S., Ohara, Y., Namba, T., Negishi, T., and Hayatsu, H. 1980. Inhibition of the mutagenicity of amino acid pyrolysis products by hemin and other biological pyrrole pigments. *Biochem. Biophys. Res. Commun.* 92: 662.

Becher, G., Knize, M. G., Nes, I. F., and Felton, J. S. 1988. Isolation and identification of mutagens from a fried Norwegian meat product. *Carcinogenesis* 9: 247.

Commoner, B., Vithayathil, A. J., Dolara, P., Nair, S., Madyastha, P., and Cuca, G. C. 1978. Formation of mutagens in beef and beef extract during cooking. *Science* 201: 913.

Degawa, M., Yamaya, C., and Hashimoto, Y. 1988. Hepatic cytochrome P-450 isozyme(s) induced by dietary carcinogenic aromatic amines preferentially in female mice of DBA/2 and other strains. *Carcinogenesis* 9: 567.

Felton, J. S., Knize, M. G., Shen, N. H., Lewis, P. R., Andresen, B. D., Happe, J., and Hatch, F. T. 1986. The isolation and identification of a new mutagen from fried ground beef: 2-amino-1-methyl-6-phenylimidazo[4,5-*b*]pyridine (PhIP). *Carcinogenesis* 7: 1081.

Fujii, K., Nomoto, K., Ishidate, M., and Nakamura, K. 1987. Chronic toxicity of charred fish meat in Wistar rats. *Nutrition & Cancer* 9: 185.

Grivas, S., Nyhammar, T., Olsson, K., and Jägerstad, M. 1985. Formation of a new mutagenic DiMeIQx compound in a model system by heating creatinine, alanine and fructose. *Mutat. Res.* 151: 177.

Grivas, S., Nyhammar, T., Olsson, K., and Jägerstad M. 1986. Isolation and identification of the food mutagens IQ and MeIQx from a heated model system of creatinine, glycine and fructose. *Food Chem.* 20: 127.

Ha, Y. L., Grimm, N. K., and Pariza, M. W. 1987. Anticarcinogens from fried ground beef: heat-altered derivatives of linoleic acid. *Carcinogenesis* 8: 1881.

Hashimoto, Y., Shudo, K., and Okamoto, T. 1980a. Metabolic activation of a mutagen, 2-amino-6-methyldipyrido[1,2-*a*:3′,2′-*d*]imidazole. Identification of 2-hydroxyamino-6-methyldipyrido[1,2-*a*:3′,2′-*d*]imidazole and its reaction with DNA. *Biochem. Biophys. Res. Commun.* 92: 971.

Hashimoto, Y., Shudo, K., and Okamoto, T. 1980b. Activation of a mutagen, 3-amino-1-methyl-5*H*-pyrido[4,3-b]indole. Identification of 3-hydroxyamino-1-methyl-5*H*-pyrido[4,3-*b*]indole and its reaction with DNA. *Biochem. Biophys. Res. Commun.* 96: 355.

Hashimoto, Y., Shudo, K., and Okamoto, T. 1982. Modification of nucleic acids with muta-carcinogenic heterocyclic amines *in vivo*. Identification of modified bases in DNA extracted from rats injected with 3-amino-1-methyl-5*H*-pyrido[4,3-*b*]indole and 2-amino-6-methyldipyrido[1,2-*a*:3′,2′-*d*]imidazole. *Mutat. Res.* 105: 9.

Hashimoto, Y., Kawachi, E., Shudo K., Sekiya, T., and Sugimura, T. 1987. Transforming activity of human c-Ha-*ras*-1 proto-oncogene generated by the binding of 2-amino-6-methyldipyrido[1,2-*a*:3′,2′-*d*]imidazole and 4-nitroquinoline N-oxide: direct evidence of cellular transformation by chemically modified DNA. *Jpn. J. Cancer Res.* (Gann) 78: 211.

Hayatsu, H., Arimoto, S., Togawa, K., and Makita, M. 1981. Inhibitory effect of the ether extract of human feces on activities of mutagens: inhibition by oleic and linoleic acids. *Mutat. Res.* 81: 287.

Hayatsu, H., Oka, T., Wakata, A. Ohara, Y., Hayatsu, T., Kobayashi, H., and Arimoto, S. 1983. Adsorption of mutagens to cotton bearing covalently bound trisulfocopper phthalocyanine. *Mutat. Res.* 119: 233.

Hayatsu, H., Hayatsu, T., and Ohara, Y. 1985a. Mutagenicity of human urine caused by ingestion of fried ground beef. *Jpn. J. Cancer Res.* (Gann) 76: 445.

Hayatsu, H., Hayatsu,. T., Wataya, Y., and Mower, H. F. 1985b. Fecal mutagenicity arising from ingestion of fried ground beef in the human. *Mutat. Res.* 143: 207.

Hayatsu, H., Hayatsu, T., Zheng, O. L., Ohara, Y., and Arimoto S. 1988. Problems in monitoring mutagenicity of human urine. In *Methods for Detecting DNA Damaging Agents in Humans:* Applications in Cancer Epidemiology and Prevention. (Ed.) Bartsch, H., Hemminki, K., and O'Neill, I. K. IARC Scientific Publ. No. 89. International Agency for Research on Cancer, Lyon. In press.

Ichinose, H., Ozaki, N., Nakahara, D., Naoi, M., Wakabayashi, K., Sugimura, T., and Nagatsu, T. 1988. Effects of heterocyclic amines in food on dopamine metabolism in nigro striatal dopaminergic neurons. *Biochem. Pharmacol.* 37: 3289.

Ikeda, M., Yoshimoto, K., Yoshimura, T., Kono, S., Kato, H., and Kuratsune, M. 1983. A cohort study on the possible association between broiled fish intake and cancer. *Gann* 74: 640.

Ishida, Y., Negishi, C., Umemoto, A., Fujita, Y., Sato, S., Sugimura, T., Thorgeirsson, S. S., and Adamson, R. H. 1987. Activation of mutagenic and carcinogenic heterocyclic amines by S-9 from the liver of a rhesus monkey. *Toxic. in vitro* 1: 45.

Ishizaka, Y., Ochiai, M., Ishikawa, F., Sato, S., Miura, Y., Nagao, M., and Sugimura, T. 1987. Activated N-*ras* oncogene in a transformant derived from a rat small intestinal adenocarcinoma induced by 2-aminodipyrido[1,2-*a*:3′,2′-*d*]imidazole. *Carcinogenesis* 8: 1575.

Jägerstad, M., Olsson, K., Grivas, S., Negishi, C., Wakabayashi, K., Tsuda, M., Sato, S., and Sugimura, T. 1984. Formation of 2-amino-3,8-dimethylimidazo[4,5-*f*]quinoxaline in a model system by heating creatinine, glycine and glucose. *Mutat. Res.* 126: 239.

Kada, T., Kato, M., Aikawa, K., and Kiriyama, S. 1984. Adsorption of pyrolysate mutagens by vegetable fibers. *Mutat. Res.* 141: 149.

Kasai, H., Yamaizumi, Z., Wakabayashi, K., Nagao, M., Sugimura, T., Yokoyama S., Miyazawa, T., Spingarn, N. E., Weisburger, J. H., and Nishimura, S. 1980a. Potent novel mutagens produced by broiling fish under normal conditions. *Proc. Jpn. Acad.* 56B: 278.

Kasai, H., Yamaizumi, Z., Wakabayashi, K., Nagao, M., Sugimura T., Yokoyama S., Miyazawa, T., and Nishimura, S. 1980b. Structure and chemical synthesis of Me-IQ, a potent mutagen isolated from broiled fish. *Chem. Lett.* 1391.

Kasai, H., Yamaizumi, Z., Shiomi, T., Yokoyama, S., Miyazawa, T., Wakabayashi, K., Nagao, M., Sugimura, T., and Nishimura, S. 1981. Structure of a potent mutagen isolated from fried beef. *Chem. Lett.* 485.

Kato, R. and Yamazoe, Y. 1987. Metabolic activation and covalent binding to nucleic acids of carcinogenic heterocyclic amines from cooked foods and amino acid pyrolysates. *Jpn. J. Cancer Res.* (Gann) 78: 297.

Kato, T., Ohgaki, H., Hasegawa, H., Sato, S., Takayama, S., and Sugimura, T. 1988a. Carcinogenicity in rats of a mutagenic compound, 2-amino-3, 8-dimethylimidazo[4,5-*f*]quinoxaline. *Carcinogenesis* 9: 71.

Kato, T., Migita, H., Ohgaki, H., Sato, S., Takayama, S., and Sugimura, T. 1988b. Induction of tumors in the Zymbal gland, oral cavity, colon, skin and mammary gland of F344 rats by a mutagenic compound, 2-amino-3,4-dimethylimidazo[4,5-*f*]quinoline. In press. *Carcinogenesis.*

Kosuge, T., Tsuji, K., Wakabayashi, K., Okamoto, T., Shudo, K., Iitaka, Y., Itai, A., Sugimura, T., Kawachi, T., Nagao, M., Yahagi, T., and Seino, Y. 1978. Isolation and structure studies of mutagenic principles in amino acid pyrolysates. *Chem. Pharm. Bull.* 26: 611.

Manabe, S., Yanagisawa, H., Guo, S.-B., Abe, S., Ishikawa, S., and Wada, O. 1987. Detection of Trp-P-1 and Trp-P-2, carcinogenic tryptophan pyrolysis products, in dialysis fluid of patients with uremia. *Mutat. Res.* 179: 33.

Matsukura, N., Kawachi, T., Morino, K., Ohgaki, H., Sugimura, T., and Takayama, S. 1981. Carcinogenicity in mice of mutagenic compounds from a tryptophan pyrolyzate. *Science* 213: 346.

Matsumoto, T., Yoshida, D., Mizusaki, S., and Okamoto, H. 1977. Mutagenic activity of amino acid pyrolyzates in *Salmonella typhimurium* TA98 *Mutat. Res.* 48: 279.

Nagao, M., Honda, M., Seino, Y., Yahagi, T., and Sugimura, T. 1977a. Mutagenicities of smoke condensates and the charred surface of fish and meat. *Cancer Lett.* 2: 221.

Nagao, M., Honda, M., Seino, Y., Yahagi, T., Kawachi, T., and Sugimura, T. 1977b. Mutagenicities of protein pyrolysates. *Cancer Lett.* 2: 335.

Nagao, M., Ishikawa, F., Tahira, T., Ochiai, M., and Sugimura, T. 1987. Activation of rat and human c-raf(-1) by rearrangement. In *Oncogenes and Cancer.* (Ed.) Aaronson, S. T., Bishop, J. M., Sugimura, T., Terada, M., Toyoshima, K., and Vogt, P. K. p.75. Japan Sci. Soc. Press, Tokyo/ VNU Sci. Press, Utrecht.

Nakayasu, M., Nakasato, F., Sakamoto, H., Terada M., and Sugimura, T. 1983. Mutagenic activity of heterocyclic amines in Chinese hamster lung cells with diphtheria toxin resistance as a marker. *Mutat. Res.* 118: 91.

Negishi, C., Wakabayashi, K., Tsuda, M., Sato, S., Sugimura, T., Saito, H., Maeda, M., and Jägerstad, M. 1984. Formation of 2-amino-3,7,8-trimethylimidazo[4,5-*f*]quinoxaline, a new mutagen, by heating a mixture of creatinine, glucose and glycine. *Mutat. Res.* 140: 55.

Negishi, C., Wakabayashi, K., Yamaizumi, Z., Saito, H., Sato, S., Sugimura, T., and Jägerstad, M. 1985. Identification of 4, 8-DiMeIQx, a new mutagen. Selected abstracts of papers presented at the 13th annual meeting of the environmental mutagen society of Japan, 12–13 Oct. 1984, Tokyo (Japan). *Mutat. Res.* 147: 267.

Ohgaki, H., Matsukura, N., Morino, K., Kawachi, T., Sugimura, T., and Takayama, S. 1984a. Carcinogenicity in mice of mutagenic compounds from glutamic acid and soybean globulin pyrolysates. *Carcinogenesis* 5: 815.

Ohgaki, H., Kusama, K., Matsukura, N., Morino, K., Hasegawa, H., Sato, S., Takayama, S., and Sugimura, T. 1984b. Carcinogenicity in mice of a mutagenic compound, 2-amino-3-methylimidazo[4,5-*f*]quinoline, from broiled sardine, cooked beef and beef extract. *Carcinogenesis* 5: 921.

Ohgaki, H., Hasegawa, H., Suenaga, M., Kato, T., Sato, S., Takayama, S., and Sugimura, T. 1986. Induction of hepatocellular carcinoma and highly metastatic squamous cell carcinomas in the forestomach of mice by feeding 2-amino-3,4-dimethylimidazo[4,5-*f*]quinoline. *Carcinogenesis* 7: 1889.

Ohgaki, H., Hasegawa, H., Suenaga, M., Sato, S., Takayama, S., and Sugimura, T. 1987. Carcinogenicity in mice of a mutagenic compound, 2-amino-3,8-dimethylimidazo[4,5-*f*]quinoxaline (MeIQx) from cooked foods. *Carcinogenesis* 8: 665.

Pariza, M. W., Ashoor, S. H., Chu, F. S., and Lund, D. B. 1979. Effects of treatment of temperature and time on mutagen formation in pan-fried hamburger. *Cancer Lett.* 7: 63.

Sato, H., Takahashi, M., Furukawa, F., Miyakawa, Y., Hasegawa, R.,

Toyoda, K., and Hayashi, Y. 1987. Initiating activity in a two-stage mouse skin model of nine mutagenic pyrolysates of amino acids, soybean globulin and proteinaceous food. *Carcinogenesis* 8: 1231.

Shioya, M., Wakabayashi, K., Sato, S., Nagao, M., and Sugimura, T. 1987 Formation of a mutagen, 2-amino-1-methyl-6-phenylimidazo[4,5-*b*]pyridine(PhIP) in cooked beef, by heating a mixture containing creatinine, phenylalanine and glucose. *Mutat. Res.* 191: 133.

Snyderwine, E. G., Roller, P. P., Adamson, R. H., Sato, S., and Thorgeirsson, S. S. 1988a. Reaction of the *N*-hydroxylamine and *N*-acetoxy derivatives of 2-amino-3-methylimidazo[4,5-*f*]quinoline (IQ) with DNA. Synthesis and identification of *N*-(deoxyguanosin-8-yl)-IQ. *Carcinogenesis.* 9: 1061.

Snyderwine, E. G., Yamashita, K., Adamson, R. H., Sato, S., Nagao, M., Sugimura, T., and Thorgeirsson, S. S. 1988b. Use of the ^{32}P−postlabeling method to detect DNA adducts of the 2-amino-3-methylimidazo[4, 5-*f*]quinoline (IQ) in monkeys fed IQ: Identification of the N-(deoxyguanosin-8-yl)-IQ adduct. *Carciongenesis.* 9: 1739.

Sugimura, T. 1979. Naturally occurring genotoxic carcinogens. In *Naturally Occurring Carcinogens-Mutagens and Modulators of Carcinogenesis.* (Ed.) Miller, E. C., Miller, J. A., Hirono, I., Sugimura, T., and Takayama, S., p.241. Japan Sci. Soc. Press, Tokyo/Univ Park Press, Baltimore.

Sugimura, T. 1982. Mutagens, carcinogens, and tumor promoters in our daily food. *Cancer* 49: 1970.

Sugimura, T. 1985. Carcinogenicity of mutagenic heterocyclic amines formed during the cooking process. *Mutat. Res.* 150: 33.

Sugimura, T. 1986. Studies on environmental chemical carcinogenesis in Japan. *Science* 233: 312.

Sugimura, T., Nagao M., Kawachi, T., Honda, M., Yahagi, T., Seino, Y., Sato, S., Matsukura, N., Matsushima, T., Shirai, A., Sawamura, M., and Matsumoto, H. 1977a. Mutagen-carcinogens in food, with special reference to highly mutagenic pyrolytic products in broiled foods. In *Origins of Human Cancer.* Hiatt, H. H., Watson, J. D., and Winsten J. A., p. 1561. Cold Spring Harbor Laboratory, Cold Spring Harbor, NY.

Sugimura, T., Kawachi, T., Nagao, M., Yahagi, T., Seino, Y., Okamoto, T., Shudo, K., Kosuge, T., Tsuji, K., Wakabayashi, K., Iitaka, Y., and Itai, A. 1977b. Mutagenic principle(s) in tryptophan and phenylalanine pyrolysis products. *Proc. Jpn. Acad.* 53: 58.

Sugimura, T., Sato, S., and Wakabayashi, K. 1988. Mutagens/carcinogens in pyrolysates of amino acids and proteins and in cooked foods: heterocyclic aromatic amines. In *Chemical Induction of Cancer,*

Structural Bases and Biological Mechanisms. (Ed.) Woo, Y-T., Lai, D. Y., Arcos, J. C., and Argus, M. F., Vol. IIIC, p.681. Academic Press, Inc., New York.

Takahashi, M., Furukawa, F., Nagano, K., Miyakawa, Y., Kokubo, T., and Hayashi Y. 1983. Long-term *in vivo* carcinogenicity test of fish meat pyrolysate in Syrian golden hamsters. *Gann* 74: 633.

Takahashi, M., Wakabayashi, K., Nagao, M., Yamamoto, M., Masui, T., Goto, T., Kinae, N., Tomita, I., and Sugimura, T. 1985. Quantification of 2-amino-3-methylimidazo[4,5-*f*]quinoline (IQ) and 2-amino-3,8-dimethylimidazo[4,5-*f*]quinoxaline (MeIQx) in beef extracts by liquid chromatography with electrochemical detection (LCEC). *Carcinogenesis* 6: 1195.

Takahashi, M., Furukawa, F., Miyakawa, Y., Sato, H., Hasegawa, R., and Hayashi, Y. 1986. 3-Amino-1-methyl-5*H*-pyrido[4,3-*b*]indole initiates two-stage carcinogenesis in mouse skin but is not a complete carcinogen. *Jpn. J. Cancer Res.* (Gann) 77: 509.

Takayama, S., Katoh, Y., Tanaka, M., Nagao, M., Wakabayashi, K., and Sugimura, T. 1977. *In vitro* transformation of hamster embryo cells with tryptophan pyrolysis products. *Proc. Jpn. Acad.* 53B: 126.

Takayama, S., Hirakawa, T., Tanaka, M., Kawachi, T., and Sugimura, T. 1979. *In vitro* transformation of hamster embryo cells with a glutamic acid pyrolysis product. *Toxicol. Lett.* 4: 281.

Takayama, S., Masuda, M., Mogami, M., Ohgaki, H., Sato, S., and Sugimura, T. 1984a. Induction of cancers in the intestine, liver and various other organs of rats by feeding mutagens from glutamic acid pyrolysate. *Gann* 75: 207.

Takayama, S., Nakatsuru, Y., Masuda, M., Ohgaki, H., Sato, S., and Sugimura, T. 1984b. Demonstration of carcinogenicity in F344 rats of 2-amino-3-methylimidazo[4,5-*f*]quinoline from broiled sardine, fried beef and beef extract. *Gann* 75: 467.

Takayama, S., Nakatsuru, Y., Ohgaki, H., Sato, S., and Sugimura, T. 1985a. Carcinogenicity in rats of a mutagenic compound, 3-amino-1,4-dimethyl-5*H*-pyrido[4,3-*b*]indole, from tryptophan pyrolysate. *Jpn. J. Cancer Res.* (Gann) 76: 815.

Takayama, S., Nakatsuru, Y., Ohgaki, H., Sato, S., and Sugimura, T. 1985b. Atrophy of salivary glands and pancreas of rats fed on diet with amino-methyl-α-carboline. *Proc. Jpn Acad.* 61B: 277.

Takayama, S., Nakatsuru, Y., and Sato, S. 1987. Carcinogenic effect of the simultaneous administration of five heterocyclic amines to F344 rats. *Jpn. J. Cancer Res.* (Gann) 78: 1068.

Tanaka, T., Barnes, W. S., Williams, G. M., and Weisburger, J. H. 1985. Multipotential carcinogenicity of the fried food mutagen 2-amino-3-methylimidazo[4,5-*f*]quinoline in rats. *Jpn. J. Cancer Res.* (Gann) 76: 570.

Tohda, H., Oikawa, A., Kawachi, T., and Sugimura, T. 1980. Induction of sister-chromatid exchanges by mutagens from amino acid and protein pyrolysates. *Mutat. Res.* 77: 65.

Tsuda, M., Takahashi, Y., Nagao, M., Hirayama, T., and Sugimura, T. 1980. Inactivation of mutagens from pyrolysates of tryptophan and glutamic acid by nitrite in acidic solution. *Mutat. Res.* 78: 331.

Tsuda, M., Nagao, M., Hirayama, T., and Sugimura, T. 1981. Nitrite converts 2-amino-α-carboline, an indirect mutagen, into 2-hydroxy-α-carboline, a non-mutagen and 2-hydroxy-3-nitroso-α-carboline, a direct mutagen. *Mutat. Res.* 83: 61.

Tsuda, M., Wakabayashi, K., Hirayama, T., and Sugimura, T. 1983. Inactivation of potent pyrolysate mutagens by chlorinated tap water. *Mutat. Res.* 119: 27.

Tsuda, M., Negishi, C., Makino, R., Sato, S., Yamaizumi, Z., Hirayama, T., and Sugimura, T. 1985. Use of nitrite and hypochlorite treatments in determination of the contributions of IQ-type and non-IQ-type heterocyclic amines to the mutagenicities in crude pyrolyzed materials. *Mutat. Res.* 147: 335.

Wakata, A., Oka, N., Hiramoto, K., Yoshioka, A., Negishi, K., Wataya, Y., and Hayatsu, H. 1985. DNA strand cleavage *in vitro* by 3-hydroxy-amino-1-methyl-5*H*-pyrido[4,3-*b*]indole, a direct-acting mutagen formed in the metabolism of carcinogenic 3-amino-1-methyl-5*H*-pyrido[4,3-*b*]indole. *Cancer Res.* 45: 5867.

Yamamoto, T., Tsuji, K., Kosuge, T., Okamoto, T., Shudo, K., Takeda, K., Iitaka, Y., Yamaguchi, K., Seino, Y., Yahagi, T., Nagao, M., and Sugimura, T. 1978. Isolation and structure determination of mutagenic substances in L-glutamic acid pyrolysate. *Proc. Jpn. Acad.* 54B: 248.

Yamashita, K., Umemoto, A., Grivas, S., Kato, S., Sato, S., and Sugimura, T. 1988. Heterocyclic amine-DNA adducts analyzed by ^{32}P-postlabeling method. *Nucleic Acids Symp. Ser. 19.* IRL Press, Oxford. 111.

Yanagisawa, H., Manabe, S., Kitagawa, Y., Ishikawa, S., Nakajima, K., and Wada, O. 1986. Presence of 2-amino-3,8-dimethylimidazo[4,5-*f*]quinoxaline (MeIQx) in dialysate from patients with uremia. *Biochem. Biophys. Res. Commun.* 138: 1084.

Yokota, M., Narita, K., Kosuge, T., Wakabayashi, K., Nagao, M., Sugimura, T., Yamaguchi, K., Shudo, K., Iitaka, Y., and Okamoto, T. 1981. A potent mutagen isolated from a pyrolysate of L-ornithine. *Chem. Pharm. Bull.* 29: 1473.

Yoshida, D., Matsumoto, T., Yoshimura, R., and Matsuzaki, T. 1978. Mutagenicity of amino-α-carbolines in pyrolysis products of soybean globulin. *Biochem, Biophys. Res. Commun.* 83: 915.

4

Relative Exposure to Nitrite, Nitrate, and N-Nitroso Compounds from Endogenous and Exogenous Sources

Joseph H. Hotchkiss

Cornell University
Ithaca, New York

INTRODUCTION

The role that nitrite (NO_2^-), nitrate (NO_3^-), and NOC[1] might play in the etiology of cancer remains unclear. Many widely consumed foods contain appreciable amounts of NO_3^- and a few contain smaller amounts of NO_2^-. Trace amounts of carcinogenic N-nitrosamines (nitrosamines) occur in even fewer foods. The occurrence of nitrosamines in nitrite-cured meats results from the use of NO_2^- as a color fixative, flavor preservative, and antimicrobial agent, but nitrosamines also occur in products to which

---

[1]Abbreviations: N-nitroso compounds, NOC; N-nitrosodimethylamine, NDMA; N-nitrosodiethylamine, NDEA; N-nitrosodiethanolamine, NDELA; N-nitroso-methylbenzylamine, NMBzA; NMOR, N-nitrosomorpholine; N-nitrosoproline, NPRO; N-nitrosothiazolidine, NTHZ; N-nitrosothiazolidine carboxylic acid, NTHZCA; N-nitroso-2-methylthiazolidine carboxylic acid, NMTHZCA; N-nitrosomethylurea, NMU; N-nitrosonornicotine; NNN; N-nitrosoanatabine, NAT; N-nitrosoanabasine; NAB; 4-(methylnitrosoamino)-1-(3-pyridyl)-1-butanone, NNK; nonvolatile nitroamines, NVNA; volatile nitrosamines, VNA; tobacco specific nitrosamines, TSNA.

NO_2^- has not been added. Research has quantified the volatile nitrosamine content of many Western foods, but nonvolatile nitrosamines and N-nitrosamides (nitrosamides) have not been extensively measured. Epidemiological data have suggested that ingestion of NO_3^- correlates with increased risk of some cancers due to the in vivo (endogenous) formation of NOC, but other data have contradicted these findings.

Complicating the uncertainties is the fact that normal endogenous biological processes result in the formation of NO_3^- and NOC in humans. Exposure to NO_3^- from the diet and from endogenous synthesis appears, under most circumstances, to be about equal, although there are large intra- and interindividual differences. Other evidence indicates that humans are exposed to NO_2^- through two or more routes of endogenous synthesis and that this represents the largest source of overall exposure. The in vivo formation of noncarcinogenic N-nitrosamino acids has been conclusively demonstrated in humans and, while less conclusive, it is also likely that carcinogenic NOC are formed in the stomach and possibly elsewhere. While exposure to volatile nitrosamines is well quantified for Western diets, the quantitative data for endogenous exposure are less clear. It is probable that exposure from endogenous synthesis of NOC is greater than dietary exposure. Recent data concerning NO_2^-, NO_3^-, and NOC are reviewed in this paper, and the relative human exposure from exogenous and endogenous sources will be compared to the extent allowed by current data. Readers interested in a detailed review of the issues concerning exogenous exposure to NO_3^-, NO_2^-, and NOC are directed to the 1981 report by National Academy of Sciences (National Academy of Sciences 1981).

Nitroso Compound Formation

NOC can be divided into two classes (Fig. 4.1): the nitrosamines and the nitrosamides (and related compounds). Nitrosamines are N-nitroso derivatives of secondary amines, whereas nitrosamides are N-nitroso derivatives of substituted ureas, amides, carbamates, guanidines, and similar compounds (Mirvish, 1975). This classification is of more than a chemical interest; there are significant biological and environmental differences between nitrosamines and nitrosamides. These differences derive from differences in the relative stability of each class, their rate or ease of formation, and their biological activity. Nitrosamines are quite stable compounds, while many nitrosamides have half-lives on the order of minutes, particularly at pH > 6.5. Both classes are potent carcinogens, but by dif-

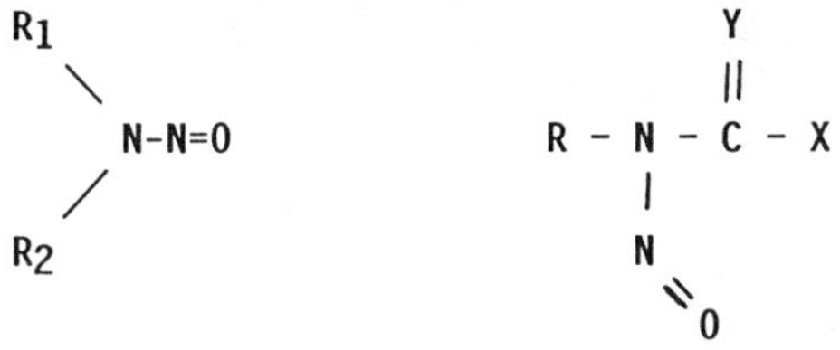

$$R_1 \diagdown$$
$$N-N=O$$
$$R_2 \diagup$$

N-Nitrosamine

$$\begin{array}{c} Y \\ \| \\ R - N - C - X \\ | \\ N \\ \diagdown \\ O \end{array}$$

N-Nitrosamide*

*where:

Y	X	Compound
O	alkyl, aryl	N-Nitrosamide
O	NH$_2$, NHR, NR$_2$	N-Nitrosourea
O	RO	N-Nitrosocarbamate
NH	NH$_2$, NHR, NR$_2$	N-Nitrosoguanidine

FIG. 4.1 Generalized structures of N-nitrosamines and N-nitrosamides and related compounds.

ferent chemical mechanisms. Carcinogenic NOC can be formed by N-nitrosation of amines and amides that are ubiquitous in foods, biological systems, and the environment.

Nitrosation most commonly occurs when chemical species which are related to nitric acid (HNO$_2$) react with nucleophiles such as amines, amides, alcohols, or anions (Challis, 1981). Carriers of NO$^+$ or NO, including H$_2$O$^+$, O-alkyl, NO$_2^-$, NO$_3^-$, or halides can be nitrosating agents depending on the reaction conditions (Fig. 4.2). The classical N-nitrosation reaction occurs when two moles of HNO$_2$ react with one mole of unprotonated secondary amine (Fig. 4.3). The reaction is second order in nitrous acid and third order overall, because nitrous anhydride is the nitrosating agent. Because of the opposing requirements of unprotonated amine (favored by higher pH) and nitrous acid formation (favored by lower pH), N-nitrosation occurs at some optimum pH, on either side of which the rate decreases rapidly. This maximum rate depends, in large part, on the basicity of the amine-more basic amines (e.g., dialkylamines) are less reactive, while weaker base amines (e.g., diphenylamine) nitrosate more readily at a given pH. Dialkylamines have an optimum pH for nitrosation of 2.5 to 3.5, which is near the pH of the mammalian stomach. Amides and related compounds do not have optimum pHs and nitrosate more rapidly as the pH decreases (Mirvish, 1975).

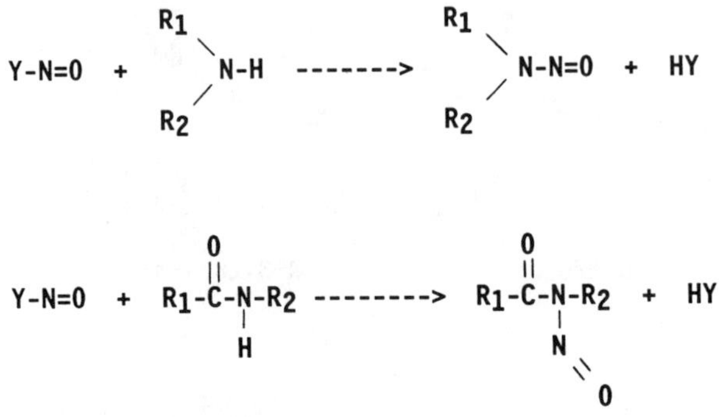

FIG. 4.2 Nitrosation of amines and amides Y = NO_2, NO_3, H_2O^+, SCN^- halides.

$$(NO_3^-) \downarrow$$

$$2NO_2^- \overset{2H^+}{\rightleftharpoons} 2HNO_2 \rightleftharpoons N_2O_3 + H_2O$$

$$N_2O_3 + R_2N\text{-}H \longrightarrow R_2N\text{-}N = O + HNO_2$$

$$\text{RATE} = K\ (\text{AMINE})\ (\text{NITROUS ACID})^2$$

FIG. 4.3 Acidic nitrosation of amines. The reaction is second order in nitrite and overall third order.

It is useful to review the chemistry of nitrogen in order to understand the ease with which NOC can be formed. Nitrogen exists in eight oxidation states from −3 to +5 (Fig. 4.4). NOC can form when secondary amines or substituted amides (oxidation state −3) react with oxides of nitrogen (NO_x) in oxidation states +3 or +4. While only NO_x in these oxidation states are capable of nitrosation, there are several common biological and chemical mechanisms through which nitrogen in other oxidation states can be converted to +3 or +4. For example, combustion leads to the formation of small amounts of nitric oxide (NO), which can be oxidized by air to nitrogen dioxide (NO_2) and other nitrosating agents. NO_3^-, which is

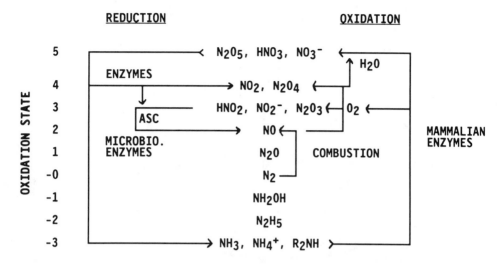

FIG. 4.4 The oxidation states of nitrogen and common oxidations and reductions. Oxidation states $+3$ and $+4$ are nitrosating agents.

the end product of the oxidation of nitrogenous compounds, can be recycled through reduction by commonly occurring microorganisms. In this way NO_3^- ($+5$) serves as a reservoir for NO_2^- ($+3$), which is an indirect nitrosating agent.

The reactions and equilibria formed by nitrosating agents and their precursors are complex (Fig. 4.5). NO_2^-, in acid, is in equilibrium (*1*) with nitrous acid, which is, in turn, in equilibrium (*2*) with nitrous anhydride (N_2O_3). NOC form (*5*) in the presence of unprotonated amines or amides. In the presence of ascorbic acid, N_2O_3 is reduced (*6*) to nitric oxide (NO) and ascorbate oxidized to dehydroascorbate (see Fig. 4.6). If aerobic, NO is oxidized to dinitrogentetroxide (N_2O_4; *7,8*). N_2O_4 is in equilibrium with the other NO_x compounds with oxidation states of $+3$ or $+4$ (*3,4*). In this way, NO, which is not a direct nitrosating agent, is recycled to a nitrosating agent. Ascorbate-mediated inhibition of nitrosation is, therefore, dependent on an excess of ascorbate. If the ascorbate is used up, then nitrosation can proceed. Nitrosating equivalence is permanently lost from the system in two ways; NO_2 and NO are gases and may be lost to the atmosphere (*10,11*). N_2O_4 can also react with water to form NO_3^- ($+5;9$). Licht et al. (1988a,b) have calculated the equilibrium constants for many of these reactions and have developed a model in order to predict the amount of nitrosamine that may form under given set of conditions, particularly those in the stomach.

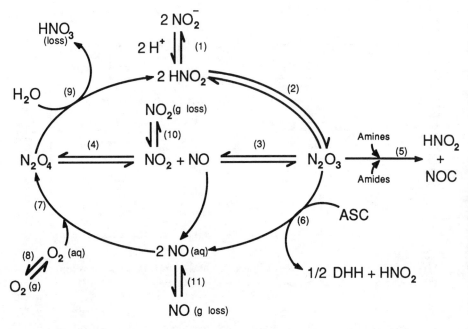

FIG. 4.5 Reactions and equilibria of oxides of nitrogen. Nitrosation equivalence is lost from the system via reaction 9 and equilibria 10 and 11. N_2O_3 and N_2O_4 are nitrosating agents.

The precursors to NOC occur widely in both the environment and in biological systems. It is not surprising that low-level amounts of nitrosamines have been widely found in many foods and other environments. Most Western foods, occupational, and general environments have been surveyed for those nitrosamines which can be easily analyzed by gas chromatography. Nitrosamines which are not volatile or stable enough for gas chromatography and nitrosamides cannot be analyzed directly. Human exposure to these compounds cannot, therefore, be assessed until improved analytical methodology is developed.

Biological Activity

The biological activity of NOC has been reviewed in depth (Preussmann and Stewart, 1984), and only a few basic comments are germane. Just under 300 NOC have been assayed for carcinogenicity, and over 90% have

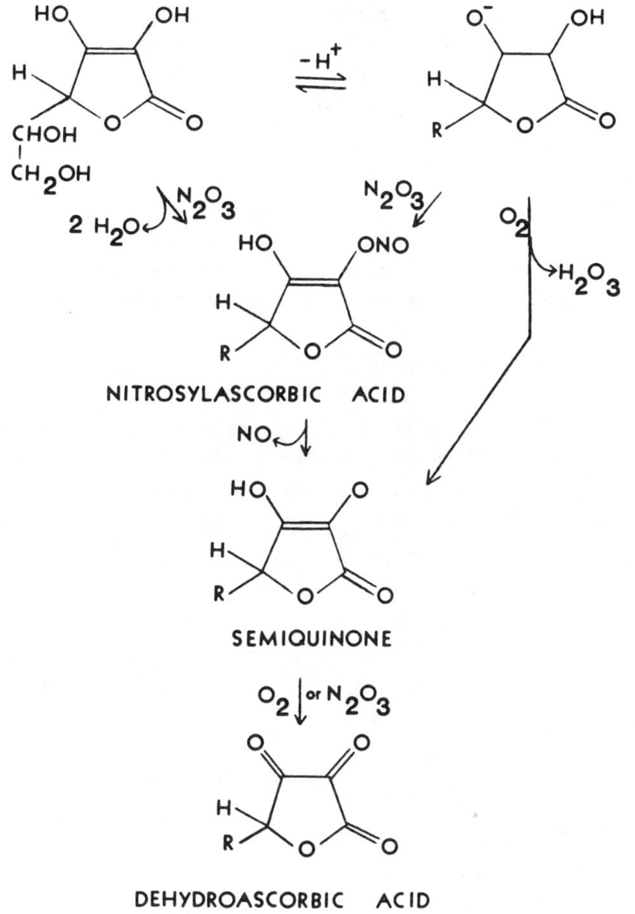

FIG. 4.6 Reaction between ascorbic acid and dinitrogen trioxide to produce nitric oxide and dehydroascorbic acid. The nitric oxide is not a nitrosating agent but can be oxidized to one by molecular oxygen.

been positive (Preussmann and Stewart, 1984). The most widely tested NOC, NDEA, has been shown to be carcinogenic in 40 species (Lijinsky, 1987). There are important distinctions between nitrosamines and nitrosamides; nitrosamines must first be activated to carcinogens by oxidative enzymes (i.e., $P_{450's}$), whereas nitrosamides are direct-acting carcinogens. Nitrosamines often produce tumors at a site(s) distant from the point of application. Within a given species, nitrosamines often show selectivity based on chemical structure for the organ in which tumors are produced. For example, in the rat, NMBzA is a potent esophageal carcinogen, while NDMA is primarily a liver carcinogen. However, there are large interspecies differences in the organs affected by the same NOC. The method of dosing the animals can also influence the tumor pattern and incidence, which indicates that there are distinct pharmacological affects. Unfortunately, the target organ in man for a given NOC cannot be predicted with any reasonable certainty. Nitrosamides can produce tumors at the site of application as well as in distant sites. Readers interested in the structure-activity relationships of NOC are directed to a recent review by Lijinsky (1987).

These differences in biological activity have important implications when considering the possible involvement of NOC in human cancer. First, nitrosamides are less likely than nitrosamines to be found in the environment or in foods because of their inherent instability. Nitrosamides, on the other hand, are more likely to be related to some forms of human cancer through endogenous formation. The potential for formation of nitrosamides in the acid environment of the human stomach has attracted considerable interest (Mirvish, 1983). Second, the types of human cancers that might be associated with a given nitrosamine cannot be predicted from animal data. The only human cancer linked to NOC is oral cancer resulting from the use of tobacco snuff (Winn. 1984).

EXPOSURE TO EXOGENOUSLY FORMED NITRATE AND NITRITE

Human exposure to NO_3^- comes from two sources: (1) exogenous sources, mainly food and water, and (2) endogenous formation due to the in vivo oxidation of more reduced NO_x compounds that are ingested or inhaled (e.g., tobacco smoke, air pollution) and the de novo synthesis of NO_3^- from more reduced forms of nitrogen. Exogenous sources have been studied in detail. Exposure to NO_2^- also originates from exogenous sources including ingestion, primarily from foods to which NO_2^- has been intentionally added, and from endogenous synthesis. NO_2^- is formed in vivo through the reduction of ingested NO_3^- by oral microorganisms. Recent evidence indicates that NO_2^-, like NO_3^-, may also be formed via oxidation of more reduced nitrogen compounds within the body. Exogenous sources of exposure are dealt with in this section; endogenous formation will be discussed in a later section.

Food and Water

For most U.S. residents, food is the major source of exogenous exposure to NO_3^- and NO_2^- (White, 1975; 1976). Contaminated water can also be a significant source of NO_3^- for those using such water. NO_3^- is nearly ubiquitous and occurs in many foods, but estimates indicate that the majority of a U.S. resident's dietary NO_3^- comes from vegetables, with a small portion coming from cured meats (Table 4.1). Breads, dairy products, and fruits and fruit juices contribute minor amounts (National Academy of Sciences, 1981). The amount of NO_3^- contained in a given vegetable will depend on several variables including variety, cultural and harvesting practices, fertilizer type, application rate, and time in relation to harvest. NO_3^- contents of greater than 2 g/kg fresh weight have been reported (White, 1975).

Few studies have been published in which human intake or exposure to NO_3^- has been directly measured either in the food consumed or through NO_3^- excretion. Stephany and Schuller (1980) reported the results of a study conducted in The Netherlands in which 201 duplicate portions of food taken over a single day were assayed for NO_3^- and NO_2^-. The average intake of NO_3^- and NO_2^- was 1.8 and 0.06 mmol/day/person, respectively (range = 1.2 to 11.5 and 0.03 to 0.87 mmol/person/day). The wide range indicated that some individuals were consuming more than six times the average amounts of NO_3^-, at least on the day of the survey. Knight et al. (1987) estimated the NO_3^- and NO_2^- intakes of 747 people in the U.K. by surveying their eating habits using mean frequency and por-

TABLE 4.1   Dietary Sources Nitrate (U.S.)

Source	µMol/Day/Person	%
Vegetables	1050 (4200)[a]	87 (97)[a]
Fruits, juices	69	6
Water	32 (2850)[b]	3 (68)[b]
Cured meat	26	2
Baked goods, cereals	26	2
Others	13	<1
Total	1216	100

[a]Vegetarian diet.
[b]Nitrate-rich water.
Source: National Academy of Science (1981).

TABLE 4.2   Dietary Sources Nitrite (U.S.)

Source	μMol/Day/Person	%
Cured meat	6.5 (26)[a]	39 (71)[a]
Baked goods, cereals	5.7	34
Vegetables	2.6 (10)[b]	16 (62)[b]
Fresh meats	1.3	8
Others	0.65	4
Total	16.8	101

[a]High cured meat diet.
[b]Vegetarian diet.
Source: National Academy of Science (1981).

tion size data. These date indicated a mean intake of 1.5 and 0.03 mmol/ person/day for NO_3^- and NO_2^-, respectively, from food. Drinking water was estimated to contribute and additional 0.21 mmol of NO_3^-/person/ day. Only means and not ranges were reported. The National Academy of Sciences (1981) surveyed the literature and estimated the mean daily intake of NO_3^- for U.S. residents to be 1.2, 1.3, and 4.3 mmol/person/day for average, high cured meat, and vegetarian diets, respectively. Vegetables contributed from 83 to 97% of the NO_3^-, depending on the type of diet considered. The NO_3^- intake from water could add as much as 2.6 mmol/day/ person if nitrate-rich water was consumed daily. NO_2^- consumption was estimated to be 0.02 and 0.04 mmol/person/day for average and high cured meat diets, respectively (Table 4.2). Cured meats contributed from 39 to 71% of daily NO_2^- intake, with the balance coming from baked goods (15 to 34%), vegetables (7 to 16%), and fresh meats (3.5 to 7.7%). These estimates were based on published per capita consumption data and literature values for NO_3^- and NO_2^- content of foods.

Other estimates of NO_3^- and NO_2^- exposure have been made. One of the most cited estimates is that of White (1975,1976) who concluded that diet contributed 1.6 and 0.05 mmol/day/person of NO_3^- and NO_2^-, respectively, based on consumption data. Hartman (1982) has surveyed the world-wide literature and found a range of values from a high of 4.5 to a low of <0.1 mmol NO_3^-/person/day. Considerations of the mean exposure to NO_3^- and/or NO_2^- do not take into account the possible effect of peak exposures when very high levels are ingested due to the consumption of specific nitrate-rich foods. Direct measurements of urinary excretion of NO_3^- would more accurately indicate exposure, after corrections for metabolic losses.

The published data on dietary exposure to NO_3^- and NO_2^- lead to three basic conclusions:

1. There is a large intra- and interindividual variability in NO_3^- and NO_2^- exposure. A single individual may, because of daily changes in diet, ingest amounts of NO_3^- and/or NO_2^- that vary by more than three to six fold.

2. An average Western diet contains 1 to 2 mmol of NO_3^-/person/day. Higher vegetable consumption and/or nitrate-rich water can substantially increase these values.

3. Vegetables and cured meats represent the largest dietary sources of NO_3^- and NO_2^-, respectively. As is discussed below, vegetables may also be the largest contributor of NO_2^- through in vivo reduction of NO_3^-. Water can be a significant source of NO_3^- in those populations consuming nitrate-rich water.

EXPOSURE TO ENDOGENOUSLY FORMED NITRATE AND NITRITE

The pharmacology and metabolism of NO_2^- and NO_3^- has been studied in detail and reviewed (Tannenbaum and Young, 1980; Hartman, 1983), but only recently has the endogenous formation of NO_3^- been conclusively demonstrated. In man, ingested NO_3^- is absorbed in the upper digestive tract and is excreted in the urine and sweat and, to a very limited extent, in feces (Bartholomew and Hill, 1984).

Ingested NO_3^- is catabolized, and only 50 to 55% of a labeled oral dose can be recovered as NO_3^- from humans (Wagner et al., 1983a; Leaf et al., 1987). Experiments in rats indicate that a portion of the nitrogen from NO_3^- can be recovered in more reduced forms including ammonia and urea, which suggests that the microorganisms of the anaerobic gut are responsible for the reduction (Wang et al., 1981). Dull and Hotchkiss (1984a) have treated ferrets with a combination of antibiotics in order to reduce the microbial load in the gut and found that the amount of NO_3^- excreted by the ferret is inversely proportional to the number of microorganisms in the feces. Witter et al. (1981) compared the NO_3^- balance in conventional and germ-free rats and showed that intestinal microorganisms decrease the output of NO_3^-. They later showed that NO_3^- is a product of the mammalian host and not the microflora of the gut (Witter et al., 1982).

Importantly, from the standpoint of the endogenous formation of NOC, NO_3^- is concentrated and secreted in human saliva where a portion is reduced by oral microorganisms to NO_2^- (Tannenbaum et al. 1976). Saliva from the salivary duct contains only NO_3^-, whereas saliva from the mouth contains NO_3^- and NO_2^-. The NO_3^- content of human saliva has been reported to be as high as 200 mg/L (Boyland and Walker, 1974). The NO_3^- and NO_2^- content of human saliva peaks approximately 1 hour after ingestion of NO_3^-, although there appears to be wide interindividual variability.

Spiegelhalder et al. (1976) found that the NO_2^- level of saliva was directly proportional to the amount of NO_3^- ingested and that, on the average, 25% of an oral dose of NO_3^- appeared in the saliva, but again there were wide interindividual differences. They further concluded that 20% of the salivary NO_3^- (5% of the total oral dose) was reduced to NO_2^- by the oral microorganisms. The interindividual variability may have been due to differences in the numbers and types of oral microorganisms containing NO_3^- reductase activity (Ishiwata et al., 1975). Oral NO_3^- reductase activity has only been demonstrated in man and may not occur in common laboratory species (Tannenbaum and Young, 1980).

Green et al. (1981a) conclusively demonstrated the endogenous formation of NO_3^- in both germ-free and conventional rats. Using ^{15}N-labeled NO_3^-, they showed that the excretion of $^{14}N-NO_3^-$ remained constant, regardless of overall NO_3^- balance. We have performed similar balance experiments in conventional flora ferrets (Dull and Hotchkiss, 1984a). When the animals consumed less than 6.3 μmol NO_3^-/day, they excreted as much as 10.3 μmol more NO_3^- than they took in. However, when the NO_3^- dose became large enough so that 65% of the oral NO_3^- lost to catabolism was greater than the endogenously synthesized NO_3^-, the animals excreted less NO_3^- than they took in (Fig. 4.7). When the oral dose was made up of $^{15}N-NO_3^-$, the excretion of $^{14}N-NO_3^-$ exceeded intake, even though the overall NO_3^- excretion was less than the intake (Table 4.3). This explains why some balance studies in which NO_3^- intake was greater than endogenous synthesis have failed to detect endogenous synthesis.

Green et al. (1981b) have shown that man also synthesizes NO_3^-. During an investigation into human NO_3^- balance, Wagner and Tannenbaum (1982) found that the synthesis of NO_3^- was increased fivefold during an episode of intestinal diarrhea. The effect could be duplicated in rats by treating them with inflammatory agents such as lipopolysaccharide (LPS). These findings led Marletta and coworkers to investigate the source of this endogenously formed NO_3^-. They demonstrated that macrophages synthesize large amounts of NO_2^- and NO_3^- in the ration of 3:2 in culture

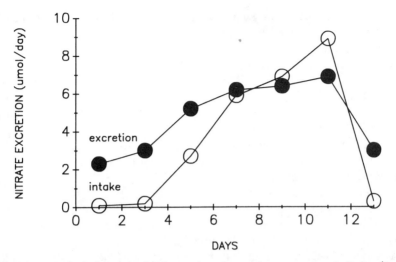

FIG. 4.7 Nitrate balance in the ferret given increasing amounts of nitrate. (*From Dull and Hotchkiss, 1984a.*)

TABLE 4.3 Nitrate Balance in the Ferret[a]

Time (hr)	$^{14}NO_3^-$		$^{15}NO_3^-$		Total NO_3^-
	In	Out	In	Out	Out/In
−48–24	0.8	240	0	0	300
0–24	0.8	230	0	0	288
0–6	11	800	5400	1500	0.43
6–12	0.8	280	0	270	688
12–18	0.8	400	0	140	675
18–24	0.8	370	0	50	525
24–36	0.8	170	0	0	213
36–48	0.8	190	0	0	238
48–60	0.8	150	0	0	188

[a]nmol/hr.

(Stuehr and Marletta, 1985). NO_2^- which was formed in vivo would be oxidized to NO_3^- and would not appear as NO_2^- in the urine. Further work by this group has shown that when 15 mM morpholine was added to the macrophage culture medium, there was a 1% conversion to N-nitrosomorpholine. This suggests that macrophages may be capable of synthesizing NOC in vivo.

The source of the nitrogen is less clear. Wagner et al. (1983b), Saul and Archer (1984), and Dull and Hotchkiss (1984b) all showed that nitrogen from ammonia was incorporated into NO_3^- but the degree of incorporation was less than would be expected if ammonia were the direct precursor. More recently, Hibbs et al. (1987) and Iyengar et al. (1987) have independently found that L-arginine was the only amino acid necessary for the synthesis of NO_2^- and NO_3^- by stimulated macrophages in culture. Analysis of the culture medium showed that the imino nitrogen was removed from the arginine, leaving NO_2^- and citrulline as products. Hibbs et al. (1987) suggested that the production of NO_2^- might be linked to the cytotoxicity of macrophages.

The quantity of NO_3^- formed endogenously is a significant proportion of overall NO_3^- exposure. Wagner et al. (1983a) estimated on the basis of NO_3^- balance studies that normal healthy adults endogenously formed 1.0 mmol NO_3^-/day. Leaf et al. (1987) conducted NO_3^- balance studies in humans using ^{15}N isotopes of NO_3^- and found that endogenous formation of NO_3^- equaled 1.2 mmol/person/day. As pointed out above, these values are nearly equal to estimates to NO_3^- intake by U.S. residents and indicate that approximately one-half of the NO_3^- exposure comes from endogenous processes.

EXPOSURE TO EXOGENOUSLY FORMED N-NITROSO COMPOUNDS

NOC have not been directly linked to any human cancer, but there is considerable indirect evidence that exposure may represent an increased risk for developing human cancer (Yoo et al., 1988). Humans are exposed to exogenously formed carcinogenic NOC by ingestion, inhalation, and dermal contact. The quantity and type of NOC to which any individual is exposed depends on several lifestyle and occupational factors, the most important of which are occupational environment, tobacco and/or cosmetics use, types of food consumed, and contact with other known sources such as rubber products or pesticides (Preussmann and Eisenbrand, 1984).

The largest individual exposures come from two easily controlled sources—occupational environments and tobacco usage. Ambient air in leather tanneries and rubber manufacturing industries have contained >100 μg/m^3 of NDMA and up to 27 μg/m^3 of NMOR (Rounbehler et al., 1979; Spiegelhalder and Preussmann, 1982). Proper controls have reduced these values to <0.1 μg/m^3. Estimates of daily exposure for individuals working in these areas were, at one time, as high as 3.8 μg/day/person (Preussmann et al., 1981). Industrial cutting fluids have been shown to contain large amounts of NDELA.

Tobacco usage presents the second largest individual exposure to NOC and the largest average exposure for populations using tobacco products. Tobacco products including snuff (Brunnemann et al, 1983a), smoke (Brunnemann et al., 1983b), and chewing tobacco (Brunnemann et al., 1985) contain large concentrations of carcinogenic NOC. Some samples of smokeless tobacco contained over 2×10^5 μg of total nitrosamines per kg (Table 4.4). The use of smokeless tobacco (snuff, chewing tobacco, etc.), and by extension NOC, has been shown to be strongly associated with oral cancer in humans (Winn, 1984).

NOC in tobacco products fall into three categories: volatile, nonvolatile, and tobacco-specific. The first two types occur in products in addition to tobacco, and the third type are nitroso derivatives of tobacco alkaloids and occur only in tobacco. Hoffman and Brunnemann (1983) and Hecht and coworkers (1987) have carried out extensive investigations of the NOC that occur in tobacco smoke and smokeless tobacco products. NOC are found preformed in cured tobacco and also are formed during smoking. Preussmann and Eisenbrand (1984) have estimated that a 20 cigarette/day smoker is exposed to 16 to 86 μg of a combination of at least eight nitrosamines.

Food and drink may represent the broadest exposure to NOC, albeit at much lower levels than the previous two sources. The occurrence of NOC in foods has recently been reviewed in detail (Hotchkiss, 1987). Most Western-style foods have been analyzed for volatile nitrosamines. For example, Spiegelhalder et al. (1980) analyzed nearly 3000 German foods, and Gough et al. (1977) surveyed 500 foods available in the U.K. The results showed that only two foods, fried bacon and beer, consistently contained volatile nitrosamines above 1 μg/kg. Nitrosamines are formed in bacon as an indirect result of the addition of NO_2^- to the bacon and are found in beer as a result of their formation during the kilning (drying) of the wet malt prior to the brewing operation. Other foods such as dried milk, chesses, fish products, and other cured meats have occasionally been found positive for volatile nitrosamines at levels above 1 μg/kg.

TABLE 4.4 Nitrosamine Content of Smokeless Tobacco[a]

Samples	NO$_3^-$ (%)	VNA (ppb)			
		NDMA	NDEA	NPYR	NMOR
U.S.	2.68	46.5	ND	93.8	19.5
	2.95	85.1	ND	291	29.4
Canada	1.56	72.8	ND	321	21.9
	4.68	23.0	ND	337	32.8
Sweden	2.22	ND	ND	12.2	ND
	2.13	ND	ND	20.2	9.1
F.R.G.	1.41	ND	ND	ND	ND
	1.17	ND	ND	ND	ND
U.S.S.R.	0.74	ND	ND	8.82	ND
	0.82	ND	ND	4.33	ND
India	0.66	ND	1.85	4.48	ND
	0.80	0.56	ND	2.70	ND

[a]ND = not detected (in the case of VNA < 0.2 ppb, NVNA < 1 ppb, TNSA < 5 ppb). All values are based on dry weight of tobacco.
Source: Brunnemann et al. (1985).

Despite these large surveys of foods, new reports that foods contain trace amounts of volatile nitrosamines appear. For example, dried chilies used for seasoning foods have been reported to contain detectable amounts of volatile NOC (Tricker et al., 1988). Some foods contain small amounts of nitrosamines as a result of migration from processing or packaging contact surfaces (Hotchkiss and Vecchio, 1983; Sen et al., 1987).

While most foods have been surveyed for volatile nitrosamines, the occurrence of other, less volatile NOC remains unanswered due to lack of analytical methodology for this class compound. For example, it was nearly 15 years after the discovery of the first nitrosamine in fried bacon that the occurrence of NTHZ was confirmed, due to analytical difficulties (Gray et al., 1982). Since then other less volatile nitrosamines such as NTHZCA (Sen et al. 1986) and the 2-methyl and 2-hydroxymethyl (Massey et al., 1985) derivatives of NTHZCA have been found in foods. Recent reports from several laboratories suggest that some foods contain unknown nonvolatile NOC. For example, Massey, et al. (1987) used an indirect assay that was selective for the nitroso group to determine that beer has an apparent nitroso content of 20 to 500 μg N-NO/kg. This does not directly establish that beer contains unknown nitroso compounds, but it

NVNA (ppb)		TSNA (ppb)				
NDELA	NPRO	NNN	NAT	NAB	NNK	Total
890	14000	9040	32500	2050	680	44270
4260	30500	28000	33300	1660	3260	66220
2720	16600	79100	152000	4000	5800	240100
1180	8800	50400	170000	4800	3200	228400
300	3120	3660	2200	130	950	6940
230	4680	4140	2180	150	1030	7500
50	700	2130	500	50	40	2720
50	550	1420	300	30	30	1810
40	ND	520	300	30	110	960
40	180	520	170	10	130	830
40	190	540	450	50	130	1170
110	410	850	300	70	230	1450

does support other evidence that nonvolatile NOC may occur in beer (Ahmed et al., 1985).

Other consumer products such as cosmetics, vulcanized rubber products (e.g., nursing nipples, tires, gloves, etc.), new automobile interiors, drugs, pesticides, packaging materials, and some drinking waters have been shown, on occasion, to contain carcinogenic nitrosamines (Hotchkiss and Cassens, 1987). With some exceptions, such as rubber nursing nipples which can contain volatile NOC at 100 to 800 µg/kg, and cosmetics, the amounts are <10 µg/kg. Nitrosamines can migrate from rubber nipples to foods and the mouths of infants during suckling (Havery and Fazio, 1982). Cosmetics can be a source of significant exposure depending on the specific product and its use. NDELA and NPABA are especially prevalent in cosmetics (Fig. 4.8). Several of these products have been shown to contain substantial amounts of one or more NOC.

Reports on the volatile nitrosamine content of foods and consumer products must not be viewed as representing current levels. In nearly all cases, changes in manufacturing processes and/or ingredients have resulted in substantial reductions in the volatile nitrosamine content of the product. For example, beer, which at one time was estimated to contribute over 60% of the dietary intake of volatile nitrosamines, has only a

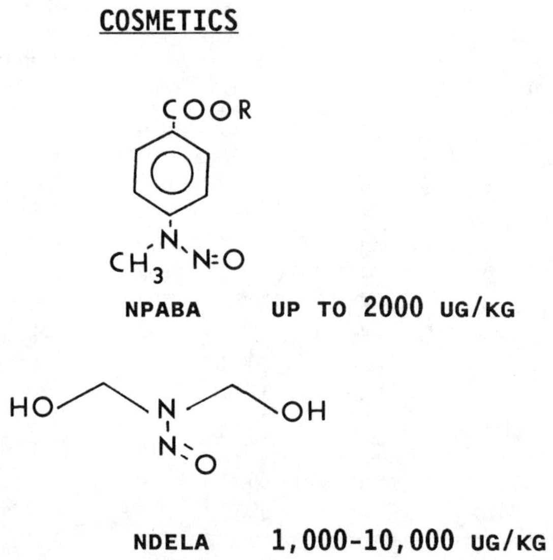

COSMETICS

NPABA   UP TO 2000 UG/KG

NDELA   1,000-10,000 UG/KG

FIG. 4.8 Structures of some N-nitrosamines reported as contaminants in cosmetic products.

small fraction of the nitrosamine content that it did when these estimates were made (Havery et al., 1981).

Relative Exposure of Exogenous Nitrosamines

The National Academy of Sciences (1981) estimated the daily intake of preformed nitrosamines for U.S. residents based on the data available in 1980 (Table 4.5). As the committee pointed out, these numbers are not absolute but are indicators of *relative* exposures. Clearly, cigarette smoke represents at least a 15- to 100-fold higher exposure to volatile nitrosamines than does food and drink. In reality, tobacco represents an even larger exposure compared to foods, because smokeless tobacco was not included in this estimate, and there is no doubt that the nitrosamine content of food, particularly beer, has decreased substantially since these estimates were made (Havery and Fazio, 1985).

Further caveats must be made when interpreting these relative exposure data. First, they are only for the volatile nitrosamines, which may be only a small portion of the total NOC from a given source. It is likely that other NOC will be found in these and other products as analytical methodology for nonvolatile NOC improves. Also, little is known about the relative im-

TABLE 4.5 Estimated U.S. Exposure to Nitrosamines

Source	NA	µg/Person/Day
Cigarette smoke	NDMA	
	NDEA	17
	NEMA	
	NPYR	
	NDELA	
	NNN	
	NAT	
	NNK	
Automobile interiors	NDMA	0.50
	NMOR	
	NDEA	
Cosmetics	NDELA	0.41
Beer	NDMA	0.34
Fried bacon	NDMA	0.17
	NPRY	
Scotch	NDMA	0.03
Smokeless tobacco	Several	?
Rubber products	Dialkyl	?
Packaging	NMOR	?
Cheese	NDMA	?
Dried foods	NDMA	?
Fish	NDMA	?
Cooking	NDMA	?
Drugs	Several	?
Water	NDMA	?
Occupational environment	NDMA	?
	NMOR	?
Endogenous formation	?	?

Source: National Academy of Science (1981).

portance of route of exposure and susceptibility of man to nitrosamine carcinogenicity compared to laboratory animals. These data do not take into account the wide differences in potency among the different nitrosamines reported in Table 4.5.

ENDOGENOUS FORMATION OF NITROSO COMPOUNDS

The chemistry of nitrosation suggests that NOC might form in the acidic environment of the stomach. Four lines of investigation have indicated that this is, indeed, the case:

1. NOC can form in vitro under conditions which are intended to mimic the human stomach.
2. Tumors can be formed in laboratory animals by feeding NO_2^- and amines. The tumors are characteristic of those expected from the intact nitrosamine.
3. Epidemiological studies have suggested that populations consuming larger amounts of the precursors to NOC are at higher risk for some types of cancer.
4. Endogenously formed NOC compounds have been found in various biological fluids from man and animals.

In Vitro Simulated Gastric Nitrosation Studies

Several studies have investigated the formation of NOC under conditions which were intended to simulate the human stomach in order to determine the feasibility of endogenous nitrosation. Such studies have led to different conclusions. One of the earliest studies was that of Sen et al. (1969), who tested the in vitro formation of NDEA in gastric fluid from several species of animals including man. Human and rabbit gastric juices produced greater amounts of NDEA than did that from the rat, no doubt because the rat's gastric fluid has a pH of 4 to 5 compared to 1 to 2 for the human. Other studies have used artificial gastric juices. Groenen et al. (1982) tested the potential of several dozen different foods to form volatile nitrosamines and nitrosoamino acids under gastric-like conditions in which the NO_2^- levels (1.4 mM) were similar to those that might occur in man. Only fish and seafood products formed nitrosamines. The authors concluded that gastric formation of NDMA "might far exceed" that found preformed in foods. Sen et al. (1985) conducted a similar study

($[NO_2^-]$ = 1.4 mM) with fish and made the opposite conclusion. Coulston and Dunne (1980) developed what has become known as the Nitrosation Assay Procedure (NAP), which is intended to determine the potential of drugs to be nitrosated in the stomach. Walters et al. (1987) have improved the method and reported that several common drugs can form NOC under gastric-like conditions.

While not conclusive, in vitro nitrosation studies can indicate the potential for endogenous nitrosation and can help identify individual NOC which might form mutagenic compounds in the stomach. For example, Piacek-Llanes and Tannenbaum (1982) identified a potent mutagen derived from the intentional nitrosation of fava beans. This legume constitutes a significant portion of the diet of some populations that have an elevated risk of gastric cancer.

Studies That Demonstrate Carcinogenicity from Feeding Precursors

Some of the first studies to investigate the endogenous formation of NOC were conducted by Sander et al. (1968) and Sander and Burkle (1969). They demonstrated endogenous formation both by direct chemical analysis of stomach contents and the production of characteristic tumors from feeding NO_2^- and amines. Later studies by Mirvish and coworkers demonstrated similar effects with a variety of amines or amides and NO_2^- (Greenblatt et al., 1971; Mirvish et al., 1972). In one study by Greenblatt and Mirvish (1973), the numbers of lung adenomas per mouse were roughly proportional to the piperazine dose and the square of the NO_2^- dose, as would be predicted by the kinetic equation for nitrosation (see Fig. 4.3). In vivo formation of mutagenicity (Whong et al., 1979) and acute toxicity (Lijinsky and Greenblatt, 1972) have been demonstrated in similar feeding experiments.

These experiments clearly indicate that endogenous nitrosation can occur, but the levels of precursors, particularly NO_2^-, were much larger than possible in environmental situations and are difficult to extrapolate to man. In general, tumors have been produced only from amines which have relatively low pKas and are, therefore, readily nitrosated.

Epidemiological Studies That Relate Nitrate to Cancer

Epidemiological studies that associate an increased risk of cancer, particularly gastric cancer, with a higher NO_3^- intake have been controversial. For example, Hartman (1983) found a positive correlation between level of NO_3^- ingestion and gastric cancer mortality in 12 countries. Others have found that populations who consume high levels of NO_3^- have a higher risk of gastric cancer (Cuello et al., 1976; Jensen, 1982).

The data of Forman et al. (1985) appear to contradict these findings. They measured the NO_3^- content of saliva from individuals living in high and low gastric cancer risk areas of the United Kingdom and found that the former population had significantly lower concentrations of salivary NO_3^- and NO_2^- than did the low-risk populations. This suggests that NO_3^- is a protective factor, not a risk factor. These data may reflect differences in vitamin C intake from vegetables (i.e., high vegetable diets would tend to be high NO_3^- diets) and that vitamin C is protective (Forman, 1987). This implies that NO_3^- from vegetables may be less of a risk than NO_3^- from sources that do not contain ascorbic acid, such as drinking water. Al-Dabbagh et al. (1986) conducted a cohort study of workers in the NO_3^- fertilizer industry in the United Kingdom. The fertilizer workers had elevated levels of salivary NO_3^- but did not show any excess cancer mortality in general or for several specific cancers, including stomach. Presumably, both groups had similar ascorbic acid intakes.

Studies That Measure NOC in Biological Fluids

Direct chemical analyses of gastric contents as well as whole animal analyses have demonstrated endogenous nitrosation. For example, Mirvish et al. (1980) demonstrated the formation of NMU in the stomachs of rats. NO_2^- was added to the diet or drinking water at levels as high as 0.4% and methyl urea at 0.01%. These levels have little relationship to levels found in foods, and the premixing of NO_2^- and amide in the diet does not seem to preclude formation prior to ingestion. Later, Mirvish et al. (1983) improved the earlier work of Iqbal et al. (1980), which demonstrated that morpholine could be nitrosated in vivo by inhalation of NO_2.

The most conclusive evidence that endogenous nitrosation occurs in humans would come from direct analysis of biological fluids for NOC after ingestion of normal levels of precursors. As in the tumorgenicity studies cited above, the major limitation is the high level of precursors used in order that the resulting NOC can be detected. Nitrosamines are metabolized at very high rates, often to untraceable products. The metabolic products of NDMA, for example, are molecular nitrogen, formaldehyde, and carbonium ions, none of which could be analyzed at the levels at which endogenous nitrosation might occur. Gombar et al. (1987) have studied the pharmacokinetics of NDMA in beagle dogs. The mean half-life for elimination of a very large dose (1.0–5.0 mg/kg) was 73 minutes with a systematic clearance rate of 43 mL/min/kg. Even at these extremely large doses, no NDMA could be detected in the urine. These data indicate that the formation of NDMA at the levels that might be expected from endogenous concentrations of precursors (Zeisel et al., 1988) would be difficult to detect in biological fluids.

Garland et al. (1986) developed an analytical technique for NDMA in urine based on mass spectrometry and sensitive to 5 ng/L. Using this technique, they suggested that humans excrete 38 ng/day. The source of the NDMA was not determined, but changes in the amounts excreted correlated positively with changes in the amount of atmospheric nitrogen dioxide (NO_2). This suggests that the NDMA could have been endogenously formed from inhaled NO_x compounds but did not present direct evidence for endogenous formation. Neither ascorbic acid nor tocopherol influenced this excretion.

The direct detection of endogenously formed NOC in humans was not demonstrated until Ohshima and Bartsch (1981) developed the NPRO model. They dosed a volunteer with 5.24 mmol of NO_3^- followed 30 minutes later by 4.35 mmol of proline. Over the next 24 hr the excretion of NPRO rose from 21 nmol to over 100 nmol. A 5.7 mmol bolus dose of vitamin C returned NPRO excretion to the level found before the precursor dose. As expected, NPRO excretion was second order in NO_3^- and first order in proline. Ohshima et al. (1984) have shown that normal human urine contains other N-nitrosoamino acids including NTHZCA and NMTHZCA.

Several studies have since been conducted using this basic model. For example, Hoffmann and Brunnemann (1983) and Ladd et al. (1984) each demonstrated that smokers have a higher capacity to form NPRO than nonsmokers. The reason for this is not clear, but it could be related to the higher thiocyanate levels in the saliva of smokers (Ladd et al., 1984). Wagner et al. (1985) investigated the effect of vitamins C and E on the endogenous formation of NPRO. Their subjects had basal NPRO excretions of 26 nmol day, which was increased to 100 nmol/day after administration of NO_3^- followed by proline. When $^{15}[N]NO_3^-$ was used, the $^{15}[N]$-nitrogen was incorporated into the NPRO.

NPRO formation has been demonstrated in the rat (Ohshima et al. 1982), but the higher pH and physiological differences in the rat's stomach may make the data less applicable to humans (Sen et al. 1969). We have shown that the ferret, with its acidic stomach, also endogenously forms and excretes NPRO (Dull et al., 1986). The ferret may have advantages as a model due to the closer similarity to the human GI tract (Pfeiffer, 1970). Ohshima et al. (1983) have attempted to model a relationship between

NPRO formation in rats with the endogenous formation of NDMA (a carcinogen) in man.

Urinary excretion of NPRO is also being used in molecular epidemiology studies. Lu et al. (1986) compared the 24-hr excretion of NPRO by residents of high- and low-risk esophageal cancer areas in China. The excretion of NPRO and other nitrosoamino acids (and NO_3^-) was significantly higher in the high-risk areas. They also demonstrated that 0.6 mmol of ascorbic acid reduced the NPRO excretion. Kamiyama et al. (1987) have observed that subjects from low gastric cancer risk areas of Japan had lower nitrosation ability after being challenged with proline than subjects from high-risk areas. There were, however, no differences in the unchallenged excretion of NPRO. Chen et al. (1987) found no correlation between nitrosation potential after proline challenge and stomach cancer for two regions in China.

Urinary nitrosoamino acids (or hypothetically, other NOC) may come from several sources (Fig. 4.9):

In vivo formation in the stomach from ingested (exogenous) precursors including NO_3^-, NO_2^-, and proline.

In vivo formation in the stomach from endogenouly formed precursors.

In vivo formation at sights other than the stomach.

The ingestion of N-nitrosoamino acids, which can be found in the food.

N-nitrosoamino acids, which are in the diet in such a way as not to be directly analyzable in the food. For example, peptides which are N-terminal in proline could be nitrosated. NPRO might then appear in the urine after in vivo proteolysis.

These last two sources of urinary NPRO have caused some confusion. Stitch et al. (1984) reported that the consumption of nitrite-cured meats led to an increase in urinary excretion of NPRO in humans. They suggested that the NPRO was preformed in the meat and not endogenously formed because the excretion could not be reduced by consuming large amounts of vitamin C. Later these same workers (Dunn and Stitch, 1984) reported that the NPRO could not be directly analyzed in the cured meats but that enzymic digestion of the meat gave substantially higher amounts of NPRO. Kubacka et al. (1984) have shown that peptides which are N-terminal in proline can be nitrosated.

We have investigated the source of this excess urinary NPRO when ferrets are consuming nitrite-cured meat diets. NPRO excretion increased

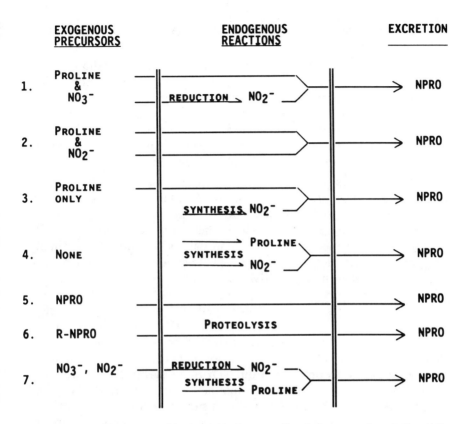

FIG. 4.9 Possible sources of urinary N-nitrosoproline in human urine. 4, 5, and 6 may not be affected by ASC.

13-fold when ferrets were switched from a semi-purified diet to a cured meat diet. Using stable isotopes of NO_2^- and proline, we showed that a majority of the NPRO was formed in the cured meat before ingestion, and less than 17% was formed in the stomach. These data show that the exposure to NOC due to consumption of cured meats may be higher than direct analysis of the food indicates (Perciballi et al., 1989).

Tannenbaum (1987) has recently discussed the NPRO model and its shortcomings. Three basic forms of the NPRO test have evolved.:

1. NO_3^- and proline are sequentially administered and NPRO excretion monitored by collecting 24-hr urine. This form of the model has the least intraindividual variability and is most useful under highly controlled dietary conditions in which the effect of a single variable

is sought. There is a large interindividual variability in this form of the test.

2. Only proline (or another nitrosatable amino acid) is administered. This form is designed to test the nitrosation capacity of a population and has been used in biochemical epidemiology studies. It presumes that populations who have a higher capacity to form NPRO without administration of the nitrate are at a greater risk of developing some forms of cancer. The test is often repeated with a large vitamin C dose in order to show that the NPRO is formed in vivo.

3. No precursors (proline or NO_3^-) are administered and the urine is collected, most often in 24-hr segments. This is most often done in epidemiology studies to determine the exposure of a population to NOC without regard to whether they were endogenously or exogenously formed. Differences in urinary NPRO may reflect simply differences in diet. Vitamin C is sometimes administered as a control for preformed dietary NPRO.

Data from these three types of investigations have led to what is called the "hypothesis of gastric cancer." Mirvish (1983) has discussed this hypothesis in detail and suggested that dietary NO_3^- coupled to a diet deficient in vitamin C is a key risk factor. According to this hypothesis, nitrosamides may be produced from NO_2^- in the stomach. This would be more likely to occur in individuals that have higher intakes of NO_3^- and lower intakes of inhibitors of nitrosation such as vitamin C. Data which directly support this hypothesis are not convincing at present. Tannenbaum (1987) has suggested that the NPRO model may not be an adequate test of the hypothesis due to the reasons detailed above.

The NPRO test is most useful under controlled conditions in order to determine the effect of some known variable, such as vitamin C dose, on nitrosation capacity, especially in humans. The NPRO test has the distinct disadvantage of not being an overall indicator of general exposure to carcinogenic NOC, especially those formed endogenously.

FACTORS AFFECTING ENDOGENOUS NITROSATION

Several factors could influence the endogenous formation of NOC. Unfortunately, many of these factors have not been adequately researched. A primary factor is the amount of NO_3^- ingested. As discussed above, several studies have shown that the quantity of NPRO excreted is positively correlated with NO_3^- intake. However, not all individuals respond in the same manner. Interindividual difference in response to the nitrate-proline challenge varies by as much as tenfold when the same amount of precurcors are administered (Fig. 4.10; Wagner et al., 1985; Leaf et al., 1987). Day-to-day intraindividual variability in NPRO excretion is greater than interindividual differences for persons not challenged with NO_3^- and proline. This probably reflects daily differences in diet.

In addition to NO_3^- intake, the temporal relationship between the NO_3^- and proline administration have been shown to influence individual response to nitrate-proline challenge (Wagner et al., 1985).

Other, pharmacological factors such as the rate of NO_3^- absorption, stomach emptying rate, peak salivary nitrite concentratioin, and activity of salivary NO_3^- reductase will also influence individual responses. The oral reductase activity will depend on the numbers and types of microorganisms present in the mouth.

Gastric pH might influence inter- and intraindividual differences in nitrosation capacity in two ways. As pointed out above, pH can influence the rate of nitrosation by several orders of magnitude (Mirvish, 1975). The pH of the normal human stomach varies over at least three pH units. This would be expected to influence the amount of NOC formed before the stomach emptied. A second pH-related influence occurs in the achlorhydric stomach. At the higher pH of the achlorhydric stomach, colonization

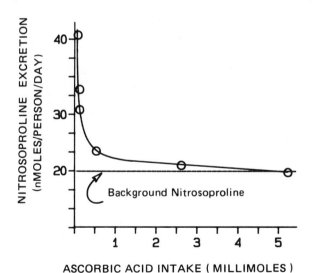

FIG. 4.10 Individual excretion of N-nitrosoproline by seven individuals receiving the same dose of proline and nitrate. The line represents the mean of the data.

of the stomach by nitrate-reducing bacteria might lead to greatly elevated levels of NO_2^-, which may overcome the reduced rate of nitrosation due to the elevated pH.

The presence of inhibitors and/or catalysts in the stomach also influences the endogenous formation of NOC. For example, we have determined the effect of different doses of ascorbic acid on the formation of NPRO in humans. As little as 0.05 mmol of vitamin C reduced the excretion of NPRO, but doses as high as 5.68 mmol did not lower the excretion to the same levels seen when no NO_3^- or proline was administered (Fig. 4.11). Catalysts may also influence the endogenous formation of NOC.

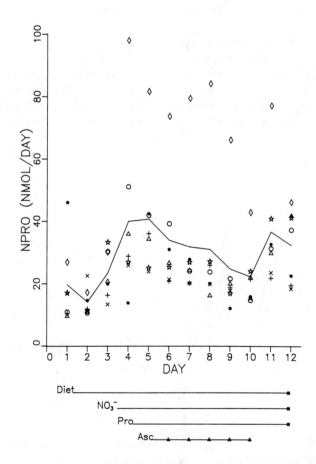

FIG. 4.11 Effect of ascorbic acid on the endogenous formation of N-nitroso-proline in humans. (*From Leaf et al., 1987.*)

Ladd et al. (1984) found that the increased formation of NPRO in smokers correlated with salivary thiocyanate. Thiocyanate has been shown to be a potent in vitro catalyst of nitrosation. Other catalysts and/or inhibitors such as carbonyl compounds, phenolics, or metals could influence endogenous nitrosation.

RELATIVE EXPOSURE/RISKS FROM ENDOGENOUS VERSUS EXOGENOUS NITROSO COMPOUNDS

Nitrate

The human balance studies of Wagner et al. (1983a) which were confirmed by Leaf et al. (1987) clearly indicated that NO_3^- is synthesized through a de novo pathway in humans. This synthesis amounts to 1 to 2 mmol/person/day. This level of endogenous synthesis can increase substantially as the immune system is stimulated.

The data concerning exposure to NO_3^- from ingestion is less clear because there are no surveys where actual excretion amounts are monitored. Data that are available usually come from dietary surveys and extrapolations from literature values for the NO_3^- content of foods. These data indicate that mean daily intake of NO_3^- is approximately equal to or slightly larger than endogenous synthesis. The data also indicate that individual diets vary considerably both within and between individuals. Mean data do not factor in the effects of high short-term exposures or the effects of individual lifestyle variables which might result in high NO_3^- intakes.

Nitrite

Assuming a 5% reduction of NO_3^- to salivary NO_2^-, exposure to NO_2^-, through endogenous reduction would be 0.05×2.4 mmol NO_3^-/day/person = 120 µmol/day/person. This compares to 20 µmol/day/person estimated to come from the diet. This does not include the NO_2^- that may be endogenously formed by the immune system. This NO_2^- is oxidized to NO_3^- and would not be detected in vivo as NO_2^-. Clearly, the major exposure to NO_2^- comes from endogenous sources, although exogenous NO_3^- significantly contributes to this exposure.

Preformed N-nitroso Compounds

Few estimates of exposure to preformed nitrosamines have been made. The most comprehensive was that of the National Academy of Sciences (1981). Their estimates for U.S. residents ranged from a high of 17 µg/day/person from cigarette smoke to a low of 0.17 µg/person/day from bacon consumption. An average exposure for all identified sources of volatile nitrosamines estimated in this work would be 18.7 µg/person/day. Cigarette smoking would contribute 87% of the exposure with all others <5% each. For nonsmokers, the exposure would be 1.65 µg/person/day with 30, 25, 21, and 10% coming from automobile interiors, cosmetics, beer, and fried bacon, respectively. These estimates do not include several other known sources or recent discoveries of NOC contamination in products such as vulcanized rubber.

All such data must be viewed as rough estimates. As pointed out above, the data upon which they are made may not reflect current levels. For example, the estimates for beer assume a NDMA concentration of 1.0 µg/L, which may be higher than current values, and we have previously pointed out that the estimate for bacon consumption is in error (Vecchio et al., 1986). These data also do not incorporate more recent findings that foods may contain NOC in addition to those included in the 1981 estimates. For example, recent evidence has shown that fried bacon as well as other smoked and nitrite-cured meats and fish contain NTHZCA and other nonvolatile NOC and that food contact surfaces can contribute nitrosamines to foods. There may be other unknown less volatile NOC in these or other environmental materials. Despite these shortcomings, these data are useful for comparing one source of exposure to another and as a benchmark for determining the relative exposure from endogenous nitrosation.

Endogenously Formed N-Nitroso Compounds

The types and quantity of carcinogenic NOC that may be formed endogenously cannot be directly determined because of the rapid metabolism of the compounds. Two indirect approaches and one direct one to quantifying the endogenous formation of carcinogenic NOC are being pursued:

1. Biological markers of NOC exposure, such as alkylated DNA or specific protein adducts, are being sought.

2. Animal experiments in which the rapid metabolism of carcinogenic NOC is slowed so that the compounds can be detected are being developed (Perciballi et al., 1989).

3. Kinetic models which incorporate several of the variables which influence endogenous nitrosation are being developed in order to predict the amount of a given NOC that might be formed in vivo.

The first approach is to develop analytical methods which are capable of detecting adducts formed by the reactive intermediate resulting from carcinogenic NOC. For example, metabolic activation of NDMA to electrophilic methyl carbonium ions results in the alkylation of bases in DNA. These alkylated bases are excised by the DNA repair mechanisms and eventually appear in the urine. An increase above background would, presumably, be related to the original amount of NDMA activated.

Another similar approach would be to assay for protein adducts. This type of adduct may be in higher amounts because proteins are more abundant than DNA (Tannenbaum and Skipper, 1984). This approach has the disadvantage that DNA adducts are more likely to be indicative of carcinogenesis than are protein adducts.

Hecht et al. (1987) have investigated the binding of tobacco-specific NOC to both DNA and hemoglobin. The products of the metabolism of the N-nitroso derivatives of the two major tobacco alkaloids were found to bind to an unidentified site in hemoglobin after the NOC was injected into rats. These adducts could be detected up to 6 weeks after treatment. Green et al. (1984) have conducted similar experiments in animals and found hemoglobin adducts of 4-aminobiphenyl, which is related to exposure to cigarette smoke. These studies may be useful in determining individual exposure to tobacco products and may be extended to other NOC.

The second approach to determining the amount of NOC formed endogenously has been to partially inhibit the metabolism of NOC so that they will appear in a body fluid and can be analyzed. This approach grew out of an experiment in which NDMA was measured in the urine of an individual who had consumed beer containing a known amount of NDMA. No NDMA could be detected in the urine when a similar amount of NDMA was consumed in orange juice. It was suggested that the ethanol in the beer had sufficiently inhibited the metabolism of NDMA so that a portion (2%) was detectable in the urine.

The third approach to quantifying the amount of endogenously formed carcinogenic NOC has been to estimate formation based on in vitro kinetic models. One of the first attempts to estimate endogenous exposure to NOC was that of Tannenbaum (1980), who calculated the rate of NDMA formation based on the assumptions that the steady-state concentration of NDMA in blood is 0 to 1 μg/L, that the rate of clearance equals the rate of formation, and that the rate of clearance is as high as 0.7 μg/L/hr, These calculations indicated that 0 to 670 μg of NDMA might be endogenously formed per person/day. The upper limit of this estimation may be too high because the steady-state concentration of NDMA in blood was overestimated by at least an order of magnitude.

Ohshima et al. (1983) have developed a kinetic model for the production of tumors resulting from the endogenous formation of carcinogenic NOC in rats. The model combines experimental data on the endogenous formation of NPRO in the rat, the in vitro rate constants for the formation of several carcinogenic NOC, and the carcinogenic potency of the resulting NOC. This model was used to predict the amount of NO_2^- and amine that would be required in the daily diet of rats in order to produce a 50% tumor incidence in 2 years. Estimates of the amount of precursor ranged from a low of 2.2×10^7 to 1.5×10^{14} μmol/kg bw/day for NO_2^- with aminopyrine and pyrrolidine, respectively. The concentration of amine needed in the food ranged from 0.04 to 17,000 mmol/kg for these two amines, respectively. These data suggest the biological significance of endogenous NOC formation depends, in large part, on the basicity and carcinogenic potency of the amine.

Challis et al. (1982) have developed a kinetic model for gastric nitrosation based on the NO_2^- and amine concentrations found in gastric fluid (Milton-Thompson et al., 1982) and the in vitro nitrosation rate constants for four amines and amides. The formation of carcinogenic NOC was summed over a 24-hr period based on measured changes in gastric pH of a group of volunteers. These data predict that only very low levels of NDMA (1.6×10^{-8} μmol/L) but much higher levels (2.2 μmol/L) of NMU would be formed. Differences in nitrosation rate constants accounted for the wide differences in amount formed. However, these calculations do not take into consideration a number of variables including the presence of catalysts or inhibitors. Tannenbaum et al. (1981) have nitrosated morpholine in vitro in human gastric juice and have found a range of NMOR contents of 2 to 48 μmol/L. This suggests that the situation is much more complex than simple in vitro models would predict and that there are unknown factors influencing the rate of nitrosation both positively and negatively.

Recently, Licht et al. (1986; 1988a,b) have begun to address the complexity of endogenous nitrosation and have proposed a more complex model. Initial work developed a model based on empirical data determined in the cannulated dog's stomach for the stability and rate of loss of NO_2^-. This model predicts that the loss of NO_2^- is rapid with a half-life of less than 10 min due to direct absorption from the stomach. The most recent models were developed in order to predict the effect of several variables such as ascorbic acid and thiocyanate concentration (Licht et al., 1988a). These data show that:

1. The stoichiometry of the reaction between NO_2^- and ascorbic acid is highly dependent on the amount of oxygen present and the mass transfer rates between the gas and liquid phases. Low mass transfer rates resulted in the ascorbic acid being used up before the NO_2^- due to recycling of the NO to N_2O_4 (Eq. 7, Fig. 4.5). This indicates that low mass transfer rates should lead to less effective inhibition.

2. Ascorbic acid is used up faster in the presence of thiocyanate, which suggests that thiocyanate could reduce the effectiveness of ascorbic acid in vivo.

3. As the pH is decreased the loss of ascorbic acid increases relative to the loss of nitrosation capacity. This is due to faster recycling of NO_2^- and suggests that ascorbic acid would be a less effective inhibitor at lower gastric pHs.

4. Ascorbic acid will be less effective at higher oxygen concentrations, and high mass transfer rates favor inhibition by removing nitrosating equivalence.

5. Decreasing the oxygen concentration will favor inhibition by ascorbic acid because the rate of oxidation of NO to N_2O_4 will be decreased.

These observations were used to construct a complex kinetic model to predict the formation of NPRO under physiological conditions. The in vitro model developed from this work was used to test the in vivo formation of NPRO in a cannulated dog's stomach (Licht et al., 1988b). The in vivo formation of NPRO as well as the effects of ascorbic acid and thiocyanate were successfully predicted by the model. The model was not extended to the formation of carcinogenic NOC in humans but suggests that exposure to endogenously formed NOC would be greater than exposure to known sources of preformed NOC.

Others have also developed models in order to predict the quantity of NOC that may be endogenously formed in humans. Leach et al. (1987) found that nitrosation catalyzed by bacteria occurred at a much faster rate at neutral pHs than would chemical nitrosation at the same pH. On the basis of chemical kinetics they predicted that the amount of NOC formed in the infected achlorhydric stomach would be greater than that formed in the normal acidic stomach. This could be the reason that achlorhydric individuals are more at risk of developing gastric cancer. Again, no quantitative comparison between exogenous and endogenous exposure can be made, but these data suggest that endogenous formation is quantitatively higher.

CONCLUSIONS

Several conclusions can be drawn concerning the relative exposure to NO_3^-, NO_2^-, and N-nitroso compounds from exogenous and endogenous sources:

1. Humans are exposed to preformed volatile N-nitrosamines from many sources, but the quantity derived from tobacco products is up to 100 times greater than from any other known source with the possible exception of certain occupational settings. Several factors and modifiers influence an individual's exposure and NOC-associated risks (Fig. 4.12).

2. Man's total exposure to preformed N-nitroso compounds is unknown because analytical methods for N-nitrosamides and nonvolatile N-nitroso compounds are inadequate.

3. Exposure to carcinogenic N-nitroso compounds that are formed within the body cannot be accurately quantified, but substantial indirect evidence indicates that such exposure is as great as or greater than the exposure from exogenously formed N-nitroso compounds.

4. The major source of exposure to NO_3^- is foods, and vegetables contribute the greatest proportion of the NO_3^-. NO_3^- from foods and water is a indirect source of endogenous nitrosating agent and thus may represent a risk factor.

5. The quantity of NPRO excreted by humans can be related to the exposure to NO_3^-.

6. Exposure to NO_3^- also results from endogenous biological processes. The quantity of NO_3^- from this route of exposure is a significant proportion of overall exposure.

7. Food in general, and nitrite-cured meats in particular, represent the largest source of exogenous exposure to NO_2^-. However, the greatest overall source of NO_2^- is the reduction of NO_3^- to NO_2^- that occurs in the mouth. Thus, NO_2^- exposure is directly related to overall NO_3^- exposure.

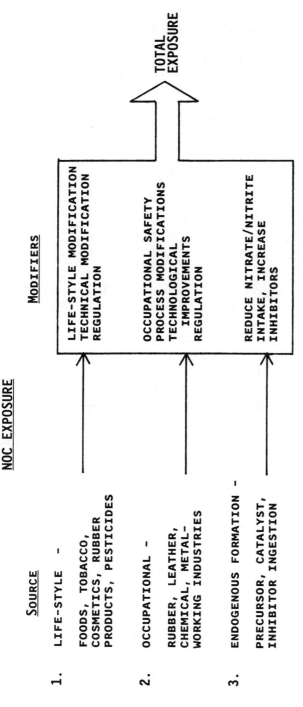

FIG. 4.12 Lifestyle and occupational exposures to N-nitroso compounds (Adapted from Preussmann and Eisenbrand, 1984.)

8. There is strong evidence that NO_3^- and NO_2^- are formed by the immune system and that stimulation of this system increases the endogenous formation of NO_3^- and NO_2^-.

REFERENCES

Ahmad, M. U., Libbey, L. M., Barbour, J. F., and Scanlan, R. A. 1985. Isolation and characterization of products from the nitrosation of the alkaloid gramine. *Food Chem. Toxic.* 23(9): 841.

Al-Dabbagh, S., Forman, D., Bryson, D., Stratton, I., and Doll, R. 1986. Mortality of nitrate fertiliser workers. *B. J. Ind. Med.* 43: 507.

Bartholomew, B. and Hill, M.J. 1984. The pharmacology of dietary nitrate and the origin of urinary nitrate. *Food Chem. Toxic.* 22(10): 789.

Boyland, E. and Walker, S.A. 1974. Effect of thiocyanate on nitrosation of amines. *Nature* 248: 601.

Brunnemann, K.D., Genoble, L., and Hoffmann, D. 1985. N-nitrosamines in chewing tobacco: An international comparison. *J. Agric. Food Chem.* 33: 1178.

Brunnemann, K.D., Masaryk, J., and Hoffman, D. 1983b. Role of tobacco stems in the formation of N-nitrosamines in tobacco and cigarette mainstream and sidestream smoke. *J. Agric. Food Chem.* 31: 1221.

Brunnemann, K.D., Scott, J.C., and Hoffmann, D. 1983a. N-nitrosoproline, an indicator for N-nitrosation of amines in processed tobacco. *J. Agric. Food Chem.* 31: 905.

Challis, B.C. 1981. The chemistry of formation of N-nitroso compounds. In *Safety Evaluation of Nitrosatable Drugs and Chemicals.* (Ed.) Gibson, G.G. and Ioannides, C., p. 16. Taylor and Francis, London.

Challis, B.C., Lomas, S.J., Rzepa, H.S., Bavin, P.M.G., Darkin, D.W., Viney, N.J., and Moore, P.J. 1982. A kinetic model for the formation of gastric N-nitroso compounds. In *Nitrosamines and Human Cancer.* Banbury Report 12, (Ed.) Magee, P.N., p. 243. Cold Spring Harbor Laboratory.

Chen, J., Ohshima, H., Yang, H., Li, J., Campbell, T.C., Peto, R., and Bartsch, H. 1987. A correlation study on urinary excretion of N-nitroso compounds and cancer mortality in China: Interim results. In *Relevance of N-Nitroso Compounds to Human Cancer: Exposures and Mechanisms.* (Ed.) Bartsch, H., O'Neill, I.K., and Schulte-Hermann, R. IARC Scientific Publications No. 84, p. 503. International Agency for Research on Cancer, Lyon.

Coulston, F. and Dunne, J.F. 1980. An in vitro test for N-nitrosatability. In *The Potential Carcinogenicity of Nitrosatable Drugs.* (Ed.) Coulston, F., and Dunne, J.F., p. 8. Ablex Publishing Co., Norwood, NJ.

Cuello, C., Correa, P., and Haenszel, W. et al. 1976. Gastric cancer in Columbia. 1. Cancer risk and suspect environmental agents. *J. Nat. Cancer Inst.* 57: 1015.

Dull, B.J. and Hotchkiss, J.H. 1984a. Nitrate balance and biosynthesis in the ferret. *Toxicol. Let.* 23: 79.

Dull, B.J. and Hotchkiss, J.H. 1984b. Activated oxygen and mammalian nitrate biosynthesis. *Carcinogenesis* 5(9): 1161.

Dull, B.J., Hotchkiss, J.H., and Vecchio, A.J. 1986. Basal N-nitrosoproline formation and excretion in the ferret. *Food Chem. Toxic.* 24(8): 843.

Dunn, B.P. and Stich, H.F., 1984. Determination of free and protein-bound N-nitrosoproline in nitrite-cured meat products. *Food Chem. Toxic.* 22(8): 609.

Forman, D. 1987. Gastric cancer, diet, and nitrate exposure. *Br. Med. J.* 294: 528.

Forman, D., Al-Dabbagh, S., and Doll, R. 1985. Nitrates, nitrites and gastric cancer in Great Britain. *Nature* 313: 620.

Garland, W.A., Kuenzig, W., Rubio, F., Kornychuk, H., Norkus, E.P., and Conney, A.H. 1986. Urinary excretion of nitrosodimethylamine and nitrosoproline in humans: Interindividual and intraindividual differences and the effect of administered ascorbic acid and alpha-tocopherol. *Cancer Res.* 46: 5392.

Gombar, C.T., Pylypiw, H.M., and Harrington, G.W. 1987. Pharmacokinetics of N-nitrosodimethylamine in Beagles. *Cancer Res.* 47: 343.

Gough, T.A., McPhail, M.F., Webb, K.S., Wood, B.J., and Coleman, R.F. 1977. An examination of some foodstuffs for presence of volatile nitrosamines. *J. Sci. Food Agric.* 28: 345.

Gray, J.I., Reddy, S.K., Price, J.F., Mandagere, A., and Wilkens, W.F. 1982. Inhibition of N-nitrosamines in bacon. *Food Technol.* 36(6): 39.

Green, L.C., Ruiz de Luzuriaga, K., Wagner, D.A., Rand, W., Istfan, N., Young, V.R., and Tannenbaum, S.R. 1981b. Nitrate biosynthesis in man. *Proc. Nat. Acad. Sci.* 78(12): 7764.

Green, L.C., Skipper, P.L., Turesky, R.J., Bryant, M.S., and Tannenbaum S.R. 1984. In vivo dosimetry of 4-aminobiphenyl in rats via a cysteine adduction hemoglobin. *Cancer Res.* 44: 4254.

Green, L., Tannenbaum, S.R., and Goldman, P. 1981a. Nitrate synthesis in the germfree and conventional rat. *Science* 212: 56.

Greenblatt, M. and Mirvish, S. S. 1973. Dose-response studies with concurrent administration of piperazine and sodium nitrite to strain A mice. *J.Natl. Cancer Inst.* 50: 119.

Greenblatt, M., Mirvish, S., and So, B.T. 1971. Nitrosamine studies: Induction of lung adenomas by concurrent administration of sodium nitrite and secondary amines in Swiss mice. *J. Natl. Cancer Inst.* 46: 1029.

Groenen, P.J., Luten, J.B., Dhont, J.H., de Cock-Bethbeder, M.W., Prins, L.A., and Vreeken, J.W. 1982. Formation of volatile N-nitrosamines from food products, especially fish, under simulated gastric conditions. In *N-Nitroso Compounds: Occurrence and Biological Effects.* (Ed.) Bartsch, H., O'Neill, I.K., Castegnaro, M., and Okada, M., IARC Scientific Publications No. 41, p. 99. International Agency for Research on Cancer, Lyon.

Hartman, P.E. 1982. Nitrates and nitrites: Ingestion, pharmacodynamics, and toxicology. Ch. 6. In *Chemical Mutagens,* Vol. 7 (Ed.) de Serres, F.J., and Hollander, A., p. 211. Plenum Publishing Corp.

Hartman, P.E. 1983. Review: Putative mutagens and carcinogens in foods. I. Nitrate/nitrite ingestion and gastric cancer mortality. *Environ. Mutat.* 5: 111.

Havery, D.C. and Fazio, T. 1982. Estimation of volatile N-nitrosamines in rubber nipples for babies' bottles. *Food Chem. Toxic.* 20: 939.

Havery, D.C. and Fazio, T. 1985. Human exposure to nitrosamines from foods. *Food Technol.* 39(1): 80.

Havery, D.C., Hotchkiss, J.H., and Fazio, T. 1981. Nitrosamines in malt and malt beverages. *J. Food Sci.* 46(2): 501.

Hecht, S.S., Carmella, S.G., Trushin, N., Foiles, P.G., Lin, D., Rubin, J.M., and Chung, F.-L. 1987. Investigations on the molecular dosimetry of tobacco-specific N-nitrosamines. In *Relevance of N-Nitroso Compounds to Human Cancer: Exposures and Mechanisms,* (Ed.) Bartsch, H., O'Neill, I.K., and Schulte-Hermann, R. IARC Scientific Publications No. 84, p. 219. International Agency for Research on Cancer, Lyon.

Hibbs, J.B., Taintor, R.R., and Vavrin, Z. 1987. Macrophage cytotoxicity: Role for 1-arginine deiminase and imino nitrogen oxidation to nitrite. *Science* 235: 473.

Hoffman, D. and Brunnemann, K.D. 1983. Endogenous formation of N-nitrosoproline in cigarette smokers. *Cancer Res.* 43: 5570

Hotchkiss, J.H. 1987. A review of current literature on N-nitroso compounds in foods. *Adv. Food Res.* 31: 53.

Hotchkiss, J.H. and Cassens, R.G. 1987. Nitrate, nitrite, and nitroso compounds in foods. *Food Technol.* 41(4): 127.

Hotchkiss, J.H. and Vecchio, A.J. 1983. Analysis of direct contact paper and paperboard food packaging for N-nitrosomorpholine and morpholine. *J. Food Sci.* 48(1): 240.

Iqbal, Z.M., Dahl, K., and Epstein, S.S. 1980. Role of nitrogen dioxide in the biosynthesis of nitrosamines in mice. *Science* 207: 1475.

Ishiwata, H., Tanimura, A., and Ishidate, M. 1975. Studies on in vivo formation of nitroso compounds (III). Nitrite and nitrate concentrations in human saliva collected from salivary ducts. *J. Food Hyg. Soc.* 16: 89.

Iyengar, R., Stuehr, D.J., and Marletta, M.A. 1987. Macrophage synthesis of nitrite, nitrate, and N-nitrosamines: Precursors and role of the respiratory burst. *Proc. Natl. Acad. Sci.* 84: 6369.

Jensen, O.M. 1982. Nitrate in drinking water and cancer in Northern Jutland, Denmark, with special reference to stomach cancer. *Ecotoxicol. Environ. Safety* 6: 258.

Kamiyama, S., Ohshima, H., Shimada, A., Saito, N., Bourgade, M.-C., Ziegler, P., and Bartsch, H. 1987. Urinary excretion of N-nitrosamino acids and nitrate by inhabitants in high- and low-risk areas for stomach cancer in northern Japan. In *Relevance of N-Nitroso Compounds to Human Cancer: Exposures and Mechanisms,* (Ed.) Bartsch, H., O'Neill, I.K., and Schulte-Hermann, R., IARC Scientific Publications No. 84, p. 492. International Agency for Research on Cancer, Lyon.

Knight, T.M., Forman, D., Al-Dabbagh, S.A., and Doll, R. 1987. Estimation of dietary intake of nitrate and nitrite in Great Britain. *Food Chem. Toxicol.* 25(4): 277.

Kubacka, W., Libbey, L.M., and Scanlan, R.A. 1984. Formation and chemical characterization of some nitroso dipeptides N terminal in proline. *J. Agric. Food Chem.* 32: 401.

Ladd, K.F., Newmark, H.L., and Archer, M.C. 1984. N-nitrosation of proline in smokers and nonsmokers. *J. Nat. Cancer Inst.* 73(1): 83.

Leach, S.A., Thompson, M., and Hill, M. 1987. Bacterially catalysed N-nitrosation reactions and their relative importance in the human stomach. *Carcinogenesis* 8(12): 1907.

Leaf, C.D., Vecchio, A.J., Roe, D.A., and Hotchkiss, J.H. 1987. Influence of ascorbic acid dose on N-nitrosoproline formation in humans. *Carcinogenesis* 8(6): 791.

Licht, W.R., Fox, J.G., and Deen, W.M. 1988a. Effects of ascorbic acid and thiocyanate on nitrosation of proline in the dog stomach. *Carcinogenesis* 9(3): 373.

Licht, W.R., Schultz, D.S., Fox, J.G., Tannenbaum, S.R., and Deen, W.M.

1986. Mechanisms of nitrite loss from the stomach. *Carcinogenesis* 7(10): 1681.

Licht, W.R., Tannenbaum, S.R., and Deen, W.M. 1988b. Use of ascorbic acid to inhibit nitrosation: Kinetic and mass transfer considerations for an in vitro system. *Carcinogenesis* 9(3): 365.

Lijinsky, W. 1987. Structure-activity relations in carcinogenesis by N-nitroso compounds. *Canc. Metas. Rev.* 6: 301.

Lijinsky, W. and Greenblatt, M. 1972. Carcinogenic dimethylnitrosamine produced in vivo from nitrite and aminopyrine. *Nature New Biol.* 236: 177.

Lu, S.-H., Ohshima, H., Fu, H.-M., Tian, Y., Li, F.-M., Blettner, M., Wahrendorf, J., and Bartsch, H. 1986. Uriny excretion of N-nitrosamino acids and nitrate by inhabitants of high- and low-risk areas for esophageal cancer in Northern China: Endogenous formation of nitrosoproline and its inhibition by vitamin C. *Cancer Res.* 46: 1485.

Massey, R.C., Crews, C., Dennis, M.J., McWeeny, D.J., Startin, J.R., and Knowles, M.E. 1985. Identification of a major new involatile N-nitroso compound in smoked bacon. *Anal. Chim. Acta* 174: 327.

Massey, R.C., Key, P.E., McWeeny, D.J., and Knowles, M.E. 1987. An investigation of apparent total N-nitroso compounds in beer. In *Relevance of N-Nitroso Compounds to Human Cancer: Exposures and Mechanisms,* (Ed.) Bartsch, H., O'Neill, I.K., and Schulte-Hermann, R. IARC Scientific Publications No. 84, p. 219. International Agency for Research on Cancer, Lyon.

Milton-Thompson, G.J., Lightfoot, N.F., Ahmet, Z., Hunt, R.H., Barnard, J., Bavin, P.M.G., Brimblecombe, R.W., Darkin, D.W., Moore, P.J., and Viney, N. 1982. Intragastric acidity, bacteria, nitrite and N-nitroso compounds, before, during and after cimetidine treatment. *Lancet.* i: 1091.

Mirvish, S.S. 1975. Formation of N-nitroso compounds: Chemistry, kinetics, and in vivo occurrence. *Tox. Appl. Pharm.* 31: 325.

Mirvish, S.S. 1983. The etiology of gastric cancer—Intragastric nitrosamide formation and other theories. *J. Nat. Cancer Inst.* 71(3): 630.

Mirvish, S.S., Greenblatt, M., and Kommineni, V.R.C. 1972. Nitrosamide formation in vivo: Induction of lung adenomas in Swiss mice by concurrent feeding of nitrite and methylurea or ethylurea. *J. Nat. Cancer Inst.* 48: 1311.

Mirvish, S.S., Karlowski, K., Birt, D.F., and Sams, J.P. 1980. Dietary and other factors affecting nitrosomethylurea (NMU) formation in the rat stomach. In *N-Nitroso Compounds: Analysis, Formation and Occurrence,* (Ed.) Walker, E.A., Castegnaro, M., Griciute, L., and Borzsonyi, M.

IARC Scientific Publications No. 31, p. 271. International Agency for Research on Cancer, Lyon.

Mirvish, S.S., Sams,. J.P., and Issenberg, P. 1983. The nitrosating agent in mice exposed to nitrogen dioxide: Improved extraction method and localization in the skin. *Cancer Res.* 43: 2550.

National Academy of Science. 1981. *The Health Effect of Nitrate, Nitrite, and N-Nitroso Compounds.* National Academy Press, Washington, DC.

Ohshima, H. and Bartsch, H. 1981. Quantitative estimation of endogenous nitrosation in humans by monitoring N-nitrosoproline excreted in the urine. *Cancer Res.* 41: 3658.

Ohshima, H., Bereziat, J.-C., and Bartsch, H. 1982. Monitoring N-nitros-amino acids excreted in the urine and feces of rats as an index for endogenous nitrosation. *Carcinogenesis* 3(1): 115.

Ohshima, H., Mahon, G.A.T., Wahrendorf, J., and Bartsch, H. 1983. Dose-response study of N-nitrosoproline formation in rats and a deduced kinetic model for predicting carcinogenic effects caused by endogenous nitrosation. Cancer Res. 43: 5072.

Ohshima, H., O'Neill, I.K., Friesen, M., Bereziat, J.-C., and Bartsch, H. 1984. Occurrence in human urine of new sulphur-containing N-nitros-amino acids N-nitrosothiazolidine 4-carboxylic acid and its 2-methyl derivative, and their formation. *J. Cancer Res. Clin. Oncol.* 108: 121.

Perciballi, M., Conboy, J.J., and Hotchkiss, J.H. 1989. Origin of excess urinary N-nitrosoproline in the ferret. *Food Chem. Toxicol.* (in press).

Pfeiffer, C.J. 1970. Surface topology of the stomach in man and the laboratory ferret. *J. Ultrastruc. Res.* 33: 252.

Piacek-Llanes, B.G. and Tannenbaum, S.R. 1982. Formation of an activated N-nitroso compound in nitrite-treated fava beans (*Vicia faba*). *Carcinogenesis* 3(12): 1379.

Preussmann, R. and Eisenbrand, G. 1984. N-Nitroso carcinogens in the environment. Ch. 13. In *Chemical Carcinogens,* Vol. 2, (Ed.) Searle, C.E. p. 829. ACS Monograph 182, American Chemical Society, Washington, DC.

Preussmann, R., Spiegelhalder, B., and Eisenbrand, G. 1981. Reduction of human exposure to environmental N-nitroso compounds. Ch. 16. In *N-Nitroso Compounds,* (Ed.) Scanlan, R.A. and Tannenbaum S.R. ACS Symposium Series 174., p. 217. American Chemical Society, Washington, DC.

Preussmann, R. and Stewart, B.W. 1984. N-nitroso carcinogens. Ch. 12. In *Chemical Carcinogens,* Vol. 2, (Ed.) Searle, C.E., p. 643. ACS Monograph 182, American Chemical Society, Washington, DC.

Rounbehler, D.P., Krull, I.S., Goff, E.U., Mills, K.M., Morrison, J., Edwards, G.S., Fine, D.H., Fajen, J.M., Carson, G.A., and Rheinhold, V. 1979. Exposure to N-nitrosodimethylamine in a leather tannery. *Food Cosmet. Toxicol.* 17: 487.

Sander, J. and Burkle, G. 1969. Induction of malignant tumors in rats by simultaneous feeding of nitrite and secondary amines. *Z. Krebsforsch.* 73: 54.

Sander, J., Schweinsberg, F., and Menz, H.-P. 1968. Studies on the formation of carcinogenic nitrosamines in the stomach. *Hoppe-Seylers Z. Physiol. Chem.* 349: 1691.

Saul, R.L. and Archer, M.C. 1984. Oxidation of ammonia and hydroxylamine to nitrate in the rat and in vitro. *Carcinogenesis* 5(1): 77.

Sen, N.P., Baddoo, P.A., and Seaman, S.W. 1986. N-nitrosothiazolidine and N-nitrosothiazolidine-4-carboxylic acid in smoked meats and fish. *J. Food Sci.* 51(3): 821.

Sen, N.P., Baddoo, P.A., and Seaman, S.W. 1987. Volatile nitrosamines in cured meats packaged in elastic rubber nettings. *J. Agric. Food Chem.* 35: 346.

Sen, N.P., Smith, D.C., and Schwinghamer, L. 1969. Formation of N-nitrosamines from secondary amines and nitrite in human and animal gastric juice. *Food Cosmet. Toxicol.* 7: 301.

Sen, N.P., Tessier, L., Seaman, S. W., and Baddoo, P.A. 1985. Volatile and nonvolatile nitrosamines in fish and the effect of deliberate nitrosation under simulated gastric conditions. *J. Agric. Food Chem.* 33: 264.

Spiegelhalder, B., Eisenbrand, G., and Preussmann, R. 1976. Influence of dietary nitrate on nitrite content of human saliva: Possible relevance to in vivo formation of N-nitroso compounds. *Food Cosmet. Toxicol.* 14: 545.

Spiegelhalder, B., Eisenbrand, G., and Preussman, R. 1980. Volatile nitrosamines in food. *Oncology* 37: 211.

Spiegelhalder, B. and Preussmann, R. 1982. Nitrosamines and rubber. In *N-Nitroso Compounds: Occurrence and Biological Effects,* (Ed.) Bartsch, H., O'Neill, I.K., Castegnaro, M., and Okada, M. IARC Scientific Publications No. 41, p. 231. International Agency for Research on Cancer, Lyon.

Stephany, R.W. and Schuller, P.L. 1980. Daily dietary intakes of nitrate, nitrite and volatile N-nitrosamines in The Netherlands using the duplicate portion sampling technique. *Oncology* 37: 203.

Stich, H.F., Hornby, A.P., and Dunn, B.P. 1984. The effect of dietary factors on nitrosoproline levels in human urine. *Int. J. Cancer* 33: 625.

Stuehr, D.J. and Marletta, M.A. 1985. Mammalian nitrate biosynthesis: Mouse macrophages produce nitrite and nitrate in response to *Escherichia coli* lipopolysaccharide. *Proc. Natl. Acad. Sci.* 82: 7738.

Tannenbaum, S.R. 1980. A model for estimation of human exposure to endogenous Ni-nitrosodimethylamine. *Oncology* 37: 232.

Tannenbaum, S.R. 1987. Endogenous formation of N-nitroso compounds: A current perspective. In *Relevance of N-Nitroso Compounds to Human Cancer: Exposures and Mechanisms*, (Ed.) Bartsch, H., O'Neill, I.K., and Schulte-Hermann, R. IARC Scientific Publications No. 84, p. 292. International Agency for Research on Cancer, Lyon.

Tannenbaum, S.R., Moran, D., Falchuk, K.R., Correa, P., and Cuello, C. 1981. Nitrite stability and nitrosation potential in human gastric juice. *Cancer Let.* 14: 131.

Tannenbaum, S.R. and Skipper, P.L. 1984. Biological aspects to the evaluation of risk: Dosimetry of carcinogens in man. *Fund. Appl. Toxic.* 4: S367.

Tannenbaum, S.R., Weisman, M., and Fett, D. 1976. The effect of nitrate intake on nitrate formation in human saliva. *Food Cosmet. Toxicol.* 14: 549.

Tannenbaum, S.R. and Young, V.R. 1980. Endogenous nitrite formation in man. *J. Environ. Path. Toxicol.* 3: 357.

Tricker, A.R., Siddiqi, M., and Preussmann, R. 1988. Occurrence of volatile N-nitrosamines in dried chillies. *Cancer Lett.* 38: 271.

Vecchio, A.J., Hotchkiss, J.H., and Bisogni, C.A. 1986. N-nitrosamine ingestion from consumer-cooked bacon. *J. Food Sci.* 51(3): 754.

Wagner, D.A., Shuker, D.E., Bilmazes, C., Obiedzinski, M., Baker I., Young, V.R., and Tannenbaum, S.R. 1985. Effect of vitamins C and E on endogenous synthesis of N-nitrosamino acids in humans: Precursor-product studies with [^{15}N]nitrate. *Cancer Res.* 45: 6519.

Wagner, D.A., Schultz, D.S., Deen, W.M., Young, V.R., and Tannenbaum, S.R. 1983a. Metabolic fate of an oral dose of ^{15}N-labeled nitrate in humans: Effect of diet supplementation with ascorbic acid. *Cancer Res.* 43: 1921.

Wagner, D.A. and Tannenbaum, S.R. 1982. Enhancement of nitrate biosynthesis by *Escherichia coli* lipopolysaccharide. In *Nitrosamines and Human Cancer*. Banbury Report 12, (Ed.) Magee, P.N., p. 437. Cold Spring Harbor Laboratory.

Wagner, D.A., Young, V.R., and Tannenbaum, S.R. 1983b. Mammalian nitrate biosynthesis: Incorporation of $^{15}NH_3$ into nitrate is enhanced by endotoxin treatment. *Proc. Natl. Acad. Sci.* 80: 4518.

Walters, C.L., Gillatt, P.N., Palmer, R.C., Smith, P.L.R., and Reed, P.I. 1987. In vitro and in vivo formation of N-nitrosomethylcyclohexylamine from bromhexin and sodium nitrite, and DNA methylation in rats. In *Relevance of N-Nitroso Compounds to Human Cancer: Exposures and Mechanisms,* (Ed.) Bartsch, H., O'Neill, I.K., and Schulte-Hermann, R. IARC Scientific Publications No. 84, p. 351. International Agency for Research on Cancer, Lyon.

Wang, C.F., Cassens, R.G., and Hoekstra, W.G. 1981. Fate of ingested ^{15}N-labeled nitrate and nitrite in the rat. *J. Food Sci.* 46: 745.

White, J.W. 1975. Relative significance of dietary sources of nitrate and nitrite. *J. Agric. Food Chem.* 23: 886.

White, J.W., 1976. Correction: Relative significance of dietary sources of nitrate and nitrite. *J.Agric. Food Chem.* 24: 202.

Whong, W.-Z., Speciner, N.D., and Edwards, G.S. 1979. Mutagenicity detection of in vivo nitrosation of dimethylamine by nitrite. *Environ. Mutagen.* 1: 277.

Winn, D.M. 1984. Tobacco chewing and snuff dipping: An association with human cancer. In *N-Nitroso Compounds: Occurrence, Biological Effects and Relevance to Human Cancer.* (Ed.) O'Neill, I.K., Von Borstel, R.C., Miller, C.T., Long, J., and Bartsch, H. IARC Scientific Publications No. 57 p. 837. International Agency for Research on Cancer, Lyon.

Witter, J.P., Balish, E., and Gatley, S.J. 1982. Origin of excess urinary nitrate in the rat. *Cancer Res.* 42: 3654.

Witter, J.P., Gatley, S.J., and Balish, E. 1981. Evaluation of nitrate synthesis by intestinal microorganisms in vivo. *Science* 213: 449.

Yoo, J.S.H., Guengeri, F.P., and Yang, C.S. 1988. Metabolism of N-nitrosodialkylamines by human liver microsomes. *Cancer Res.* 48(6): 1499.

Zeisel, S.H., daCosta, K.A., and LaMont, J.T. 1988. Mono-, di- and trimethylamine in human gastric fluid: Potential substrates for nitrosodimethylamine formation. *Carcinogenesis* 9(1): 179.

5
Anticarcinogens and Tumor Promoters in Foods

**David E. Williams, R. H. Dashwood,
Jerry D. Hendricks, and George S. Bailey**
Oregon State University
Corvallis, Oregon

INTRODUCTION

Epidemiological studies utilizing human populations from different geographical locations and dietary customs strongly suggest that food constituents play an important modulatory role in the incidence of some cancers (see Table 5.1). Recently, increasing attention has been focused on dietary modifiers of carcinogenesis and a large number of animal studies have examined the effect of factors such as fat levels (saturated and polyunsaturated), antioxidants (natural and synthetic), plant constituents (retinoids, phenolics, protease inhibitors, indoles, isothiocyanates, etc.), and trace elements such as selenium. In many cases the findings from these epidemiological studies are consistent with the results from animals studies. Some guidelines to reduce the risk of certain cancers by modifying the diet have resulted from the above studies (Table 5.2), but to date, no "ideal" dietary compound has been found which provides universal inhibition against all cancers. Since cancer is a complicated multistage disease affected by a wide variety of factors which are still relatively obscure, complete chemoprevention may not be possible.

Some progress has been made in recent years in our understanding of the basic mechanisms by which dietary constituents inhibit or promote

TABLE 5.1 Epidemiological Associations Between Dietary Components and Some Human Cancers

	Association	
Organ site	Positive	Negative
Breast	Fats, protein, sugar	Se, low fat
Pancreas	Protein, sugar, ethanol fried meats? fats	Se, low fat, fruits, vegetables
Lung		Vit. A, Se
Stomach	Salted, pickled, smoked fish, fava beans, nitrate	Milk, crucifers, vit. C, E
Prostate	Fats, protein	Vit. A, Se
Colon/Rectum	Fats, protein, Se?, fiber?	Crucifers, milk, Se? pentosans, fiber?, A
Larynx		Vit. A, C
Bladder		Vit. A, Se
Esophagus	Ethanol	Milk, fruits, green and yellow vegetables

Source: Diet, nutrition, and cancer (1982) (National Academy Press)

TABLE 5.2 Dietary Recommendations of the 1982 National Academy of Sciences Committee on Diet, Nutrition, and Cancer

Recommendations
1. Reduce intake of both saturated and unsaturated fat.
2. Include fruit, vegetables, and whole grain cereal products in daily diet, especially citrus fruits and carotene-rich and cabbage family vegetables.
3. Minimize consumption of cured, pickled, and smoked food.
4. Drink alcohol only in moderation.

Source: Linder (1985).

cancer, though we are still not at the point of being able to evaluate the potential of a given compound to affect human cancer in various organs or under different exposure regimens. Dietary constituents can reduce initiation by inhibiting formation of ultimate carcinogens by altering the balance of activation versus detoxication biochemical pathways of procarcinogens or by directly blocking or reducing DNA damage in target cells. Other compounds acting as anti-promoters are capable of interfering with progression of cancer development at some stage subsequent to initiation. Evidence indicates that some compounds, notably antioxidants, can repress either the initiation or promotion phases of carcinogenesis.

A number of excellent reviews are available on diet and cancer (Ames, 1983; Graham, 1984; Fiala et al., 1985; Wattenberg, 1985; Weisburger, 1987). In this paper we will present brief summaries from the literature on anticarcinogens and promoters in food according to chemical class (antioxidants, vitamins and trace elements, plant phenolic, indoles, and other nonnutrients and n-3 fatty acids for anticarcinogens and chlorinated hydrocarbon contaminants, steroids and special lipids, and dietary protein and amino acids for tumor promoters). We will discuss current studies concerning the probable mechanisms of action of anticarcinogens, drawing from results on both mammalian models and our own studies with the rainbow trout. Finally, we will discuss an important but perhaps not frequently presented topic, that is, the effect of exposure protocol on the action of a dietary constituent on tumor development. In particular, many "anticarcinogens" become tumor promoters on reversal of exposure protocol. There is thus a clear need to quantitate the relative potencies of a given compound for these opposing activities, so that risk-benefit estimates can be made. We discuss an approach by our laboratory for quantitative analysis of anticarcinogenic potency.

ANTICARCINOGENESIS BY FOOD COMPONENTS AND ADDITIVES

Antioxidants

As aerobic organisms, we are susceptible to oxidative stress and damage by reduced species of molecular oxygen, including hydrogen peroxide, superoxide anion radical, and the very reactive hydroxyl radical. Sources of these reactive oxygen species include the mitochondrial electron transport system, cellular peroxidases, monooxygenases, and the autooxidation of flavins, thiols, and lipids. Added to this burden of endogenously produced prooxidants are numerous xenobiotics, many of which are carcinogens, which result in increased oxidative damage. In fact, oxidative damage may be an important mechanism by which carcinogenesis is initiated and promoted (reviewed in Cerutti, 1985; Vuillaume, 1987; Marnett, 1987; Perera et al., 1987).

The cell has evolved a number of protective mechanisms to reduce the damage produced by prooxidants. Enzymes such as catalase, superoxide dismutase, glutathione peroxidase, glutathione transferase, and DT-diaphorase all function to inactive potentially damaging prooxidants and, as will be discussed in following sections, some dietary antioxidants appear to function as inhibitors primarily through their ability to induce one or more of these enzyme systems. In addition, there are a number of natural dietary components, such as vitamins E and C, β-carotene, selenium, and others, as well as synthetic additives such as 2-(3)-tert-butyl-4-hydroxyanisole (BHA), which are effective antioxidants and have been demonstrated to have anticarcinogenic properties. These synthetic and natural antioxidants will be discussed separately below, but in many cases their mechanism of action as modulators of carcinogenesis may be similar.

Oxidation of lipid and protein components is one of the major destablizing processes in foods, resulting in decreased nutritional value and consumer acceptance. A number of synthetic antioxidants (Fig. 5.1) are utilized as food additives, including the phenolic antioxidants BHA and BHT (3,5-di-tert-butyl-4-hydroxytoluene), propyl gallate, and ethoxyquin.

BHA and BHT.   Phenolic antioxidants are widely used in foods to prevent lipid peroxidation (approved concentrations of 0.001–0.02%), and the estimated daily intake in the United States is 3 mg and 14 mg/day for BHA and BHT, respectively. Results from a number of studies have demonstrated that both BHA and BHT can be effective as inhibitors of carcinogenesis in a number of rodent target organs (lung, colon, forestomach, mammary gland, and liver) induced by a variety of chemical carcinogens (benzo(a)pyrene (BP), 7,12-dimethylbenz(a)anthracene (DMBA), dibenz(a,h)anthracene, diethylnitrosamine (DEN), 4-nitroquinoline-N-oxide, uracil mustard, urethane, methylazoxymethanol acetate, aflatoxin B1 (AFB1), and trans-5-amino-3-[2-(5-nitro-2-furyl)-vinyl]-1,2,4-oxadiazole (reviewed in Wattenberg, 1986; Ito and Hirose, 1987).

Such studies point to a major complication in the potential use of antioxidants for deliberate chemoprevention. Table 5.3 summarizes tumor studies involving postinitiation treatment using several antioxidants. These studies have revealed that net response to antioxidants can include inhibition, no effect, or tumor promotion, depending on the carcinogen, animal, and organ examined.

A similarly diffuse pattern of response is evident for studies administering antioxidants before or during carcinogen exposure (Ito and Hirose, 1987). This complicated response modality raises serious ques-

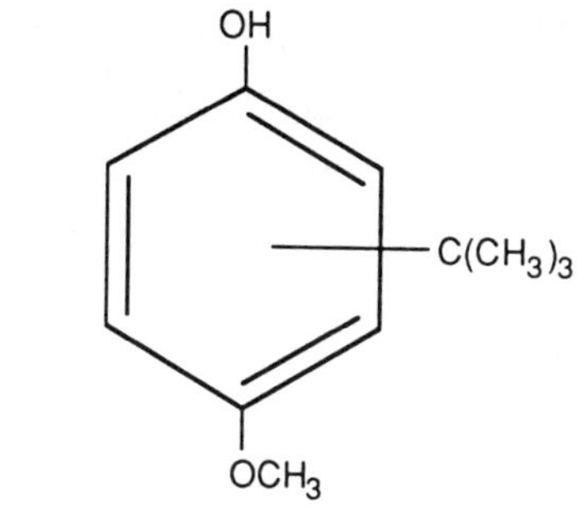

BHA
(mixture of 2- and 3- tert-butyl- 4- methoxyphenonl)

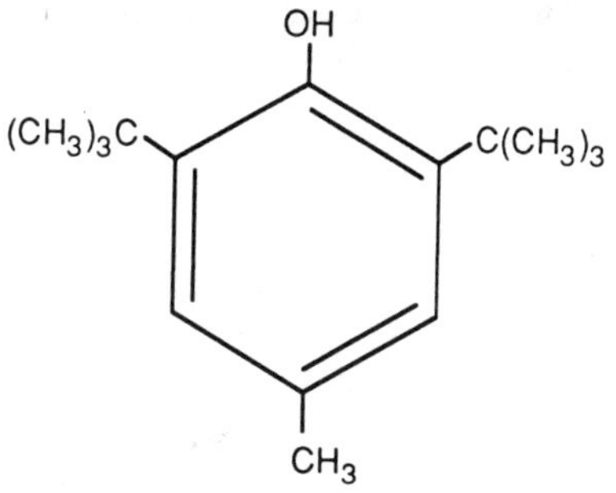

BHT

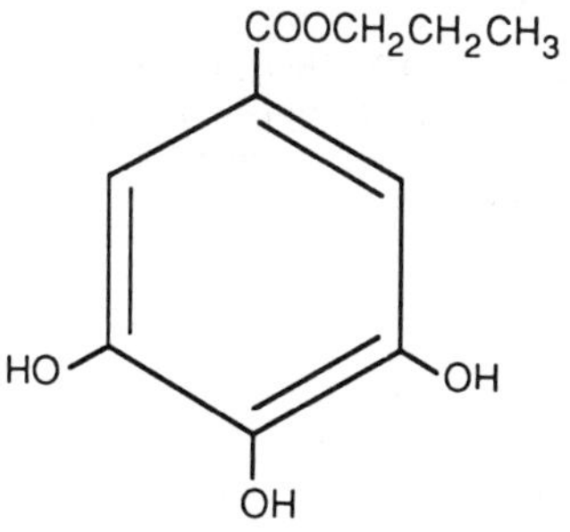

Propyl Gallate

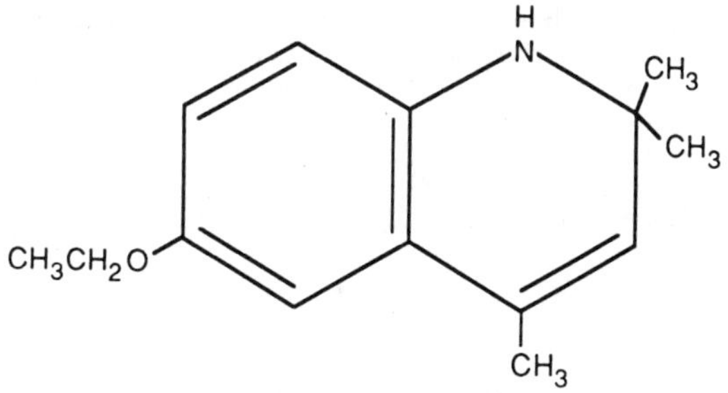

Ethoxyquin

FIG. 5.1 Structures of synthetic antioxidant food additives which modulate experimental carcinogenesis.

tions on the possible use of antioxidants as chemopreventive agents. Specifically, human antioxidant consumption may indeed reduce the promotion of prior initiation events in some organs but could simultaneously promote tumor response in other organs or enhance initiation from certain classes of carcinogens present at the time of antioxidant treatment. Thus, there are potential risks, as well as benefits, to be derived from antioxidant exposure. A major challenge for experimentalists is to attempt to quantify the relative risks and benefits. Especially lacking is further information on the dose-response nature of these opposing activities.

TABLE 5.3 Modifying Effect of Antioxidants on the Second Stage of Carcinogenesis in Animals

Organ	Initiator[a]	Species	Antioxidant[a]					
			BHA	BHT	EQ	SA	SE	E
Forestomach	MNNG	Rat	+[b]	0	0	0	−	0
	DBN	Rat	+	0	0	0	0	
	MNU	Rat	+	0		+		
Gland. stom.	MNNG	Rat	0	0	+	0	0	0
Colon	DMH	Rat	0	−	+	+		
	DMH	Mouse		+				
Liver	DEN	Rat	−	0	−	0		
	DBN	Rat	0	0	0	0		
	DHPN	Hamster	−	−				
Kidney	DHPN	Hamster	0	0				
Mammary	DMBA	Rat	−	−	−	0		0
Ear duct	DMBA	Rat	0	−	−	0		−

[a]Abbreviations are as follows: BHA, butylated hydroxyanisole; BHT, butylated hydroxytoluene; EQ, ethoxyquin; SA, sodium ascorbate; SE, selenium; E, vitamin E; MNNG, N-methyl-N′-nitro-N-nitrosoguanidine; DBN, dibutylnitrosamine; MNU, N-methyl-N-nitrosourea; DMH, dimethylhydrazine; DEN, diethylnitrosamine; DHPN, dihydroxydi-N-propylnitrosamine; DMBA, 7,12-dimethylbenz[a]anthracene.
[b]+ indicates inhibition; 0 indicates no effect; − indicates tumor enhancement.
Source: Ito and Hirose (1987).

A few studies performed recently have also questioned the carcinogenic status of BHA and BHT. BHA fed to F344 rats at a level of 2% of the diet produced significant increases in papilloma and squamous cell carcinoma of the forestomach (Ito et al., 1983). Dietary levels of 0.5 and 2.0% produced a dose-related increase in hyperplasia of the forestomach. The same laboratory reported that Syrian golden hamsters fed 1% BHA developed severe hyperplasia in the forestomach after 4 weeks, and the 3-tert BHA isomer was identified as the agent primarily responsible. Little effect was observed in an analogous study with a diet of 1% BHT (Hirose et al., 1986). In a study by Witschi (1986) the increased tumor development observed following continuous feeding of 0.05 and 0.5% BHT varied with strain (C3H and BALB/c mice), tissue, and carcinogen. In liver of C3H mice, spontaneous tumors were increased to a greater degree by 0.05% BHT, compared to the 0.5% diet. This surprising inverse relationship with BHT dose has also been observed in other rodent systems. No effect of BHT on spontaneous liver tumors was observed in BALB/c mice. The effect of BHT was carcinogen-dependent in the gastrointestinal tract, enhancing dimethylhydrazine-induced tumor development, but not tumors initiated with methylnitrosourea. In a study which examined a wider dose range for BHT (Powell et al., 1986), no observable effect was seen at a dose of 25 mg/kg/day, a dose at least 100 times the average intake in the United States.

In summary, BHA and BHT are effective inhibitors against a wide variety of spontaneous and chemically induced tumors. However, these compounds appear to have an epigenetic promoting effect at very high doses in some tissues, the mechanism of which is not yet understood but which may be related to tissue hyperplasia, similar to the promoting effect of phenobarbital. The results from studies to date would suggest that the carcinogenic properties of BHA and BHT may not be of major human health concern at the levels consumed in the average diet. In addition, the major site of carcinogen activity in these rodent models is the forestomach, an organ which is not present in humans. The dual action of phenolic antioxidants as both tumor inhibitors and enhancers may be of greater concern for chemoprevention. These "ambivalent modulators" will be discussed later together with other examples of protocol-dependent tumor enhancement by some anticarcinogens. The mechanism of action of phenolic antioxidants as inhibitors of carcinogenesis appears to be due to their ability to induce various detoxifying enzymes, especially the glutathione-S-transferases.

Propyl Gallate and Ethoxyquin. Compared to the phenolic oxidants, relatively few tumor studies have been performed with these compounds. Ethoxyquin has been reported to inhibit AFB1-induced hepatocarcinogenesis in rats (Cabral and Neal, 1983). Rats fed a diet containing 0.5% ethoxyquin and then treated with ciprofibrate had a lower incidence of hepatic tumors, fewer tumors per animal, and reduced tumor size compared to controls (Rao et al., 1984). The inhibitory action of ethoxyquin (and BHA) in this system was probably a direct function of their ability to scavenge active oxygen species and other free radicals produced from H_2O_2 following peroxisome proliferation by ciprofibrate. Propyl gallate, BHA, BHT, and especially ethoxyquin are very efficient inhibitors of lipid peroxidation in vitro at concentrations expected in tissues from humans consuming 1–10 mg per day (Kahl and Hilderbrandt, 1986). In addition to a direct antioxidant function, ethoxyquin also appears to act via induction of detoxification enzymes, especially glutathione-S-transferase. Male F344 rats fed diets containing 0.5% ethoxyquin, 0.45% BHT, 0.45% BHA, or 0.1% oltipraz for 2 weeks prior to an i.p. dose of 1 mg/g AFB1 displayed 91,

85, 65, and 76%, respectively, lower covalent DNA adduction compared to controls (Kensler et al., 1985). All four antioxidants were effective inducers of glutathione reductase, glutathione-S-transferase, UDP-glucuronyl transferase, and epoxide hydrolase. An excellent correlation ($r = 0.95$) between inhibition of DNA binding and induction of glutathione-S-transferase was observed. In a subsequent study, prefeeding male Fischer rats for 1 week on a diet containing 0.4% ethoxyquin, prior to treatment with AFB1, again significantly reduced covalent DNA binding as well as reducing, by greater than 95%, focal areas positively staining for γ-glutamyl transpeptidase (Kensler et al., 1986). The reduction in aflatoxin-DNA adducts and preneoplastic foci was accompanied by a greater than fivefold induction of multiple forms of glutathione-S-transferase in vitro and a 4.5-fold increase in biliary elimination of aflatoxin in vivo as the glutathione conjugate.

Vitamins and Trace Elements

α-Tocopherol (Vitamin E).   Vitamin E (Fig. 5.2) is the term given to the tocopherols (from the Greek "bringing forth in childbirth") of which the α-isomer is the most biologically active. Tocopherols are found predominantly in vegetable oils, cereal grain products, fish, meat, eggs, dairy products, and green leafy vegetables (IFT Expert Panel and Committee on Public Information, 1977). A number of studies have documented that vitamin E is the major lipid-soluble antioxidant in mammalian cells, and there is a strong inverse correlation with vitamin E levels in mammalian tissues and lipid peroxidation (Kornbrust and Mavis, 1980). The results from a number of animal studies and human epidemiological studies suggest an anticarcinogenic role for vitamin E. For example, dietary levels of 0.36–1.5% vitamin E (as DL-α-tocopherol acetate) inhibited the induction of γ-glutamyltranspeptidase-positive foci in rat liver after initiation with DEN and partial hepatectomy (Ura et al., 1987). Topical application of vitamin E (as D-γ-tocopherol) was an effective inhibitor of 12-O-tetradecanoylphorbol-13-acetate promotion of DMBA-induced skin papillomas in mice (Perchellet et al., 1985). Perhaps more striking is the ability of vitamin E to regress established epidermoid carcinomas in the buccal pouch of Syrian hamster initiated with DMBA (Shklar et al., 1987).

As mentioned above, epidemiological studies in general support the results from animal studies suggesting that vitamin E is an anticarcinogen. A recent study from Finland employing 21,172 men from six different geographical areas demonstrated that men with higher blood levels of vitamin E had a lower risk of subsequently developing cancer (Knekt et al., 1988).

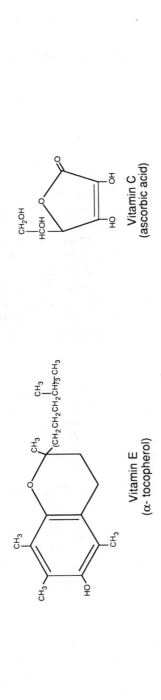

Vitamin E
(α- tocopherol)

Vitamin C
(ascorbic acid)

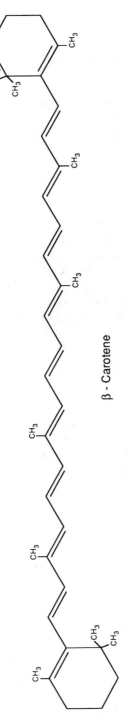

β - Carotene

FIG. 5.2 Structures of vitamin E, vitamin C, and beta-carotene.

109

The RDAs (National Academy of Sciences, 1973) for vitamin E are 4–5 IU (1 mg of DL-α-tocopherol acetate = 1 IU) for infants, 7–12 for children, and 12–15 for adults. The estimated average daily intake in the U.S. is about 14 mg. Although more evidence is required to fully evaluate the potential of vitamin E as an anticarcinogen, there is relatively little risk associated with megadoses, as vitamin E displays little toxicity in mammalian studies.

Vitamin C (ascorbic acid). Vitamin C (Fig. 5.2) is also an important dietary antioxidant, but definitive evidence for its role as an anti-carcinogen is lacking. In fact the results from animal studies are equivocal and difficult to interpret. For example, a study by Mirvish et al. (1975) found inhibition of carcinogenesis at one site and enhancement at another with vitamin C treatment. Epidemiological studies with human populations also are inconclusive. Case control studies have suggested that dietary vitamin C can inhibit cancer of the cervix, mouth, stomach, and larynx (Graham et al., 1977, 1981, 1982; Kolonel et al., 1981). Other studies have found no relationship between dietary vitamin C and cancer of the colon, rectum, bladder, prostate, breast, or stomach (Graham et al., 1978, 1983; Mettlin and Graham, 1979;). Perhaps a more convincing role for vitamin C is as an inhibitor of nitrosamine formation.

β-Carotene (vitamin A). β-Carotene is the provitamin form of vitamin A and is one of many carotenoids found in foods of plant origin. β-Carotene, in high concentrations primarily in yellow, orange, and green vegetables (especially pumpkins and carrots), is converted into two units of retinol (vitamin A can exist as the alcohol (retinol), aldehyde (retinal) or acid (retinoic acid) which along with various synthetic analogues are collectively referred to as retinoids). Foods of animal origin provide vitamin A predominantly as retinal esters. β-Carotene can be taken in megadoses, as the degree of conversion to retinol in vivo can be regulated, but excess intake of retinol or retinal can be toxic. Vitamin A functions in vision, tissue growth, differentiation, and reproduction. It has also been observed that β-carotene is an excellent free radical trapping agent and, in fact, is the most efficient scavenger known of the very reactive singlet oxygen (Ames, 1983).

A number of epidemiological studies of β-carotene have been published. A study of Norwegian men in 1975 (Bjelke, 1975) found a negative correlation between estimated β-carotene dietary intake and lung cancer at all levels of smoking. A large prospective dietary study from Japan indicated that β-carotene could provide protection against cancer of the lung, stomach, colon, prostate, and cervix (Hirayama, 1979). Perhaps the most striking study was that reported by Shekelle et al. (1981) in which a sevenfold lower risk of developing lung cancer was noted between the group consuming the highest dietary β-carotene, compared to the group consuming the lowest. Interestingly, β-carotene did not reduce the risk for any other cancers, and when the intake of dietary retinol was calculated, no protective effect was observed. In a recently published population-based incident case-control study of lung cancer in white males in six different locations in New Jersey (Ziegler et al., 1986), consumption of β-carotene, but not retinoids, was associated with reduced risk of lung cancer. The protective effect of β-carotene was most pronounced in smokers. Two separate prospective blood studies have demonstrated an inverse relationship between blood levels of vitamin A and cancer (Wald et al., 1980; Kark et al., 1982). In a study of serum samples from Georgia, a fivefold higher cancer risk was found in the group with the lowest serum vitamin A levels, compared to the group with the highest levels. A number of retrospective studies have documented lower blood levels of vitamin A and/or β-carotene in cancer patients compared to controls (Wahil et al., 1962; Basu et al., 1976, Ibrahim et al., 1977).

The protective effect of β-carotene has been confirmed in animal studies. Dietary supplementation of β-carotene reduced the onset, tumor incidence, and time to death of mice injected with tumor cells (Rettura et al., 1982). Supplementation with β-carotene also has been demonstrated to decrease the time of appearance, incidence, and growth of skin tumors induced either chemically or by UV light (Epstein, 1977; Mathews-Roth, 1982; Santamaria et al., 1983).

Therefore, data from both epidemiological and animal studies performed to date strongly indicate an anticarcinogenic role for β-carotene, especially towards lung cancer. These studies resulted in the recommendation by the National Academy of Sciences Committee on Diet, Nutrition and Cancer to increase dietary intake of carotene-rich foods (Table 5.2). This recommendation is especially important given that it has been reported that a significant proportion of the U.S. population is consuming dietary levels below the RDA (Pao and Mickle, 1981). Since the retinoids can be toxic, vitamin A can be more safely supplied as β-carotene.

Selenium.   Dietary intake of selenium (primarily as selenite and seleno-amino acids) has been inversely correlated with cancer incidence in epidemiological studies from geographical areas of the world varying in soil selenium content (Jacobs and Griffin, 1981). The inverse relationship between dietary selenium intake and cancer incidence is especially strong for cancers of the breast, colon, rectum, prostate, and in leukocytes (Schrauzer et al., 1977). The results from animal studies strongly support epidemiological findings. Dietary levels of selenium influence the appearance and growth of tumors of the mammary gland (Ip 1981), colon (Jacobs et al., 1981), and liver (Griffin and Jacobs, 1977). Dietary supplementation with 0.2, 2.0, and 5.0 ppm selenium produced a dose-dependent decrease in the appearance of preneoplastic foci in rats exposed to AFB1 (Milks et al., 1985).

The types of cancer for which selenium exhibits the strongest anticarcinogenic effect are those in which dietary fat has been indicated as a high risk factor. A possible explanation lies in the fact that selenium functions indirectly as a lipid antioxidant through its incorporation as the prosthetic group of glutathione peroxidase, one of the most important cellular protective enzymes against lipid peroxidation. Although the inverse association between dietary selenium intake and cancer incidence is strong, the high toxicity associated with excess selenium intake may make it impractical to go beyond supplementation of deficient diets.

Plant Phenolics

Plant phenols (Fig. 5.3) are a large group of compounds (e.g., the caffeic, ellagic, tannic, anthraflavic, ferulic, and chlorogenic acids, chrysin, apigenin, quercetin, myricetin, robinetin, and luteolin) found naturally in fruits and vegetables. The total daily intake of plant phenols in the human diet may approach 1 g (Brown, 1980). Topical administration of ellagic acid to mice just prior to the application of (+)-7,8-dihydroxy-9,10-epoxy-7,8,9,10-tetrahydrobenzo[a]pyrene (BP 7,8-diol-9,10-epoxide-2) produced a significant reduction in skin tumors promoted by 12-O-tetradecanoyl-phorbol-13-acetate (Chang et al., 1985). In this same study, treatment of newborn mice i.p. with ellagic acid, quercetin, or robinetin 10 min prior to i.p. dosing with BP-7,8-diol-9,10-epoxide-2 significantly inhibited the subsequent incidence of lung tumors. Interestingly, these plant phenolics had either no effect (pulmonary tumors) or a statistically insignificant effect (skin tumors) when BP was used as the initiator. Similar ngative or equivocal results for ellagic acid as an inhibitor of BP-induced skin or lung cancer were obtained in a subsequent experiment utilizing a variety of dosing regiments (Smart et al., 1986). However, previous studies (Lesca, 1983) demonstrated that ellagic acid was capable of inhibiting lung tumor formation in mice. Perhaps of more relevance for extrapolation to human populations was a study performed by Mukhtar et al. (1986) in which exposure of mice to only 3 ppm ellagic acid in the drinking water reduced the risk of developing skin tumors induced by 3-methylcholanthrene. The authors suggested that the anticarcinogenic effect of ellagic acid was

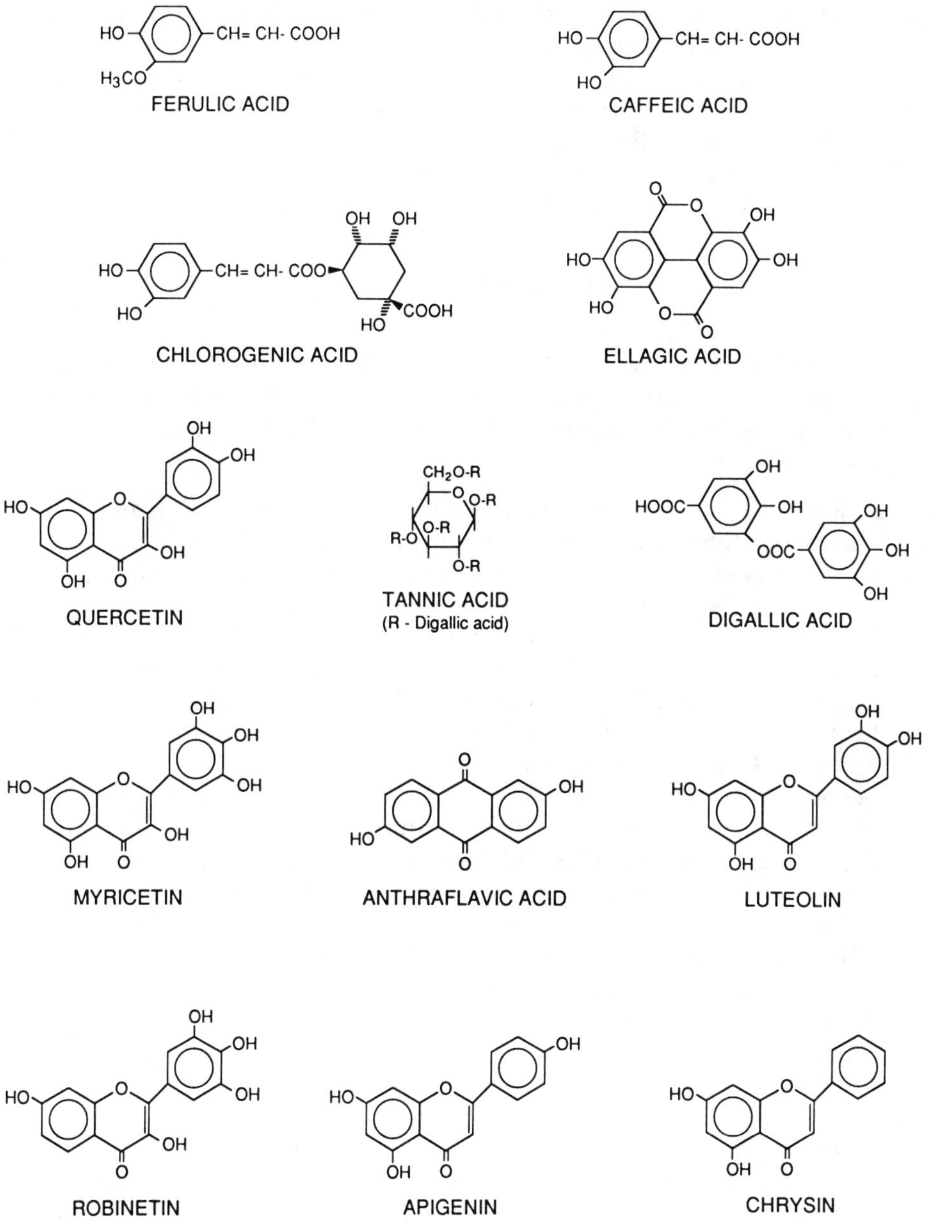

FIG. 5.3 Structure of common plant phenolics which can act as experimental anticarcinogens.

related to its ability to inhibit skin aryl hydrocarbon hydroxylase activity, the cytochrome P-450 activity thought to be involved in the bioactivation of polycyclic aromatic hydrocarbons and derivatives to the ultimate carcinogenic metabolites. In addition, plant phenols appear to inhibit tumor development with direct acting carcinogens (BP-7,8-diol-9,10-epoxide-2, methylazoxymethanol acetate, and N-methyl-N-nitrosourea) (Mori et al., 1986; Mukhtar et al., 1988).

Indoles and Other Nonnutrients

In addition to the indoles (indole-3-carbinol, indole-3-acetonitrile, and 3,3'-diindolylmethane), this section will discuss the anticarcinogenic properties of isothiocyanates, protease inhibitors, and organosulfur compounds (Fig. 5.4).

Indoles.   Indole-3-carbinol (I3C), indole-3-acetonitrile (IAN), and 3,3'-diindolylmethane (I33') are the major indoles derived from glucobrassicin, found in high concentration in cruciferous vegetables such as cabbage, cauliflower, and Brussels sprouts (Bradfield and Bjeldanes, 1987b; McDanell et al., 1988). The results from animal feeding studies either with the cruciferous vegetables, glucobrassicin, or one or more of the derived indoles generally support the hypothesis that these compounds have anticarcinogenic properties. Weanling male Fisher rats fed diets containing 25% freeze-dried cabbage exhibited a significantly reduced average number of tumors per animal following a carcinogenic dose of AFB1 (Boyd et al., 1982). In an experiment with the purified indoles, pretreatment with I3C and I33', but not IAN, inhibited the subsequent development of DMBA-induced mammary tumors in the rat (Wattenberg and Loub, 1978). In the same study, all three indoles were effective in inhibiting BP-induced tumors of the forestomach. Additional studies from Wattenberg's laboratory have indicated that glucobrassicin pretreatment 3, 2, and 1 days prior to administration of BP, protected mice against developing tumors of the lung and forestomach (Wattenberg et al., 1986). This same study observed that pretreatment of mice with glucobrassicin as little as 4 hr prior to exposure to BP inhibited mammary tumorigenesis. Our laboratory has found that pretreatment of rainbow trout fry with dietary I3C significantly reduces hepatocarcinogenesis induced by subsequent exposure to AFB1 (Nixon et al., 1984). Interestingly, whereas I3C is an effective inhibitor in trout, it appears to act primarily through mechanism(s) other than induction of Phase I and Phase II detoxication enzymes, a process thought to be important in mammalian animal models.

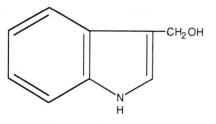

Indole- 3- carbinol
(I3C)

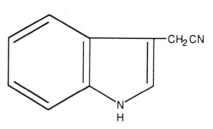

Indole- 3- acetonitrile
(IAN)

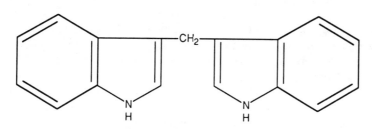

3,3'- Diindolylmethane
(I33')

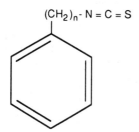

$CH_2 = CH - CH_2 - S - S - S - CH_2 - CH = CH_2$

Diallyl trisulfide

(n = 1) Benzyl isothiocyanate
(n = 2) Phenethyl isothiocyanate

FIG. 5.4 Structures of anticarcinogenic plant indoles, isothiocyanates, and organosulfur compounds.

Isothiocyanates.   The aromatic isothiocyanates (Figure 5.4), like the in-doles (see above), are naturally occurring constituents of cruciferous vegetables such as cabbage, cauliflower, and Brussels sprouts (Virtanen, 1965). Administration of benzylisothiocyanate to mice decreased by 80% the appearance of BP-induced tumors of the forestomach (Sparnins and Wattenberg, 1981). The aromatic isothiocyanates have been found to be effective only when fed in conjunction with, or administered shortly before, carcinogen exposure. Mice fed either benzyl- or phenethyl-isothio-cyanate (5000 ppm) in a diet also containing a carcinogenic dose of DMBA developed fewer forestomach and lung tumors than mice fed the carcinogen only (Wattenberg, 1977). This same study found that adminis-tration of the aromatic isothiocyanates 2–4 hr prior to dosage with DMBA resulted in inhibition, but no effect was observed if given 4 hr after DMBA exposure.

Protease Inhibitors.   Epidemiological studies with vegetarian groups, such as the Seventh-Day Adventists, have indicated that diets especially rich in seed proteins and legumes such as soybean provide protection against certain cancers, especially those of the breast, prostate, and colon (Philips, 1975). The potential beneficial effect of protease inhibitors as an-titumor agents (reviewed in Troll et al., 1984) have been confirmed in a large number of animal studies using both synthetic and natural protease inhibitors (Hozumi et al., 1972; Troll et al., 1980; Nomura et al., 1980; Becker, 1981; Corasanti et al., 1982; Yavelow et al., 1983; Weed et al., 1985).

Organosulfur Compounds.   Onions and garlic contain relatively high levels of allylic di- and tri-sulfides which have been demonstrated to in-hibit both initiation and promotion. These organosulfur compounds have been shown to inhibit tumors of the forestomach, lung, colon, esophagus, and skin, induced by three distinct chemical classes of carcinogens (Bel-man, 1983; Hayes et al., 1987; Wargovich, 1987; Sparnins et al., 1988). The major mechanism involved in the protection against initiation appears to be the ability of these compounds to induce glutathione-S-transferase activity.

N-3 Fatty Acids

A number of epidemiological and animal studies have indicated that high-fat diets increase the risk of cancer, especially of the breast, colon, and pancreas (summarized in Carroll et al., 1986). These studies prompted the National Academy of Sciences Committee on Diet, Nutrition and

Cancer to recommend reductions in dietary fats (Table 5.2). High-fat diets appear to function as promoters, and the risk is much greater for polyunsaturated fat from vegetable oils than from saturated fat or polyunsaturated fat from fish oils, which contain high levels of the n-3 fatty acids (Cohen et al., 1986a,b; Reddy and Maruyama, 1986). In fact, evidence suggests that fish oils may inhibit tumor formation under certain circumstances (Karmali et al., 1984; Jurkowski and Cave, 1985; O'Connor et al., 1985; Gabor and Abraham, 1985; Nigro et al., 1986). Although the exact mechanism by which n-3 fatty acids function as anticarcinogens is uncertain, one probable contributing effect is the reduction of prostaglandin levels. The n-3 fatty acids inhibit the production of the eicosanoids, which are thought to play an important role in tumor growth. This hypothesis is supported by the finding that synthetic inhibitors of prostaglandin synthesis, such as indomethacin, inhibit promotion by high-fat diets (Carter et al., 1983).

TUMOR PROMOTORS IN FOODS

Chlorinated Hydrocarbon Contaminants

Polychlorinated biphenyls and a number of chlorinated hydrocarbon pesticides, including dichlorodiphenyltrichloroethane (DDT), chlordane, and heptaclor, have been demonstrated to be effective co-carcinogens, promoters, and weak carcinogens in a number of studies (Peraino et al., 1975; Nishizumi, 1979; Preston et al., 1981; Pereira et al., 1982; Deml and Oesterle, 1982; Deml et al., 1983; Oesterle and Deml, 1983; Williams and Numuto, 1984; Ward, 1985; Deml and Oesterle, 1986). In the rainbow trout, polychlorinated biphenyls are not promoters but are capable of acting as co-carcinogens or enhancers. The effectiveness of chlorinated hydrocarbons and polychlorinated biphenyls in promotion is probably a function of their ability to induce hyperplasia. Again, it may be of interest that trout do not respond to the hypertrophic actions of this class of chemicals.

Steroids and Special Lipids

A number of steroids, especially synthetic (ethinyl estradiol and diethylstilbesterol) and natural (β-estradiol) sex steroids are capable of acting as co-carcinogens or promoters (Sumi et al., 1980; Cameron, 1981; Lian, et al., 1984). We have found β-estradiol to be a potent promoter of hepatocarcinogenesis in the rainbow trout model (Nunez et al., 1988; Nunez et al., in preparation). The promoting effect of natural and synthetic estrogens may be tissue-specific, as epidemiological and animal model studies suggest that estrogens may play an anticarcinogenic role in breast cancer (MacMahon et al., 1973; Wotiz et al., 1984; Grubbs et al., 1985). In addition to the sex steroids, bile acids have been demonstrated to act as promoters and may be of major significance in human colon cancers (Cameron et al., 1982). Of these two classes of steroids, the estrogens are of more concern as components of human diet.

The cyclopropenoid fatty acids, sterculic and malvalic acids, are introduced into the human diet from oils or seeds from cottonseed, kapok, and okra or from the consumption of livestock fed with diets containing high levels of cottonseed. Cyclopropenoid fatty acids produce a variety of acute and chronic effects in mammals and are potent co-carcinogens and promoters of hepatocarcinogenesis induced by AFB1 and its metabolites in rainbow trout (Lee et al., 1971; Sinnhuber et al., 1974; Hendricks et al., 1980; Schoenhard et al., 1981).

Sorbitan fatty acid ester is used in the food industry as an emulsifying agent in formation of margarine and has been shown to act as a promoter of 3-methyl-4-dimethylaminoazobenzene-induced hepatocarcinogenesis in rats (Yanagi, et al., 19895).

Dietary Protein and Amino Acids

Epidemiological studies with vegetarian groups suggest that high levels of dietary protein increase the relative risk of some cancers, especially those of the breast and colon (Correa, 1981). The findings from these epidemiological studies are consistent with the results from most animal studies which have examined the effect of dietary protein on chemically induced (Hawrylewicz et al., 1982; Appleton and Campbell, 1983; Clinton et al., 1984; Hawrylewicz et al., 1986) or spontaneous (Ross and Bras, 1973) tumor formation. Our studies on the effect of dietary protein on AFB1-induced hepatocarcinogenesis in trout confirm that high dietary protein acts as a promoter (Lee et al., 1978). The source of the protein appeared important as no difference in the incidence of trout AFB1-induced hepatocarcinogenesis was observed between the low (32%) and high (49.5%) casein diets, whereas significant differences were seen with fish protein concentrate fed at the same high and low levels. Although casein levels did not influence tumor incidence, trout fed the low casein diet had consistently smaller tumors although the size difference was not as dramatic as with the high and low fish protein concentrate. Later experiments using protein levels in the 40–70% range (trout are carnivorous) indicated little difference between these two protein sources; both were strongly promotional (unpublished results).

In summary, the studies briefly reviewed in this section indicate the presence in the human diet of a variety of components capable of promoting chemical carcinogenesis in experimental animals. Such compounds may function similarly when consumed by man. Since different cultures and individuals are likely to vary widely in varieties and quantities of tumor promoters as well as anticarcinogens consumed, this may be expected to result in profound variability in response to carcinogen exposure. This may be a major source of confounding variation in the search for human carcinogens by epidemiological methods. As indicated in the next section, the situation is further complicated by the fact that many modulators do display both promotional inhibitory activity, depending on the experimental protocol chosen.

PROTOCOL-DEPENDENT TUMOR ENHANCEMENT BY SOME ANTICARCINOGENS

Although the potential for deliberate chemoprevention by dietary anticarcinogens has great appeal, enthusiasm must be tempered by animal experiments which indicate possible adverse effects. As pointed out above, there are experimental situations in which treatment with these agents results in enhancement, rather than reduction, in final tumor response. In some cases tumor burden is merely shifted from one organ to another, so that overall animal tumor burden is not relieved. Such opposing effects can occur when the same "anti-carcinogen" is given to different animal strains or species treated with the same carcinogen, or given to the same species treated with different carcinogens, or when the timing of carcinogen and anticarcinogen exposures are reversed.

Variable Response with Different Carcinogens

Among the dietary modulators which man consumes, the antioxidants have received perhaps the greatest attention. As reviewed previously, the phenolic antioxidants BHA and BHT have been shown to effectively reduce tumor response in a wide range of models and protocols. For example, feeding of 1000 or 6000 ppm BHA or BHT 1 week before, during, and after aflatoxin B1 (AFB1) treatment provided dose-responsive reduction of preneoplastic foci and hepatocellular neoplasms in F344 rats (Williams et al., 1986). However, similar experiments examining BHA effects on nitrosamine carcinogenesis have produced mixed results. Feeding 0.5% BHA before and during 10 weeks of nitrosamine exposure reduced N-nitrosodimethylamine induced lung adenomas in A/J mice, but enhanced the response to N-nitrosopyrrolidine response (Chung et al., 1986). Prolonged feeding of 2% BHA or 1% BHT resulted in promotion of urinary bladder carcinogenesis initiated by N-butyl-N-(4-hydroxybutyl) nitrosamine in F344 rats (Imaida et al., 1983). Numerous such contrasting effects of antioxidants are demonstrated in Table 5.3, taken from a recent review by Ito and Hirose (1987). Here it is seen that, even using a single type of exposure protocol, tumor modulation by a given antioxidant can involve enhancement, inhibition, or no effect. The direction and magnitude of the effect is highly dependent on the initiating carcinogen chosen, as well as the test animal, antioxidant, and target organ examined.

This type of confounding, carcinogen-dependent modulation is not unique to antioxidants. Our laboratory has examined the effect of various modulators on the hepatocarcinogenicity of AFB1 and DEN in the rainbow trout model. As shown in Table 5.4, the effects of the modulators Aroclor 1254, beta-naphthoflavone (BNF), or I3C differ for the two carcinogens. Dietary treatment of trout before and during AFB1 exposure by any of these three compounds inhibited hepatocarcinogenesis. By comparison, DEN carcinogenesis was inhibited by I3C but enhanced by BNF or by the polychlorinated biphenyl (PCB) mixture Aroclor 1254. A significant enhancing effect of PCBs on DEN-induced preneoplastic lesions in rats has also been observed (Deml and Oesterle, 1986).

Animal Species and Target Organ Variability

An important rational for comparative studies is that modulators (if any) which can be shown to be consistently protective among various animal model species, without toxicity or enhancing effects, may receive priority attention for chemopreventive use in man. Unfortunately, such an agent has yet to be identified. Modulators which function during the initiation phase of carcinogenesis by altering procarcinogen metabolism seem especially prone to animal and organ-specific variation in effectiveness. A clear example derives from studies on BHT modulation of urethane-induced lung adenomas in mice, in which BHT pretreatment decreased tumor multiplicity by 32% in adult A/J mice, but increased tumor number 48% in SWR/J mice, 240% in C57BL/6J mice, 655% in 129/J mice, and 38%

TABLE 5.4 Effect of Exposure Protocol on Dietary Modulation of Chemical Carcinogenesis in Rainbow Trout

Experiment	Period of dietary exposure			Tumor incidence
	Preinitiation	Initiation	Postinitiation	
1[a]	Control	Control	Control	0/99 (0%)
	Control	AFB1	Control	9/99 (9%)
	BNF (500 ppm)	BNF + AFB1	Control	1/100 (1%)*
	I3C (2000 ppm)	I3C + AFB1	Control	1/99 (1%)*
	Control	AFB1	BNF (500 ppm)	30/100 (30%)*
	Control	AFB1	I3C (2000 ppm)	51/100 (51%)*
2[b]	Control	AFB1	Control	37/79 (47%)
	PCB (100 ppm)	PCB + AFB1	Control	20/77 (26%)
3[c]	Control	AFB1	Control	34/117 (29%)
	Control	AFB1	PCB (100 ppm)	40/119 (34%)
4[d]	Control	DEN	Control	112/132 (85%)
	I3C (2000 ppm)	DEN + I3C	Control	37/138 (27%)*
	BNF (500 ppm)	DEN + BNF	Control	98/98 (100%)*
	PCB (100 ppm)	DEN + PCB	Control	132/140 (94%)*
5[c]	Control	DEN	Control	44/118 (37%)
	Control	DEN	I3C (2000 ppm)	81/103 (79%)*

[a]Preinitiation diet for 8 wk, initiation 4 wk at 10 ppb AFB1, postinitiation 12 wk.
[b]Preinitiation diet for 12 wk, initiation 2 wk at 20 ppb AFB1.
[c]Initiation by embryo immersion (AFB1, 0.5 ppm, 30 min; DEN, 1500 ppm, 24 hr). Postinitiation dietary treatment for 9 mo.
[d]Preinitiation diet for 6 wk, initiation by gill uptake (250 ppm DEN, 24 hr).
*Significantly different from appropriate control ($p < 0.05$, Fisher Exact test).
Source: Bailey et al. (1987).

in 14-day old A/J mice (Malkinson and Thaete, 1986). Thus the effect was variable among strains of the same species and, most problematically, was reversed in juveniles and adults of the same strain. Similarly, while BHA was indicated above to reduce AFB1 response in rat, studies in our laboratory show that AFB1-initiated carcinogenesis in trout is refractory to BHA treatment (Goeger et al., 1986). The difference in response appears to be due to BHA enhancement of AFB1-glutathione detoxication in rats, but not in trout (Valsta et al., 1988). Clearly it would be important to know if human cells are responsive to this inductive activity.

Anticarcinogens which are effective when provided after carcinogen initiation have attracted increasing interest since, by definition, they repress the promotional phase of tumor development and thus cannot act as tumor promoters. Such compounds should also be less carcinogen-specific than the anti-initiators, and their use would not require prior knowledge of human carcinogen exposure patterns. An example is the use of the cruciferous anticarcinogen benzyl isothiocyanate, which reduced DMBA-initiated mammary carcinogenesis in Sprague-Dawley rats if given following carcinogen treatment (Wattenberg, 1981). Antiproteases such as those in raw soybean preparations are also believed to have anti-promotional activity and have been shown to survive inactivation by stomach digestion in rodents (Yavelow et al., 1983). Preparations containing the Bowman-Birk antiprotease do protect against colon carcinogenesis in mice (Weed et al., 1985). The use of such agents is problematic, however, because of their known pancreatic carcinogenicity in rats (Morgan et al., 1977; McGuinness et al., 1984). Another class of such compounds, carotenoids and retinoids with vitamin A-like activity, are effective at inhibiting tumor progression in many animal models. However, contraindications exist for these compounds as well. For example, a recent study examining the effects of four synthetic retinoids on pancreatic carcinogenesis in Lewis rats showed that postinitiation treatment by each of the four retinoids reduced azaserine-induced pancreatic tumors, but three of the four enhanced hepatocarcinoma in females (Longnecker et al., 1983). Thus, tumor burden was shifted from one organ to another. A similar effect of vitamin C was noted earlier.

Variable Response with Timing of Administration

It is important in the design of anticarcinogenesis experiments to determine the effects of a modulator on both the initiation and postinitiation phases of carcinogenesis to test for possible opposing activities. Perhaps because of expense, many tumor studies in the literature lack this sophistication. The need for such complete testing is made apparent by those studies which do test effects on both phases. As an example, treatment of mice with BHT prior to urethan exposure reduced lung adenoma response, whereas BHT given after urethan promoted the response (Malkinson and Beer, 1984). Studies with rainbow trout in our laboratory show that this sort of reversal in effect with reversal in carcinogen-modulator exposure order is not uncommon. As shown in Table 5.4, dietary BNF or I3C given before and during AFB1 initiation reproducibly reduced tumor response in trout, whereas both compounds promoted tumor response when given after AFB1. The same effect has been seen when this experiment was conducted in F344 rats (Selivonchick and Bailey, unpublished results). I3C also inhibited hepatocarcinogenesis in trout when given before and during DEN exposure but promoted it when given after (Table 5.4). Interestingly, postinitiation treatment with PCB did not promote initiation by DEN or AFB1 in trout (Table 5.4). Using yet a different protocol, administration of I3C before, during and after carcinogen significantly enhanced dimethyl hydrazine-induced colon cancer in F344 rats (Pence et al., 1986). These studies indicate some possible risk associated with I3C, either casually in the diet or for deliberate chemoprevention.

MECHANISMS OF ANTICARCINOGENESIS

In the Synopsis to the First International Conference on Antimutagenesis and Anticarcinogenesis Mechanisms, Shankel et al. (1986, 1987) have stated:

> There is a strong feeling that mechanisms can be found that will offer mankind a substantial degree of cancer prevention.

> ... if cancer rates are determined in part by deficiencies in anticarcinogens, then our goal of preventing most forms of cancer may actually be attainable.

These views have received increasing support from the studies of anticarcinogenesis reviewed in the beginning of this chapter. Thus, evidence has accrued over the last decade indicating that the human diet contains not only a great variety of natural carcinogens (Sugimura, 1982, 1986; Ames, 1983; Ohgaki et al., 1987) but also many compounds anticarcinogenic in some experimental animal protocols (Wattenberg, 1982, 1983; Fiala et al., 1985; Shankel et al., 1986, 1987). However, the overall effect which such compounds may be having on present human cancer rates, and their potential for deliberate chemoprevention, remains problematic. Human protection is uncertain, not only because unreasonably high doses are often required for effect in many animals, but especially because many "anticarcinogens" exhibit promotional activity in some experiments. A full understanding of such ambivalent modulators will require further studies into mechanisms of anticarcinogenesis, including detailed investigation of the relationships between carcinogen dose, inhibitor dose, and final tumor response. Moreover, it is of fundamental importance that for naturally occurring compounds to which human exposure may be unavoidable, the potencies of inhibition versus promotion are fully characterized, down to levels commonly encountered in human diet. Because of their importance for human risk assessment, we will address these issues in more detail later in this section, with a focus on current efforts from our laboratory to provide quantitative potency information for I3C in trout. This will be preceded by a brief overview of our current understanding of anticarcinogenesis mechanisms.

Categorization of Anticarcinogens

Precursor-Conversion Inhibitors. Inhibitors of carcinogenesis have been broadly subdivided into three categories, depending upon the time at which they exert their protective effects (Wattenberg, 1983, 1985). These are summarized in Fig. 5.5, together with selected examples of dietary chemopreventative agents which operate, though not necessarily exclusively, at each level. The first category consists of agents which prevent the in situ formation of carcinogens from precursors (termed "precursor-conversion inhibitors" in Fig. 5.5.). This group includes both synthetic and naturally occurring dietary constituents, such as ascorbic acid, alpha-tocopherol, sulfamate, BHA, BHT, caffeic acid, ferulic acid, and gallic acid (Mirvish, 1981a,b; Newmark and Mergens, 1981; Kuenzig et al., 1984). For example, certain food constituents have been found to prevent the in vivo and in vitro formation of potent carcinogenic N-nitroso compounds such as dimethylnitrosamine from precursor nitrite and amines (Mergens et al., 1978; Mirvish, 1981a,b). While the ingestion of amine-containing foods treated with nitrite (e.g., fish, beans) may potentially lead to the formation of nitrosamines under acidic conditions in the stomach, these nitrosation reactions can be inhibited by the agents listed above as a result of their preferential competitive neutralization of nitrite (Weisburger and Williams, 1980). This protective effect was illustrated over a decade ago, when Tinbergen and Krol reported significant lowering of dimethylnitrosamine, nitrosopyrrolidine, and other nitrosamine levels in meats pre-

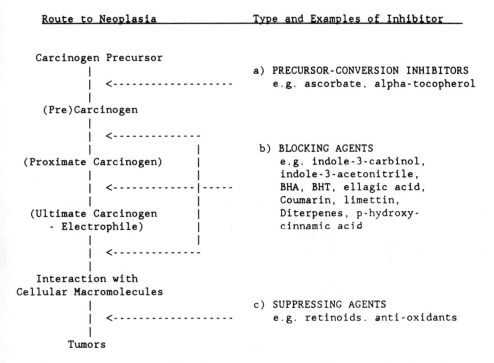

FIG. 5.5 Mechanisms of anticarcinogenesis: categorization of anticarcinogens found naturally or as synthetic additives in food. (*Adapted from Miller and Miller, 1979; Wattenberg, 1985*).

served with nitrite while at the same time being treated with ascorbic acid or erythrobate (Tinbergen and Krol, 1977). Weisburger (1979) also has discussed the contribution of this interaction between dietary constituents and nitrite to declining stomach cancer incidences in the United States, both in the indigenous population and in those who have migrated from countries where stomach cancer incidences still are high (e.g., Japan).

Blocking Agents. The second and probably most widely studied group of anticarcinogens contains agents which prevent carcinogens from damaging cellular macromolecules such as DNA (see Wattenberg, 1985 and references therein). These "blocking agents" (Fig. 5.5) have been further subdivided into compounds which augment Phase I detoxification pathways relative to activation reactions (e.g., aromatic ring hydroxylations), stimulate Phase II conjugation steps, or act directly to trap ultimate carcinogens (reactive electrophilic species). Thus, these agents act to prevent the pathway:

(pre)Carcinogen → (proximate carcinogen) → (ultimate carcinogen) → interaction with cellular macromolecules

It can be seen from Fig. 5.5. that this category of anticarcinogens contains a large and diverse group of both synthetic (e.g., BHA, BHT) and naturally occurring food constituents (e.g., I3C, ellagic acid). Insight into the first stage of blocking agent activity, the inhibition of carcinogen activation, has come not so much with food anticarcinogens as with the prototype mixed-function oxidase inducer (BNF). For example, BNF greatly stimulates cytochrome P-448 catalyzed hydroxylation of the potent food-borne hepatocarcinogen AFB1 to a less potent carcinogen, the metabolite and structural analogue AFM1. This detoxification reaction has been reported both in trout (Bailey et al., 1982) and rats (Gurtoo et al., 1985) and is presumably important in the BNF-mediated protection against AFB1 hepatocarcinogenesis in both species.

Compounds within the second subgroup of blocking agents may be broadly described as those which operate via enhancement of carcinogen detoxification systems. It should be remembered that detoxification reactions play a key role in preventing toxicity from a diverse array of xenobiotics which are ingested in foods, especially of plant origin (e.g., fruit, vegetables, nuts, and grains), as well as other sources both synthetic and natural (e.g., drugs, poisons). Detoxification reactions primarily involve metabolic transformation of xenobiotic compounds in such a way as to facilitate excretion, usually by introducing large polar groups into the molecule such as sulphates, glucuronides, and glutathione moieties (Phase II conjugation reactions). These reactions are often preceded by Phase I reactions, which frequently involve the microsomal mixed-function oxidase system. The latter serves to increase the polarity of the food constituent, drug, or xenobiotic undergoing metabolism (principally via a range of oxidative reactions, though certain reductive pathways also have been identified), thereby facilitating subsequent Phase II conjugations.

Blocking agents which modulate these Phase I (e.g., BNF, see above) and Phase II pathways (e.g., phenolic anti-oxidants, indoles) are of special interest in view of their nonselectivity, that is, they possess the ability to inhibit a range of carcinogens from diverse chemical classes. Perhaps the best studied compound of this class is the synthetic food additive BHA. The latter typifies the "broad spectrum" anticarcinogen, inhibiting carcinogenesis due to a diverse array of compounds including DEN, 4-nitroquinoline N-oxide, BP, uracil mustard, dibenz(a,h)anthracene, and urethan (Wattenberg et al., 1980; Wattenberg, 1983). It has also been suggested that the mechanism by which dietary indoles such as I3C, IAN, and I33′ inhibit carcinogen-DNA binding and tumorigenesis may be related to their potency as inducers of cytochrome P-448 monooxygenases (Wattenberg, 1983). These compounds are among a spectrum of modulators which have been shown to elevate levels of glutathione and glutathione-S-transferase in mouse liver and forestomach as a possible mechanism by which BP-induced neoplasia is inhibited in this species (Sparnins et al., 1982a,b). These findings are supported by recent observations in the rat, where I3C and related indoles, including condensation products formed after acid treatment of I3C in vitro, were found to induce hepatic cytochrome P-448 marker enzymes such as ethoxyresorufin-O-deethylase (EROD) activity (Bradfield and Bjeldanes, 1987a).

However, evidence from other reports has raised questions about the relationship between cytochrome P-448 induction and the inhibitory effects observed with I3C and related indoles. Indeed, questions have been raised as to whether such dietary constituents belong in fact to the third subgroup of blocking agents, namely, those compounds which interact with ultimate carcinogens (electrophiles) formed either directly (from direct acting carcinogens) or after metabolic activation. Thus, Shertzer (1983, 1984) has reported that I3C protects against the DNA-damaging effects of benzo(a)pyrene and N-nitrosodimethylamine after p.o. administration to mice, despite the fact that increases in monooxygenase activities were not observed. Moreover, studies from our laboratory indicate clearly that I3C inhibits AFB1-induced hepatocarcinogenesis in trout without concomitant alterations in hepatic cytochrome P-448 monooxygenase activity (Eisele et al., 1983; Nixon et al., 1984; Goeger et al., 1986; Dashwood et al., 1988), but appears to involve direct inhibition or electrophile trapping (Swanson et al., in preparation). A further example of electrophilic trapping is the common plant phenol ellagic acid, which inhibits benzo(a)pyrene-induced pulmonary adenomas in A/J mice (Lesca, 1983), apparently through direct interaction with the benzo(a)pyrene diol-epoxide as well as through alterations in carcinogen metabolism (Wood et al., 1982).

Suppressing Agents. The third category of anticarcinogens, "suppressing agents" (Fig. 5.5), consists of those agents which act principally by inhibiting tumor promotion in the two-stage mouse skin model of carcinogenesis. Suppressing agents include natural and synthetic food constituents such as selenium salts, retinoids, carotenoids, soybean protease inhibitors, BHA, benzyl isothiocyanate, and caffeine (Nomura,

1980; Wattenberg, 1981; Griffin, 1982; Seifter et al., 1982; Moon et al., 1983; Rettura et al., 1983; Sporn, 1983; Yavelow et al., 1983; McCormick et al., 1984). Because there are no widely used, consistent short-term indicators for suppressing activity, these agents generally are more difficult to identify than compounds belonging to the first two categories of anticarcinogen, with the result that they are fewer in number. Suppressing agents are believed to operate primarily by scavenging or repressing formation of promotion-associated active oxygen species, such as superoxide anion (O_2^-) and hydroxyl radicals (OH·). However, the relationship between such effects and postinitiation inhibition of nonpromoted organ carcinogenesis is poorly understood.

The retinoids are presently the most widely studied group of suppressing agents and include the compounds retinyl acetate, retinyl palmitate, 13-*cis*-retinoic acid, ethyl retinamide, and 2-hydroxyethyl-retinamide (Sporn and Newton, 1981; Moon et al., 1983; Sporn, 1983; Sporn and Roberts, 1984). From studies with various structural analogues it has become apparent that individual retinoids target specific organs or tissues (e.g., large bowel), and although their mechanism(s) of action remain unclear, it has been established that the suppressing effects induced by these agents are reversible. It should also be remembered that retinoids, but not β-carotene, possess toxic properties which may limit their use in human chemoprevention.

Quantitative Anticarcinogenesis:Assay for Pure Anti-initiating Activity

A number of food constituent anticarcinogens have been found to inhibit carcinogen-DNA adduct formation in vivo, with evidence for inhibitor-altered metabolism of the initiating agent (Fukayama and Hsieh, 1985; Ioannou et al., 1982; Kensler et al., 1985, 1986; Monroe et al., 1986; Goeger et al., 1986). However, the quantitative relationships between carcinogen dose, inhibitor dose, in vivo DNA adduction, and final tumor response are not well understood in any animal model for such blocking agents. Therefore, it has not been clear whether dietary agents which inhibit carcinogen-DNA binding in vivo operate by a combination of mechanisms, or whether some possess pure anti-initiating activity (i.e., operate as blocking agents only). Further, few studies have addressed the issue of anticarcinogen effectiveness over a broad range of carcinogen doses and tumor incidences—can one extrapolate the results of inhibitor experiments conducted at high carcinogen doses and tumor incidences down to low levels more realistic for man?

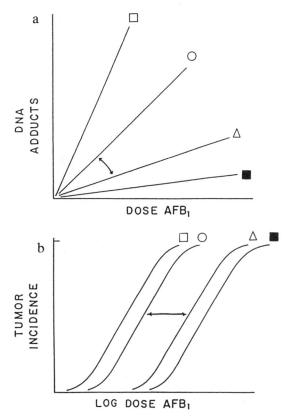

FIG. 5.6 Hypothetical curves relating dose of AFB1 to (a) DNA adducts formed in vivo, or (b) final tumor response, for groups pretreated with I3C at various doses. For example, □ = 0 ppm, ○ = 1000 ppm, △ = 3000 ppm, ■ = 4000 ppm I3C. No attempt is made in this diagram to quantitatively correlate hypothetical slopes in (a) with horizontal shifts in (b). This is the "hypothesis under test" (see text).

To address these questions, we have employed the rainbow trout model in a combined in vivo DNA binding/tumor dose-response study with AFB1 and the dietary indole I3C. An inherent component of the study design is that it assesses anticarcinogen effectiveness over a very broad range of carcinogen doses and tumor incidences, down to 1% and less. Using a range of both carcinogen and anticarcinogen doses, these studies compared inhibitor-mediated shifts in AFB1-DNA binding dose-response curves (slope changes) with corresponding horizontal displacements in tumor dose-response data (Fig. 5.6). Thus, the *hypothesis under test* can be stated as follows: For a pure anti-initiating agent, inhibitor-mediated effects on carcinogen dose actually received (DNA adducts formed) in the target organ are precisely predictive of the reduced response to the applied dose of carcinogen in tumor dose-response curves.

In this study it is important that animals are treated under identical conditions in both sets of dose-response curves (DNA binding and tumorigenicity) and that sufficient numbers of animals are used so that data may be compared on a firm statistical basis. The trout model possesses certain unique features which facilitate such detailed in vivo dose-response comparisons. These include essentially zero background

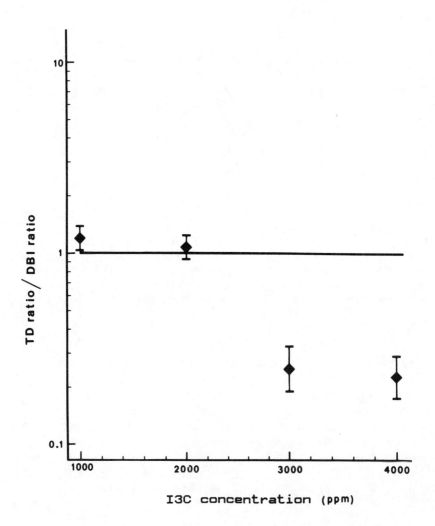

tumor incidence, persistent carcinogen-DNA adduction due to poor DNA repair activity, and a capacity for using large numbers of animals at relatively low cost.

Thus, in our studies, approximately 10,000 animals were pretreated for 4 weeks with I3C at one of five dietary dose-levels: 0, 1000, 2000, 3000, or 4000 ppm. Trout were subsequently treated with the same inhibitor level together with dietary AFB1 in the range 10 to 320 ppb. To enable quantitation of AFB1-DNA binding levels, all animals received tritium-labeled carcinogen, with the exception of negative control groups. Each AFB1-I3C dose-point consisted of triplicate groups of 150 fish, from which 15 trout were selected at random after 7 and 14 days AFB1-I3C co-treatment in order to determine AFB1-DNA adduct levels (Dashwood et al., 1988). The 120 animals remaining in each tank were returned to diet containing no AFB1 or I3C, and tumor incidences were determined at 12 months.

By comparing inhibitor-mediated shifts in AFB1-DNA binding dose-response curves with corresponding displacements in tumor dose-re-

---

FIG. 5.7 Ratio of inhibitory responses in tumor versus DNA binding dose-response curves as a function of dietary I3C concentration. In our studies, AFB1 − DNA binding levels increased linearly with AFB1 dose (corr. coeff. > 0.98), while each increase in I3C dose produced a shift towards lower slope value. These inhibitor-mediated shifts may be expressed quantitatively by the DNA binding index (DBI) ratio:

$$DBI_i/DBI_o \qquad (i)$$

where i/o is the relationship between DNA binding slope values for I3C at any dose i compared to the control value at 0 ppm I3C.

Tumor data fit a parallel straight-line relationship, each increase in inhibitor dose producing a displacement towards higher AFB1 dose (see legend, Fig. 5.6). These horizontal displacements may be expressed quantitatively by the tumor dose (TD) index:

$$TDx_o/TDx_i \qquad (ii)$$

where x = tumor incidence being compared across groups in tumor dose-response curves (e.g., 50%), TDx_o = 0 dose of AFB1 required to give that tumor response in the 0 ppm I3C group, and TDx_i = dose of AFB1 needed to produce that tumor response in the group receiving i ppm I3C.

If the hypothesis under test (see text) is sustained, a plot of (ii)/(i) (TD ratio over DBI ratio) versus I3C dose will be linear, and horizontal to the ratio of ratios value = 1. (Ratio of ratios refers to TD over DBI indices; data are means ± S.E.; for number of animals, see text).

sponse curves, a number of key issues were recognized. First, at I3C doses of 2000 ppm or lower, a direct quantitative correlation exists between I3C-mediated changes in AFB1-DNA binding slopes (i.e., carcinogen dose actually received in the target organ) and the degree of horizontal displacement towards higher carcinogen dose in tumor dose-response curves. This is evidenced by the plot of TD_{50} versus DNA binding index (DBI) ratios for data at each inhibitor level from this study (Fig. 5.7). Data points at I3C doses of 1000 and 2000 ppm were well correlated with the horizontal line shown in Fig. 5.7. Only when shifts in tumor dose-response curves are predicted precisely by I3C-altered AFB1-DNA binding values will datapoints fall on the horizontal line where the ratio of ratios = 1 (Fig. 5.7). These data constitute the first direct evidence of pure anti-initiating activity in the mechanism of anticarcinogenesis by a compound found as a natural constituent of the human diet.

Second, from the foregoing it is evident that in the absence of inhibitor (i.e., the 0 ppm I3C group), AFB1-DNA adduct levels were correlated well with corresponding tumor responses at each of the four AFB1 dose-points tested (i.e., triplicate groups tested at carcinogen doses of 10, 20, 40, and 80 ppb AFB1). These findings have important implications in view of the important suggestion (Swenberg et al., 1987) that DNA adduct levels (carcinogen dose *received*) may be a more appropriate exposure index for quantitative risk assessment than the chemical's exposure concentration (*"applied"* dose). Together with published data showing high AFB1-DNA binding/carcinogenicity correlations in other species (corr. coeff. > 0.98, D. Bechtel, personal communication), these results provide support for the "molecular dosimeter" concept discussed recently (Swenberg et al., 1987; van Zeeland, 1988).

Further, at I3C doses greater than 2000 ppm changes in AFB1-DNA binding dose-response data were not well correlated with the degree of inhibition in corresponding tumor response data (Fig. 5.7). Thus, datapoints at 3000 and 4000 ppm I3C were displaced below the horizontal line (ratio of ratios = 1) in Fig. 5.7. This indicates that fewer tumors were obtained at these I3C doses than were predicted by the extent of inhibition in AFB1-DNA binding curves. These findings will be discussed in more detail in the next section, which addresses the issue of inhibitory versus promotional potency for ambivalent modulators such as I3C.

Finally, the effect of a given level of carcinogen is to shift the entire tumor dose-response curve toward a parallel curve at higher carcinogen dose, without unusual effect at either end of the curve. That is, at least for this study, the effectiveness of a given I3C dose was independent of carcinogen dose, so that studies at high carcinogen dose could be extrapolated to low dose.

Ambivalent Modulators—Inhibitory Versus Promotional Potency

An important issue mentioned above is that the final tumor response for any modulator-inhibitor pair of compounds may differ dramatically depending upon the dosing regimen of the initiator relative to the modulator. Thus I3C can either inhibit or promote AFB1 hepatocarcinogenesis in trout, depending respectively upon whether I3C is given before/during AFB1 exposure (initiation phase) or after AFB1 (postinitiation phase) (Table 5.4). Quantitative potency information is thus needed for such ambivalent modulators in order to provide insight into the relative risks versus benefits for dietary anticarcinogens which also exhibit promoting activity. The in vivo DNA binding/tumor dose-response studies discussed in the previous paragraphs may be viewed as an initial attempt to provide information on inhibitory potency for I3C over a range of doses (see Fig. 5.8).

From Fig. 5.8 it is evident that I3C inhibited AFB1-DNA binding (broken line) and final tumor response (solid line) in a dose-dependent manner, with evidence of a plateau below 100% inhibition in both curves at high inhibitor doses. The weaker correspondence between DNA binding and tumor data at I3C doses > 2000 ppm evident in Fig. 5.7, also is reflected by the greater inhibitory response observed in the tumor inhibitory potency curve at 3000 and 4000 ppm (solid line, Fig. 5.8). Since significant deviation was observed at high I3C doses only, we have taken this to indicate the involvement of other factors (e.g., toxicity), or additional mechanisms, not present at inhibitor doses of 2000 ppm or lower. Further studies are required in order to resolve this issue.

At I3C doses below 2000 ppm there was no evidence for any significant threshold for inhibition in AFB1-DNA binding dose-response curves, the data-points forming a straight line through the origin (broken-line, Fig. 5.8). In the tumor inhibitory potency curve this linearity was less evident from the limited number of data-points available. Although each data-point in Fig. 5.8 was determined with precision using large numbers of animals (45 for each DNA binding data-point and ~300 for each tumor data-point), further studies are required to provide critical information on the question of linearity at I3C doses < 1000 ppm. Only then can we address the important issue of low dose thresholds and the implied message from the DNA binding data that even low dietary levels of I3C may have a protective effect against chemically induced neoplasia.

Similarly detailed dose-response studies will be required to provide potency information for the I3C promotional activity in vivo. In trout, this might involve pretreating animals with a range of AFB1 doses, followed

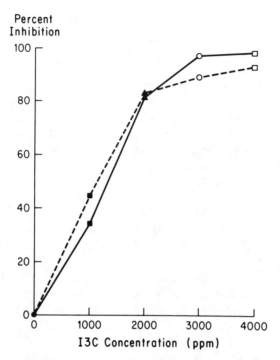

FIG. 5.8 The inhibitory potency of I3C for AFB1-DNA binding and tumorigenicity in trout. Inhibitory potencies were calculated from TD_{50} and DBI indices
(legend, Fig. 5.7) according to the formulas:

$$\text{Inhibitory potency (DNA binding)} = 1 - (DBI_i/DBI_0) \times 100$$

$$\text{Inhibitory potency (tumorigenicity)} = 1 - (TDx_0/TDx_i) \times 100$$

(For clarity, SD values have been omitted from the figure.) (-) Tumor incidence; (--)
DNA binding.

by exposure to various levels of I3C in diet. It may also be possible to
assess promotional potency using one or more putative short-term indicators, along the lines of recent studies in the rat (Pitot et al., 1987). The
design of such studies, however, will not be trivial, and may need to incorporate several protocols for postinitiation modulator treatment (e.g., feeding continuously, once weekly, on alternating weeks, etc.) to mimic
various possible patterns of human consumption. The "promotional
potency" of any modulator may well differ with each protocol chosen.

SUMMARY

Many lines of experimental evidence indicate the complex activities of tumor modulators, both naturally occurring and synthetic, which are found in the human diet. Where examined, a high proportion of modulators which exhibit anticarcinogenic behavior in some particular experiment prove to enhance tumor response using a different carcinogen, animal species, organ, or exposure protocol design. Clearly each compound of potential interest as a chemoprevention agent must be thoroughly examined in order to quantitatively estimate possible enhancement risks, as well as inhibitory benefits, to be derived from its use by man. One approach for quantitative assessment of anticarcinogenic potency is outlined in this paper. The further need for this type of research is perhaps most urgent for those modulators to which human exposure is unavoidable; it would seem highly likely that they presently impact human cancer rates, but perhaps in different directions in different cultures, populations, and individuals.

ACKNOWLEDGMENTS

The original studies from our laboratory reported in the text and Table 5.4 were partially supported by USPHS research grants ES03850, ES00210, CA34732, and CA39398. Technical Paper No. 8610, Oregon Agricultural Experiment Station, Corvallis, Oregon.

REFERENCES

Ames, B. N. 1983. Dietary carcinogens and anticarcinogens. *Science* 221: 1256–1264.

Appleton, B. S. and Campbell, T. C. 1983. Effect of high and low dietary protein on the dosing and postdosing periods of aflatoxin B1-induced hepatic preneoplastic lesion development in the rat. *Cancer Res.* 43: 2150–2154.

Bailey, G.S., Hendricks, J.D., Shelton, D.W., Nixon, J.E., and Pawlowski, N.E. 1987. Enhancement of carcinogenesis by the natural anticarcinogen indole-3-carbinol. *J. Natl. Cancer Inst.* 78: 931–934.

Bailey, G.S., Taylor, M., Selivonchick, D., Eisele, T., Hendricks, J., Nixon, J., Pawlowski, N., and Sinnhuber, R. 1982. Mechanisms of dietary modification of aflatoxin B1 carcinogenesis. In *Genetic Toxicology* Fleck, R.A. and Hollaender, A., (eds.) pp. 149-165. Plenum Press, New York.

Basu, T.K., Donaldson, D., Jenner, M., Williams, D.C., and Sakula, A. 1976. Plasma vitamin A in patients with bronchial carcinoma. *Br. J. Cancer* 33: 119-121,

Becker, F.F. 1981. Inhibition of spontaneous hepatocarcinogenesis in C3H/HeN mice by Edipro A, an isolated soy protein. *Carcinogenesis* 2: 1213-1214.

Belman, S. 1983. Onion and garlic oils inhibit tumor promotion. *Carcinogenesis* 4: 1063-1065.

Bjelke, E. 1975. Dietary vitamin A and human lung cancer. *Int. J. Cancer* 15: 561-565.

Boyd, J.N., Babish, J.G., and Stoewsand, G.S. 1982. Modification by beet and cabbage diets of aflatoxin B1-induced rat plasma α-foetoprotein elevation, hepatic tumorigenesis and mutagenicity of urine. *Fd. Chem. Toxic.* 20: 47-52.

Bradfield, C.A. and Bjeldanes, L.F. 1987a. Structure-activity relationships of dietary indoles: A proposed mechanism of action as modifiers of xenobiotic metabolism. *J. Toxicol. Environ. Health* 21: 311-323.

Bradfield, C.A. and Bjeldanes, L.F. 1987b. High performance liquid chromatographic analysis of anticarcinogenic indoles in *Brassica oleracea. J. Agric. Fd. Chem.* 35: 46-49.

Brown, J.P. 1980. A review of the genetic effects of naturally occurring flavonoids, anthraquinones and related compounds. *Mutat. Res.* 75: 243-277.

Cabral, J.R.P. and Neal, G.E. 1983. The inhibitory effects of ethoxyquin on the carcinogenic action of aflatoxin B1 in rats. *Cancer Lett.* 19: 125-132.

Cameron, R. 1981. Promotive effects of ethinyl estradiol in hepatocarcinogenesis initiated by diethylnitrosamine in male rats. *Jpn. J. Cancer Res.* (Gann) 72: 339-340.

Cameron, R.G., Imaida, K., Tsuda, H., and Ito, N. 1982. Promotive effects of steroids and bile acids on hepatocarcinogenesis initiated by diethylnitrosamine. *Cancer Res.* 42: 2426-2428.

Carroll, K.K., Braden, L.M., Bell, J.A., and Kalamegham, R. 1986. *Fat and Cancer; Cancer (Suppl.)* 58: 1818-1825.

Carter, C.A., Milholland, R.J., Shea, W., and Ip, M.M. 1983. Effect of the prostaglandin synthetase inhibitor indomethacin on 7,12-dimethylbenz(a)anthracene-induced mammary tumorigenesis in rats fed different levels of fat. *Cancer Res.* 43: 3559–3562.

Cerutti, P.A. 1985. Prooxidant states and tumor promotion. *Science* 227: 375–381.

Chang. R. L., Huang, M-T., Wood, A.W., Wong, C-Q., Newmark, H.L., Yagi, H., Sayer, J.M., Jerina, D.M., and Conney, A.H. 1985. Effect of ellagic acid and hydroxylated flavonoids on the tumorigenicity of benzo(a)pyrene and (+)-7,8-dihydroxy-9,10-epoxy-7,8,9,10-tetrahydro-benzo(a)pyrene on mouse skin and in the newborn mouse. *Carcinogenesis* 6: 1127–1133.

Chung, F.-L., Wang, M., Carmella, S.G., and Hecht, S.S. 1986. Effects of butylated hydroxyanisole on the tumorigenicity and metabolism of N-nitrosodimethylamine and N-nitrosopyrrolidine in A/J mice. *Cancer Res.* 46: 165–168.

Clinton, S.K., Imrey, P.B., Alster, J.M., Simon, J., Truex, C.R., and Visek, W.J. 1984. The combined effects of dietary protein and fat on 7,12-dimethylbenz(a)anthracene-induced breast cancer in rats. *J. Nutr.* 114: 1213–1223.

Cohen, L.A., Thompson, D.O., Maeura, Y., Choi, K., Blank, M.E., and Rose D.P. 1986a. Dietary fat and mammary cancer. I. Promoting effects of different dietary fats on N-nitrosomethylurea-induced rat mammary tumorigenesis. *J. Natl. Cancer Inst.* 77: 33–42.

Cohen, L.A., Thompson, D.O., Choi, K., Karmali, R.A., and Rose, D.P. 1986b. Dietary fat and mammary cancer. II. Modulation of serum and tumor lipid composition and tumor prostaglandins by different dietary fats: Association with tumor incidence patterns. *J. Natl. Cancer Inst.* 77: 43–51.

Corasanti, J.G., Hobika, G.H., and Markus, G. 1982. Interference with dimethylhydrazine induction of colon tumors in mice by aminocaproic acid. *Science* 216: 1020–1021.

Correa, P. 1981. Epidemiological correlations between diet and cancer frequency. *Cancer Res.* 41: 3685–3690.

Dashwood, R.H., Arbogast, D.N., Fong, A. T., Hendricks, J.D., and Bailey, G.S. 1988. Mechanisms of anti-carcinogenesis by indole-3-carbinol: Detailed in vivo DNA binding dose-response studies after dietary administration with aflatoxin B1 (AFB1). *Carcinogenesis* 9: 427–432.

Deml, E. and Oesterle, D. 1982. Sex-dependent promoting effect of polychlorinated biphenyls on enzyme-altered islands induced by diethylnitrosamine in rat liver. *Carcinogenesis* 3: 1449–1452.

Deml, E. and Oesterle, D. 1986. Enhancing effect of co-administration of polychlorinated biphenyls and diethylnitrosamine on enzyme-altered islands induced by diethylnitrosamine in rat liver. *Carcinogenesis* 7: 1697–1700.

Deml, E., Oesterle, D., and Wiebel, F.J. 1983. Benzo(a)pyrene initiates enzyme-altered islands in the liver of adult rats following single pretreatment and promotion with polychlorinated biphenyls. *Cancer Lett.* 19: 301–304.

Eisele, T.A., Bailey, G.S., and Nixon, J.E. 1983. The effect of indole-3-carbinol, an aflatoxin B1 hepatocarcinoma inhibitor, and other indole analogs on the rainbow trout hepatic mixed function oxidase system. *Toxicol. Lett.* 19: 133–138.

Epstein, J.H. 1977. Effects of β-carotene on ultraviolet induced cancer formation in the hairless mouse skin. *Photochem. Photobiol.* 25: 211–213.

Fiala, E.S., Reddy, B.S., and Weisburger, J.H. 1985. Naturally occurring anticarcinogenic substances in foodstuffs. *Annu. Rev. Nutr.* 5: 295–321.

Fukayama, M.Y. and Hsieh, D.P.H. 1985. Effect of butylated hydroxytoluene pretreatment on the excretion, tissue distribution and DNA binding of [^{14}C]aflatoxin B1 in the rat. *Fd. Chem. Toxic.* 23: 567–573.

Gabor, H. and Abraham, S. 1985. Effect of dietary menhaden oil on growth and cell loss of transplantable mammary adenocarcinoma in mice. *Proc. Am. Assoc. Cancer Res.* 26: 126.

Goeger, D.E., Shelton, D.W., Hendricks, J.D., and Bailey, G.S. 1986. Mechanisms of anti-carcinogenesis by indole-3-carbinol: effect on the distribution and metabolism of aflatoxin B1 in rainbow trout. *Carcinogenesis* 7: 2025–2031.

Graham, S. 1984. Dietary factors in the prevention of cancer. *Transplantation Proc.* 16: 392–400.

Graham, S., Dayal, H., Rohrer, T., Swanson, M., Sultz, H., Shedd, D., and Fischman, S. 1977. *J. Natl. Cancer Inst.* 59: 1611–1616.

Graham, S., Dayal, H., Swanson, M., Mittelman, A., and Wilkinson, G. 1978. *J. Natl. Cancer Inst.* 61: 709–714.

Graham, S., Haughey, B., Marshall, J., Priore, R., Byers, T., Rzepka, T., Mettlin, C., and Pontes, J. 1983. Diet in the epidemiology of carcinoma of the prostate gland. *J. Natl. Cancer Inst.* 70: 687–692.

Graham, S., Mettlin, C., Marshall, J., Priore, R., Rzepka, T., and Shedd, D. 1981. Dietary factors in the epidemiology of cancer of the larnyx. *Am. J. Epidemiol.* 113: 675–680.

Graham, S., Marshall, J., Mettlin, C., Rzepka, T., Nemoto, T., and Byers, T.

1982. Diet in the epidemiology of breast cancer. *Am. J. Epidemiol.* 116: 68–75.

Griffin, A.C. 1982. The chemopreventive role of selenium in carcinogenesis. In *Molecular Interrelations of Nutrition and Cancer,* Arnott, M.S., van Eys, J., and Wang, Y.M. (eds.), p. 401-408. Raven Press, New York.

Griffin, A.C. and Jacobs, M.M. 1977. Effects of selenium on azo dye hepatocarcinogenesis. *Cancer Lett.* 3: 177–181.

Grubbs, C.J., Farnell, D.R., Hill, D.L., and McDonough, K.C. 1985. Chemoprevention of N-nitroso-N-methylurea-induced mammary cancers by pretreatment with 17β-estraidol and progesterone. *J. Natl. Cancer Inst.* 74: 927–931.

Gurtoo, H.L., Koser, P.L., Bansal, S.K., Fox, H.W., Sharma, S.D., Mulhern, A.I., and Pavelic, Z.P. 1985. Inhibition of aflatoxin B1-hepatocarcinogenesis in rats by β-naphthoflavone. *Carcinogenesis* 6: 675–678.

Hawrylewicz, E.J., Huang, H.H., Kissane, J.Q., and Drab, E.A. 1982. Enhancement of 7,12-dimethylbenz(a)anthracene (DMBA) mammary tumorigenesis by high dietary protein in rats. *NRI* 26: 793–806.

Hawrylewicz, E.J., Huang, H.H., and Liu, J.M. 1986. Dietary protein enhancement of N-nitrosomethylurea-induced mammary carcinogenesis, and their effect on hormone regulation in rats. *Cancer Res.* 46: 4395–4399.

Hayes, M.A., Rushmore, T.H., and Goldberg, M.T. 1987. Inhibition of hepatocarcinogenic responses to 1,2-dimethylhydrazine by diallyl sulfide, a component of garlic oil. *Carcinogenesis* 8: 1155–1157.

Hendricks, J.D., Sinnhuber, R.O., Nixon, J.E., Wales, J.H., Masri, M.S., and Hsieh, D.P.H. 1980. Carcinogenic response of rainbow trout (*Salmo gairdneri*) to aflatoxin Q1 and synergistic effect of cyclopropenoid fatty acids. *J. Natl. Cancer Inst.* 64: 523–528.

Hirayama, T. 1979. Diet and cancer. *Nutr. Cancer* 1: 67–81.

Hirose, M., Masuda, A., Kurata, Y., Ikawa, E., Mera, Y., and Ito, N. 1986. Histologic and autoradiographic studies on the forestomach of hamsters treated with 2-tert-butylated hydroxyanisole, 3-tert-butylated hydroxyanisole, crude butylated hydroxyanisole, or butylated hydroxytoluene. *J. Natl. Cancer Inst.* 76: 143–149.

Hozumi, M., Ogawa, M., Sugimura, T., Takeuchi, T., and Umezawa, H. 1972. Inhibition of tumorigenesis in mouse skin by leupeptin, a protease inhibitor for actinomycetes. *Cancer Res.* 32: 1725–1728.

Ibrahim, J. Jafarey, N.A., and Zuberi, S.J. 1977. Plasma vitamin A and carotene levels in squamos cell carcinoma of oral cavity and oro-pharynx. *Clin. Oncol.* 3: 203–207.

IFT Expert Panel and Committee on Public Information. 1977. Scientific Status Summary. *Food Technol.* 31(1): 77–80.

Imaida, K., Fukushima, S., Shirai, T., Ohtani, M., Nakanishi, K., and Ito, N. 1983. Promoting activities of butylated hydroxyanisole and butylated hydroxytoluene on 2-stage urinary bladder carcinogenesis and inhibition of γ-glutamyl transpeptidase-positive foci development in the liver of rats. *Carcinogenesis* 4: 895–899.

Ioannou, Y.M., Wilson, A.G.E., and Anderson, M.W. 1982. Effect of butylated hydrosyanisole on the metabolism of benzo(a)pyrene and the binding of metabolites to DNA, in vitro and in vivo, in the forestomach, lung and liver of mice. *Carcinogenesis* 3: 739–745.

Ip, C. 1981. Factors influencing the anticarcinogenic efficacy of selenium in dimethylbenz(a)anthracene-induced mammary tumorigenesis in rats. *Cancer Res.* 41: 2683–2686.

Ito, N., Fukushima, S., Hagiwara, A., Shibata, M., and Ogiso, T. 1983. Carcinogenicity of butylated hydroxyanisole in F344 rats. *J. Natl. Cancer Inst.* 70: 343–349.

Ito, N. and Hirose, M. 1987. The role of antioxidants in chemical carcinogenesis. *Jpn. J. Cancer Res.* (Gann) 78: 1011–1026.

Jacobs, M.M., Forst, C.F., and Beams, F.A. 1981. Biochemical and clinical effects of selenium on dimethylhydrazine-induced colon cancer in rats. *Cancer Res.* 41: 4458–4465.

Jacobs, M.M. and Griffin, A.C. 1981. In *Inhibition of Tumor Induction and Development.* (Ed.) Zedek, M.S. and Lipkin, M. p. 169–188. Plenum Press, New York.

Jurkowski, J.J. and Cave, W.T., Jr. 1985. Dietary effects of menhaden oil on the growth and membrane lipid composition of rat mammary tumors. *J. Natl. Cancer Inst.* 74: 1145–1150.

Kahl, R. and Hilderbrandt, A.G. 1986. Methodology for studying antioxidant activity and mechanisms of action of antioxidant. *Fd. Chem. Toxic.* 24: 1007–1014.

Kark, J.D., Smith, A.H., and Hames, C.G. 1982. Serum retinol and the inverse relationship between serum cholesterol and cancer. *Br. Med. J.* 284: 152–154.

Karmali, R.A., March, J., and Fuchs, G. 1984. Effect of omega-3 fatty acids on growth of a rat mammary tumor. *J. Natl. Cancer Inst.* 73: 457–461.

Kensler, T.W., Egner, P.A., Trush, M.A., Bueding, E., and Groopman, J.D. 1985. Modification of aflatoxin B1 binding to DNA in vivo in rats fed phenolic antioxidants, ethoxyquin and a dithiothione. *Carcinogenesis* 6: 759–763.

Kensler, T.W., Egner, P.A., Davidson, N.E., Roebuck, B.D., Pikul, A., and Groopman, J.D. 1986. Modulation of aflatoxin metabolism, aflatoxin-N7-guanine formation, and hepatic tumorigenesis in rats fed ethoxyquin: role of induction of glutathione S-transferases. *Cancer Res.* 46: 3924–3931.

Knekt, P., Aromaa, A., Maatela, J., Aaran, R., Nikkari, T., Hakama, M., Hakulinen, T., Peto, R., Saxen, E., and Teppo, L. 1988. Serum vitamin E and risk of cancer among Finnish men during a ten-year follow-up. *Am. J. Epidemiol,* 127: 28–41.

Kolonel, L.N., Nomura, A.M.Y., Hirohata, T., Hankin, J.H., and Hinds, M.W. 1981. Association of diet and place of birth with stomach cancer incidence in Hawaiin Japanese and Caucasians. *Am. J. Clin. Nutr.* 34: 2478–2485.

Kornburst, D.J. and Mavis, R.D. 1980. Relative susceptibility of microsomes from lung, heart, liver, kidney, brain and testes to lipid peroxidation: correlation with vitamin E content. *Lipids* 15: 315–322.

Kuenzig, W., Chau, J., Norkus, E., Holowaschenko, H., Newmark, H., Mergens, W., and Conney, A.N. 1984. Caffeic and ferulic acid as blockers of nitrosamine formation. *Carcinogenesis* 5: 309–314.

Lee, D.J., Sinnhuber, R.O., Wales, J.H., and Putnam, G.B. 1978. Effect of dietary protein on the response of rainbow trout. (*Salmo gairdneri*) to aflatoxin B1. *J. Natl. Cancer Inst.* 60: 317–320.

Lee, D.J., Wales, J.H., and Sinnhuber, R.O. 1971. Promotion of aflatoxin-induced hepatoma growth in trout by methyl malvalate and sterculate. *Cancer Res.* 31: 960–963.

Lesca, P. 1983. Protective effects of ellagic acid and other plant phenols on benzo(a)pyrene-induced neoplasia in mice *Carcinogenesis* 4: 1651–1653.

Lian, D., Daoyun, Z., Jinyan, C., Juantan, W., Yuanbu, W., Shaoru, P., and Shuhua, W. 1984. A histological study of the promotive effect of diethylstilbesterol on diethylnitrosamine initiated carcinogenesis of liver in rat. *Path. Res. Pract.* 178: 339–344.

Linder, M.C. 1985. Nutrition and cancer prevention. In *Nutritional Biochemistry and Metabolism with Clinical Applications* (Ed.) Linder, M.C., p. 347–368. Elsevier, New York.

Longnecker, D.S., Kuhlmann, E.T., and Curphey, T.J. 1983. Divergent effects of retinoids on pancreatic and liver carcinogenesis in azaserine-treated rats. *Cancer Res.* 43: 3219–3225.

142   Williams et al.

MacMahon, B., Cole, P., and Brown, J. 1973. Etiology of human breast cancer. A review. *J. Natl. Cancer Inst.* 50: 21–42.

Malkinson, A.M. and Beer, D.S. 1984. Pharmacologic and genetic studies on the modulatory effects of butylated hydroxytoluene on mouse lung adenoma formation. *J. Natl. Cancer Inst.* 73: 925–933.

Malkinson, A.M. and Thaete, L.G. 1986. Effects of strain and age on prophylaxis and co-carcinogenesis of urethan-induced mouse lung adenomas by butylated hydroxytoluene. *Cancer Res.* 46: 1694–1697.

Marnett, L.J. 1987. Peroxyl free radical: potential mediators of tumor initiation and promotion. *Carcinogenesis* 8: 1365–1373.

Mathews-Roth, M.M. 1982. Antitumor activity of carotene, canthaxanthin and phytoene. *Oncology* 39: 33–37.

McCormick, D.L., Major, N., and Moon, R.C. 1984. Inhibition of 7,12-dimethylbenz(a)anthracene-induced mammary carcinogenesis by concomitant or postcarcinogen antioxidant exposure. *Cancer Res.* 44: 2858–2863.

McDanell, R., McLean, A.E.M., Hanley, A.B., Heaney, R.K., and Fenwick, G.R. 1988. Chemical and biological properties of indole glucosinolates (glucobrassicins): A review. *Fd. Chem. Toxic.* 26: 59–70.

McGuinness, E.E., Morgan, R.G.H., and Wormsley, K.G. 1984. Effects of soybean flour on the pancreas of rats. *Environ. Health Persp.* 56: 205–212.

Mergens, W.J., Kamm, J.J., Newmark, H.L., Fiddler, W., and Pensabene, J. 1978. Alpha-tocopherol: Uses in preventing nitrosamine formation. In Environmental Aspects of N-Nitroso Compounds. (Ed.) Walker, E.A., Castegnara, M., Griciute, L., and Lyle, R.E. IARC Publication No. 19, p. 119–211, Lyon, France.

Mettlin, C. and Graham, S. 1979. *Am. J. Epidemiol.* 110: 255–263.

Milks, M.M., Wilt, S.R., Ali, I.I., and Couri, D. 1985. The effects of selenium on the emergence of aflatoxin B1-induced enzyme-altered foci in rat liver. *Fundament. Appl. Toxicol.* 5: 320–326.

Miller, E.C. and Miller, J.A. 1979. Milestones in chemical carcinogenesis. *Seminars in Oncology* 6: 445–460.

Mirvish, S.S. 1981a. Ascorbic acid inhibition of N-nitroso compound formation in chemical, food and biological systems. In Inhibition of Tumor Induction and Development. (Ed.) Zedeck, M.S., and Lipkin, M. p. 101–126, Plenum Publishing Corp., New York.

Mirvish, S.S. 1981b. Inhibition of the formation of carcinogenic N-Nitroso compounds by ascorbic acid and other compounds. In *Cancer Achievements, Challenges and Prospects for the 1980's,* (Ed.) Burchenal,

J.H., and Oettgen, H.F. p. 557–588. Grune and Stratton, New York.

Mirvish, S.S., Cardesa, A., Wallcave, L. and Shubik, P. 1975. *J. Natl. Cancer Inst.* 55: 633–636.

Monroe, D.H., Holeski, C.J., and Eaton, D.L. 1986. Effects of single-dose pretreatment with 2(3)-tert-butyl-4-hydroxyanisole (BHA) on the hepatobiliary disposition and covalent binding to DNA of aflatoxin B1 in the rat. *Fd. Chem. Toxic* 24: 1273–1281.

Moon, R.C., McCormick, D.L., and Mehta, R.G. 1983. Inhibition of carcinogenesis by retinoids. *Cancer Res.* (Suppl.) 43: 2469–2475s.

Morgan, R.G.H., Levinson, D.A., Hopwood, D., Saunders, J.H.B., and Wormsley, K. G. 1977. Potentiation of the action of azaserine on the rat pancreas by raw soya bean flour. *Cancer Lett.* 3: 87–90.

Mori, H., Tanaka, T., Shima, H., Kuniyasu, T., and Takahashi, M. 1986. Inhibitory effect of chlorogenic acid on methylazoxymethanol acetate-induced carcinogenesis in large intestine and liver of hamster. *Cancer Lett.* 30: 49–54.

Mukhtar, H., Das, M., and Bickers, D.R. 1986. Inhibition of 3-methylcholanthrene-induced skin tumorigenicity in BALB/c mice by chronic oral feeding of trace amounts of ellagic acid in drinking water. *Cancer Res.* 46: 2262–2265.

Mukhtar, H., Das, M., Khan, W.A., Wang, Z.Y., Bik, D.P., and Bickers, D.R. 1988. Exceptional activity of tannic acid among naturally occurring plant phenols in protecting against 7,12-dimethylbenz(a)anthracene-, benzo(a)pyrene-, 3-methylcholanthrene-, and N-methyl-N-nitrosourea-induced skin tumorigenesis in mice. *Cancer Res.* 48: 2361–2365.

Newmark, H. and Mergens, W. 1981. α-Tocopherol (vitamin E) and its relationship to tumor induction. In *Inhibition of Tumor Induction and Development.* (Ed.) Zedeck, M.S. and Lipken, M. p. 127–168. Plenum Publishing Corp., New York.

Nigro, N.D., Bull, A.W., and Boyd, M.E. 1986. Inhibition of intestinal carcinogenesis in rats: Effect of difluoromethylornithine with piroxicam or fish oil. *J. Natl. Cancer Inst.* 77: 1309–1313.

Nishizumi, M. 1979. Effect of phenobarbital, dichlorodiphenyltrichloroethane and polychlorinated biphenyls on diethylnitrosamine-induced hepatocarcinogenesis. *Jpn. J. Cancer Res.* (Gann) 70: 835–837.

Nixon, J.E., Hendricks, J.D., Pawlowski, N.E., Pereira, C.B., Sinnhuber, R.O., and Bailey, G.S. 1984. Inhibition of aflatoxin B1 carcinogenesis in rainbow trout by flavone and indole compounds *Carcinogenesis* 5: 615–619.

Nomura, T. 1980. Timing of chemically induced neoplasia in mice revealed by the antineoplastic action of caffeine. *Cancer Res.* 40: 1332–1340.

Nomura, T., Hata, S., Enomoto, T., Tanaka, H., and Shibata, K. 1980. Inhibiting effects of antipain on urethane-induced lung neoplasia in mice. *Br. J. Cancer* 42: 624–626.

Nunez, O., Hendricks, J.D., and Bailey, G.S. 1988. Enhancement of aflatoxin B1 and N-methyl-N'-nitro-N-nitrosoguanidine hepatocarcinogenesis in rainbow trout (*Salmo gairdneri*) by 17-β-estradiol and other organic compounds. *Diseases of Aquatic Organisms,* 5: 185–196.

Nunez, O., Hendricks, J.D., Lee, B.C., and Bailey, G.S. (Submitted). Promotion of aflatoxin B1 hepatocarcinogenesis in rainbow trout (*Salmo gairdneri*) by 17-β-estradiol.

O'Connor, T.P., Roebuck, B.D., Peterson, F., and Campbell, T.C. 1985. Effect of dietary intake of fish oil and fish protein on the development of L-azaserine-induced preneoplastic lesions in the rat pancreas. *J. Natl. Cancer Inst.* 75: 959–962.

Oesterle, D. and Deml, E. 1983. Promoting effect of polychlorinated biphenyls on development of enzyme-altered islands in livers of weanling and adult rats. *J. Cancer Res. Clin. Oncol.* 105: 141–147.

Ohgaki, H., Hasegawa, H., Suenaga, M., Sato, S., Takayama, S., and Sugimura, T. 1987. Carcinogenicity in mice of a mutagenic compound, 2-amino-3,8-dimethylimidazole[4,5-f]quinoxaline (MeIQx) from cooked foods. *Carcinogenesis* 8: 665–668.

Pao, E.M. and Mickle, S.J. 1981. Problem nutrients in the United States. *Food Technol.* 35: 58–79.

Pence, B.C., Buddingh, F., and Yang, S.P. 1986. Multiple dietary factors in the enhancement of dimethylhydrazine carcinogenesis: Main effect of indole-3-carbinol. *J. Natl. Cancer Inst.* 77: 269–276.

Peraino, C., Fry, R.J.M., Staffeldt, E., and Christopher, J.P. 1975. Comparative enhancing effects of phenobarbital, amobarbital, diphenylhydantoin, and dichlorodiphenyltrichloroethane on 2-acetylaminofluorene induced hepatic tumorigenesis in the rat. *Cancer Res.* 35: 2884–2890.

Perchellet, J-P., Owen, M.D., Posey, T.D., Orten, D.K., and Schneider, B.A. 1985. Inhibitory effects of glutathione level-raising agents and D-α-tocopherol on ornithine decarboxylase induction and mouse skin tumor promotion by 12-0-tetradecanoylphorbol-13-acetate. *Carcinogenesis* 6: 567–573.

Pereira, M.A., Herren, S.L., Britt, A.L., and Khoury, M.M. 1982. Promotion by polychlorinated biphenyls of enzyme-altered foci in rat liver. *Cancer Lett.* 15: 105–190.

Perera, M.I.R., Betschart, J.M., Virji, M.A., Katyal, S.L., and Shinozuka, H. 1987. Free radical injury and liver tumor promotion. *Toxicol. Pathol.* 15: 51–59.

Philips, R.L. 1975. Role of life-style and dietary habits in risk of cancer among Seventh-Day Adventists. *Cancer Res.* 35: 3513–3522.

Pitot, H.C., Goldsworthy, T.L., Moran, S., Kennan, W., Glauert, H.P., Maronpot, R.R., and Campbell, H.A. 1987. A method to quantitate the relative initiating and promoting potencies of hepatocarcinogenic agents in their dose-response relationships to altered hepatic foci. *Carcinogenesis* 8: 1491–1499.

Powell, C.J., Connelly, J.C., Jones, S.M., Grasso, P., and Bridges, J.W. 1986. Hepatic responses to the administration of high doses of BHT to the rat: their relevance to hepatocarcinogenicity. *Fd. Chem. Toxic.* 24: 1131–1143.

Preston, B.D., Van Miller, J.P., Moore, R.W., and Allen, J.R. 1981. Promoting effects of polychlorinated biphenyls (Aroclor 1254) and polychlorinated dibenzofuran-free Aroclor 1254 on diethylnitrosamine-induced tumorigenesis in the rat. *J. Natl. Cancer Inst.* 66: 509–515.

Rao, M.S., Lalwani, N.D., Watanabe, T.K., and Reddy, J.K. 1984. Inhibitory effect of antioxidants ethoxyquin and 2(3)-tert-butyl-4-hydroxyanisole on hepatic tumorigenesis in rats fed ciprofibrate, a peroxisome proliferator. *Cancer Res.* 44: 1072–1076.

Reddy, B.S. and Maruyama, J. 1986. Effect of dietary fish oil on azoxymethane-induced colon carcinogenesis in male F344 rats. *Cancer Res.* 46: 3367–3370.

Rettura, G., Stratford, F., Levenson, S.M., and Seifter, E. 1982. Prophylactic and therapeutic actions of supplemental β-carotene in mice inoculated with C3HBA adenocarcinoma cells: lack of therapeutic action of supplemental ascorbic acid. *J. Natl. Cancer Inst.* 69: 73–77.

Rettura, G., Chandralekha, D., Listowsky, P., Levenson, S.M., and Seifter, E. 1983. Dimethylbenz(a)anthracene (DMBA) induced tumors: prevention by supplemental β-carotene. *Fed. Proc.* 42: 786.

Ross, M.H. and Bras, G. 1983. Influence of protein under- and overnutrition on spontaneous tumor prevalence in the rat. *J. Nutr.* 103: 944–963.

Santamaria, K., Bianchi, A., Arnaboldi, A., Andreoni, L., and Bermond, P.

1983. Dietary carotenoids block photocarcinogenic enhancement by benzo(a)pyrene and inhibit its carcinogenesis in the dark. *Experientia* 39: 1043-1045.

Schoenhard, G.L., Hendricks, J.D., Nixon, J.E., Lee, D.J., Wales, J.H., Sinnhuber, R.O., and Pawlowski, N.E. 1981. Aflatoxicol-induced hepatocellular carcinoma in rainbow trout (*Salmo gairdneri*) and the synergistic effects of cyclopropenoid fatty acids. *Cancer Res.* 41: 1011-1014.

Schrauzer, G.N., White, D.A., and Schneider, C.J. 1977. Cancer mortality correlation studies, 3. Statistical associations with dietary selenium intakes. *Bioinorg. Chem.* 7: 23-34.

Seifter, E., Rettura, G., and Levenson, S.M. 1982. Dietary β-carotene is an effective-tumor preventive agent. In *Proceedings of the Thirteenth International Cancer Congress,* Seattle, WA, September 8-15, p.30.

Shankel, D.M., Hartman, P.E., Kada, T., and Hollaender, A. 1987. Synopsis of the First International Conference on Antimutagenesis and anticarcinogenesis: Mechanisms. *Environ. Mutagen.* 9: 87-103.

Shankel, D.M., Hartman, P.E., Kada, T., and Hollaender, A. (Ed.) 1986. *Antimutagenesis and Anticarcinogenesis: Mechanisms.* Plenum Press, New York.

Shekelle, R.D., Liu, S., Raynor, W.J., Leper, M., Maliza, C., and Russef, A.H. 1981. Dietary vitamin A and risk of cancer in the Western Electric Study. *Lancet.* 2: 1185-1190.

Shertzer, H.G. 1983. Protection of indole-3-carbinol against covalent binding of benzo(a)pyrene metabolites to mouse liver DNA and protein. *Fd. Chem. Toxic.* 21: 31-35.

Shertzer H.G. 1984. Indole-3-carbinol protects against covalent binding of benzo(a)pyrene and N-nitrosodimethylamine metabolites to mouse liver macromolecules. *Chem. Biol. Interact.* 48: 81-90.

Shklar, G., Schwartz, J., Trickler, D.P., and Niukian, K. 1987. Regression by vitamin E of experimental oral cancer. *J. Natl. Cancer Inst.* 78: 987-992.

Sinnhuber, R.O., Lee, D.J., Wales, J.H., Landers, M.K., and Keyl, A.C. 1974. Hepatic carcinogenesis of aflatoxin M1 in rainbow trout (*Salmo gairdneri*) and its enhancement by cyclopropene fatty acids. *J. Natl. Cancer Inst.* 53: 1285-1288

Smart, R.C., Huang, M-C., Chang, R.L., Sayer, J.M., Jerina, D.M., Wood, A.W., and Conney, A.H. 1986. Effect of ellagic and 3-0-decylellagic acid on the formation of benzo(a)pyrene-derived DNA adducts in vivo and on the tumorigenicity of 3-methylchloranthracene in mice. *Carcinogenesis* 7: 1669-1676.

Sparnins, V.L., Barany, G., and Wattenberg, L.W. 1988. Effects of organosulfur compounds from garlic and onions on benzo(a)pyrene-induced neoplasia and glutathione S-transferase activity in the mouse. *Carcinogenesis* 9: 131-134.

Sparnins, V.L., Venegas, P.L., and Wattenberg, L.W. 1982a. Glutathione S-transferase activity: enhancement by compounds inhibiting chemical carcinogenesis and by dietary constituents. *J. Natl. Cancer Inst.* 68: 493-496.

Sparnins, V.L., Chuan, J., and Wattenberg, L. 1982b. Enhancement of glutathione S-transferase activity of the esophagus by phenols, lactones, and benzyl isothiocyanate. *Cancer Res.* 42: 1205-1207.

Sparnins, V.L. and Wattenberg, L.W. 1981. Enhancement of glutathione-S-transferase activity of the mouse forestomach by inhibitors of benzo(a)pyrene-induced neoplasia of the forestomach. *J. Natl. Cancer Inst.* 66: 769-771.

Sporn, M.B. 1983. Retinoids and suppression of carcinogenesis. *Hosp. Pract.* 18: 83-98.

Sporn, M.B. and Newton, D.L. 1981. Retinoids and chemoprevention of cancer. In *Inhibition of Tumor Induction and Development* (Ed.) Zedeck, M.S. and Lipkin, M. p. 71-100. Plenum Publishing Corp., New York.

Sporn, M.B. and Roberts, A.B. 1984. Role of retinoids in differentiation and carcinogenesis. *J. Natl. Cancer Inst.* 73: 1381-1386.

Sugimura, T. 1982. Mutagens, carcinogens, and tumor promotors in our daily food. *Cancer* 49: 1970-1984.

Sugimura, T. 1986. Studies on environmental chemical carcinogenesis in Japan. *Science* 233: 312-318.

Sumi, C., Yokoro, K., Kajitani, T., and Ito, A. 1980. Synergism of diethylstilbesterol and other carcinogens in concurrent development of hepatic, mammary and pituitary tumors in castrated male rats. *J. Natl. Cancer Inst.* 65: 169-175.

Swanson et al. (in preparation)

Swenberg, J.A., Richardson, F.C. Tyeryar, L., Deal, F., and Boucheron, J. 1987. The molecular dosimetry of DNA adducts formed by continuous exposure of rats to alkylating hepatocarcinogens. *Prog. Exp. Tumor Res.* 31: 42-51.

Tinbergen, B.J. and Krol, F. 1977. *Nitrite in Meat Products.* Centre for Agriculture Publ. and Documentation, Wageningen, Zeist. The Netherlands.

Troll, W., Frenkel, K., and Wiesner, R. 1984. Protease inhibitors as anticarcinogens. *J. Natl. Cancer Inst.* 73: 1245–1250.

Troll, W., Wiesner, R., Shellabarger, C.J., Holtzman, S., and Stone, J.P. 1980. Soybean diet lowers breast tumor incidence in irradiated rats. *Carcinogenesis* 1: 469–472.

Ura, H., Denda, A., Yokose, Y., Tsutsumi, M., and Konishi, Y. 1987. Effect of vitamin E on the induction and evolution of enzyme altered foci in liver of rats treated with diethylnitrosamine. *Carcinogenesis* 8: 1595–1600.

Valsta, L.M., Hendricks, J.D., and Bailey, G.S. 1988. The significance of glutathione conjugation for aflatoxin B1 metabolism in rainbow trout and coho salmon. *Fd. Chem. Toxicol.* 26: 129–135.

van Zeeland, A.A. 1988. Molecular dosimetry of alkylating agents: quantitative comparison of genetic effects on the basis of DNA adduct formation. *Mutagenesis* 3: 179–191.

Virtanen, A.I. 1965. Studies on organic sulfur compounds and other labile substances in plants. *Phytochemistry* 4: 207–228.

Vuillaume, M. 1987. Reduced oxygen species, mutation, induction and cancer initiation. *Mut. Res.* 186: 43–72.

Wahil, P.N., Bodkho, R.R., Arora, S., and Sriustana, M.C. 1962. Serum vitamin A studies in leukoplakia and carcinoma of the oral cavity. *Indian J. Pathol. Bacteriol.* 5: 10–16.

Wald, N., Iole, M., Boveham, J., and Bailey, A. 1980. Low serum vitamin A and subsequent risk of cancer. Preliminary results of a prospective study. *Lancet* 2: 813–815.

Ward, J.M. 1985. Proliferative lesions of the glandular stomach and liver in F344 rats fed diets containing Aroclor 1254. *Environ. Hlth. Persp.* 60: 89–95.

Wargovich, M.J. 1987. Diallyl sulfide, a flavor component of garlic (*Allium sativum*), inhibits dimethylhydrazine-induced colon cancer. *Carcinogenesis* 8: 487–489.

Wattenberg, L.W. 1977. Inhibition of carcinogenic effects of polycyclic hydrocarbons by benzyl isothiocyanate and related compounds. *J. Natl. Cancer Inst.* 58: 395–398.

Wattenberg, L.W. 1981. Inhibition of carcinogen-induced neoplasia by sodium cyanate, tert-butylisocyanate and benzyl isothiocyanate administered subsequent to carcinogen exposure. *Cancer Res.* 41: 2991–2994

Wattenberg, L.W. 1982. Inhibition of chemical carcinogens by minor dietary constituents. In *Molecular Interrelations of Nutrition and Cancer,*

(Ed.) Arnott, M.S., van Eys, J. and Wang, Y.M., p. 43–56. Raven Press, New York.

Wattenberg, L.W. 1983. Inhibition of neoplasia by minor dietary constituents. *Cancer Res.* (Suppl.) 43: 2448–2453.

Wattenberg, L.W. 1985. Chemoprevention of cancer. *Cancer Res.* 45: 1–8.

Wattenberg, L.W. 1986. Protective effects of 2(3)-tert-butyl-4-hydroxyanisole on chemical carcinogenesis. *Fd. Chem. Toxic.* 24: 1099–1102.

Wattenberg, L.W., Coccia, J.B., and Lam, L.K.T. 1980. Inhibitory effects of phenolic compounds on benzo(a)pyrene-induced neoplasia. *Cancer Res.* 40: 2820–2823.

Wattenberg, L.W., Hanley, A.B., Barany, G., Sparnins, V.L., Lam, L.K.T., and Fenwick, G.R. 1986. Inhibition of carcinogenesis by some minor dietary components. In *Diet, Nutrition and Cancer.* (Ed.) Hayashi, Y. et al., p. 13. VNU Science, Tokyo.

Wattenberg, L.W. and Loub, W.D. 1978. Inhibition of polycyclic aromatic hydrocarbon induced neoplasia by naturally occurring indoles. *Cancer Res.* 38: 1410–1413.

Weed, H.G., McGandy, R.B., and Kennedy, A.R. 1985. Protection against dimethylhydrazine-induced adenomatous tumors of the mouse colon by the dietary addition of an extract of soybeans containing the Bowman-Birk protease inhibitor. *Carcinogenesis* 6: 1239–1241.

Weisburger, J.H. 1979. Mechanism of action of diet as a carcinogen. *Cancer* 43: 1987–1995.

Weisburger, J.H. 1987. Mechanisms of nutritional carcinogenesis associated with specific human cancer. *ISI Atlas of Sci.:Pharmacol.* 1: 162–167.

Weisburger, J.H. and Williams, G.M. 1980. Chemical Carcinogens. In *Toxicology, The Basic Science of Poisons,* (Ed.) Doull, J., Klaassen, C.D. and Amdur, M.O., *Casavett & Doull's* Ch. 6, p. 84–138.

Williams, G.M. and Numuto, S. 1984. Promotion of mouse liver neoplasms by the organichlorine pesticides chlordane and heptachlor in comparison to dichlorodiphenyltrichloroethane. *Carcinogenesis* 5: 1689–1696.

Williams, G.M., Tanaka, T., and Maeura, Y. 1986. Dose related inhibition of aflatoxin B1 induced hepatocarcinogenesis by the phenolic antioxidants, butylated hydroxyanisole and butylated hydroxytoluene. *Carcinogenesis* 7: 1043–1050.

Witschi, H.P. 1986. Enhanced tumor development by butylated hydroxytoluene (BHT) in the liver, lung and gastro-intestinal tract. *Fd. Chem. Toxic.* 24: 1127–1130.

Wood, A.W., Huang, M.T., Chang, R.L., Newmark, H.L., Lehr, R.E., Yagi, H., Sayer, J.M. Jerina, D.M., and Conney, A.H. 1982. Inhibition of the mutagenicity of bay-region diol epoxides of polycyclic aromatic hydrocarbons by naturally occurring plant phenols: exceptional activity of ellagic acid. *Proc. Natl. Acad. Sci. USA* 79: 5513–5517.

Wotiz, H.H., Beebe, D.R., and Muller, E. 1984. Effect of estrogens on DMBA induced breast tumors. *J. Steroid Biochem.* 20: 1067–1075.

Yanagi, S., Sakamoto, M., Takahashi, S., Hasulike, A., Konishi, Y., Kumazawa, K., and Nakano, T. 1985. Enhancement of hepatocarcinogenesis by sorbitan fatty acid ester, a liver pyruvate kinase activity-reducing substance. *J. Natl. Cancer Inst.* 75: 381–384.

Yavelow, J., Finlay, T.H., Kennedy, A.R., and Troll, W. 1983. Bowman-Birk soybean protease inhibitor as an anticarcinogen. *Cancer Res.* (Suppl.) 43: 2454s–2459s.

Ziegler, R.G., Mason, T.J., Stemhagen, A., Hoover, R., Schoenberg, J.B., Gridley, G., Virgo, P.W., and Fraumeni, J.F., Jr. 1986. Carotenoid intake, vegetables, and the risk of lung cancer among white men in New Jersey. *Am. J. Epidemiol.* 123: 1080–1093.

6

A Case Study: The Safety Evaluation of Artificial Sweeteners

Ian C. Munro

Canadian Centre for Toxicology
Guelph, Ontario, Canada

INTRODUCTION

Artificial sweeteners are a group of discrete chemical substances which possess intense sweetness and which may be used in foods and medicines in place of naturally occurring sweetening agents. A list of the principal artificial sweeteners is given in Table 6.1. The sweetness of these substances ranges from 30 to 2000 times that of sucrose, and therefore only small quantities are required to produce appropriate sweetening properties. Of the substances listed in Table 6.1, only aspartame, cyclamate, and saccharin are currently used in foods. Although in the United States cyclamate has been banned from use in foods since 1970, it is used as a tabletop sweetener in Canada and as a sweetening additive in foods in many European countries. Until the introduction of aspartame as a sweetener in the early 1980s, the only sweeteners used in food were cyclamate and saccharin.

As a case study of artificial sweetener safety, cyclamate and saccharin represent interesting examples of the principal scientific issues that surround sweetener safety. They also provide an interesting lesson in the interpretation of toxicological data, since both these substances fell victim, several years ago, to intense study with a wide range of innovative but

TABLE 6.1 Artificial Sweeteners

Sweeteners	Approximate sweetness (sucrose = 1)
Acesulfame K	200
Alitame	2000
Aspartame	200
Cyclamate	30
Saccharin	300
Sucralose	600

largely invalidated approaches to safety evaluation. For example, with the advent of mutagenicity testing, both saccharin and cyclamate were extensively tested with conflicting results depending upon the test system and test conditions used. Similar conflicting results were reported over a period of years with respect to the carcinogenicity of saccharin and cyclamate.

It is interesting to note the reasons for the great interest in the safety of artificial sweeteners. In the first instance, both saccharin and cyclamate were used in food for many years (saccharin since the turn of the century and cyclamate from the early 1950s) without a great deal of supporting safety data, at least by today's standards. Additionally, during the 1960s artificial sweetener use increased dramatically with increased interest in calorie-reduced foods, resulting in high exposure of many individuals to these substances (NAS, 1985). As a result of these factors saccharin and cyclamate became targets for more exhaustive toxicological investigation. The purpose of this paper is to evaluate the nature and significance of toxicological investigations conducted on these substances with special emphasis on bladder carcinogenesis.

TOXICOLOGICAL STUDIES ON CYCLAMATE

To gain an understanding of the regulatory dilemma posed by cyclamate, it is important to appreciate the major issues that focused attention on this substance. The study which principally led to the banning of cyclamates was a carcinogenicity study conducted by the Food and Drug Research Laboratory (FDRL) in which a 10:1 combination of cyclamate and saccharin, fed in conjunction with cyclohexylamine, a metabolite of cyclamate, was alleged to have produced bladder tumors in rats (Oser et al., 1976). Largely on the basis of this study, an ad hoc committee of The Food and Nutrition Board of the National Research Council concluded in 1969 that a mixture of cyclamate/saccharin was carcinogenic (NRC, 1969). The committee was of the view that cyclamate and/or cyclohexylamine was responsible for the tumors but could not exclude a contributory role for saccharin. Based on this information cyclamate was subsequently banned from use as a food additive in the United States. Several additional studies on the carcinogenicity of cyclamate and cyclohexylamine have been conducted in mice (Rudali et al., 1969; Roe et al., 1970; Brantom et al., 1973; Homburger et al., 1973; Hardy et al., 1974, 1976; Kroes et al., 1975, 1977; Muranyi-Kovacs et al., 1975) and rats (Fitzhugh et al., 1951; Pliss, 1958; Plank, 1970; Carson and Vogin, 1972; Friedman et al., 1972; Homburger et al., 1973; Schmahl, 1973; Bar and Griepentrog, 1974; Gaunt et al., 1974a, b; Hicks et al 1975; Ikeda et al., 1975; Hicks and Chowaniec, 1977; Schmahl and Habs, 1980; Taylor et al., 1980) using both single-generation and multigeneration protocols with the overall conclusion that there is no evidence that cyclamate or its principal metabolite cyclohexylamine produces bladder cancer in these species (NAS, 1985). Additional studies in dogs, hamsters, and primates also have produced negative results. According to the National Academy of Sciences, however, there was evidence that cyclamate enhances or promotes the development of bladder cancer in rats given intravesicular doses of methylnitrosourea (MNU) (Hicks et al., 1975; Hicks and Chowaniec, 1977) and in mice given cholesterol/cyclamate combinations by bladder implantation (Bryan and Ertürk, 1970). These studies led the National Academy of Sciences in 1985 to declare a need for further studies to clarify the role of cyclamate as a promoting or cocarcinogenic agent. The Committee also noted that the significance of promotion studies in animals for humans was uncertain and that more generic research to assess the relevance of such studies to humans was required (NAS, 1985).

TOXICOLOGICAL STUDIES ON SACCHARIN

Extensive toxicology/carcinogenicity studies have been conducted as well on saccharin. The impetus for these studies arose principally from the increased usage of saccharin following the ban on cyclamates and the implied role of saccharin in the development of bladder cancer in the 1969 FDRL rat studies. Up until 1975, approximately a dozen single-generation carcinogenicity studies were conducted with saccharin in rats or mice

(Oser, 1985). Additional long-term studies were conducted using hamsters and primates. These early studies on the long-term toxicity of saccharin failed to indicate any substantial evidence for bladder carcinogenicity (Oser, 1985). The ability of saccharin to produce bladder cancer in rats only became evident with the conduct of two-generation studies in which pregnant rats and their offspring, exposed in utero and for two years following birth, developed bladder tumors. Several such studies have been conducted (Tisdel et al., 1974; Taylor et al., 1980; Arnold, et al., 1980; Schoenig et al., 1985). In most of these studies high doses of saccharin, equal to or greater than 5% of the diet, administered during gestation and to the offspring, resulted in the development of a statistically significant increase in the incidence of malignant bladder tumors. In one such study employing large number of animals (Schoenig et al., 1985), bladder tumors also were noted in animals given saccharin only from birth suggesting that previous single-generation studies may not have had sufficient statistical power to detect an increase in bladder cancer and/or that in previous studies animals were not started on saccharin early enough in life to allow tumors to develop. The data certainly suggest that saccharin administration in utero, or very early in life, is a necessary prerequisite for tumor development. In studies in which graded doses of saccharin were administered (Schoenig et al., 1985), a no-effect level for the induction of tumors was observed at approximately 1% dietary saccharin, indicating that a possible threshold exists in terms of bladder cancer risk. There appears to be a general consensus that, due to the steep dose-response curve for saccharin-induced bladder tumors, the risk of bladder cancer at low doses is remote. This conclusion is supported by the several negative epidemiological studies and the results of short-term tests for carcinogenicity (Report of an Expert Panel, 1985).

During the course of investigations into the mechanism of saccharin-induced tumors, several studies have been published indicating that saccharin, like cyclamate, may enhance the development of bladder tumors in rats initiated with a range of physical and chemical agents. Because of the importance attached to promotion studies, both from the regulatory point of view and as a basis to assess possible mechanisms of action of bladder cancer, the balance of this paper will focus on the significance of these studies.

PROMOTION STUDIES WITH SWEETENERS

Neoplasm promotion is a term used to described a phenomenon, observed in experimental carcinogenesis, in which a tumor-promoting agent is said to promote the development of site-specific tumors in animals initiated with subcarcinogenic doses of a carcinogenic agent. In the classical tumor promotion model a dose, or series of doses, of the initiating agent (a carcinogen), given at a subcarcinogenic dose and followed by treatment with the promoting agent, leads to the development of tumors. In animals treated only with initiating doses of the carcinogen or only with the promoter, no tumors or only a few tumors are seen to develop. Tumor promotion models are therefore characterized by sequential administration of the initiator and promoter.

Another form of tumor enhancement is described by experimental models in which two agents are administered simultaneously to animals. This operational model, known as cocarcinogenesis, is intended to evaluate tumor enhancing effects when two chemicals are given simultaneously as opposed to sequentially. The studies on the sweeteners saccharin and cyclamate include both promotion and cocarcinogenesis.

Concern over the tumor-promoting properties of cyclamate and saccharin arose principally out of studies conducted by Hicks et al. (1975) and Hicks and Chowaneic (1977), which were said to demonstrate that these substances promoted the development of bladder tumors in rats pretreated by intravesicular instillation of subcarcinogenic amounts of methylnitrosourea into the bladder. In addition, earlier studies by Bryan and Ertürk (1970) involving the implantation into the bladders of mice of cholesterol pellets containing saccharin or cyclamate also were said to demonstrate a tumor-enhancing effect of these sweeteners. Collectively these studies gave rise to a diverse series of investigations aimed at attempts to (a) repeat and extend this work on promotion and cocarcinogenesis and (b) identify possible mechanisms of actions by which saccharin and cyclamate might produce bladder tumor–promoting effects.

MOUSE STUDIES WITH CYCLAMATE

The first study conducted to evaluate the tumor-enhancing effect of cyclamate was that of Bryan and Ertürk (1970). In this study cholesterol or cholesterol mixed with sodium cyclamate was formed into a pellet and surgically implanted into the bladders of day-old mice. After 13 months of treatment 12% of mice given cholesterol alone and approximately 70% of the mice treated with cholesterol plus cyclamate developed bladder carcinomas. This study has been criticized on the basis that the pellets of cholesterol themselves were associated with tumors. Also, Clayson (1974) has pointed out that tumors induced with this model may be an artifact of the test system, since inert materials such as oxalate stones, glass beads, and other foreign objects are known to produce tumors when implanted in the bladder of the mouse. In addition it has been noted that due to the rapid elution rate of the cyclamate from the pellets (7 hr) cyclamate would have to be a potent carcinogen to illicit the response obtained (NAS, 1985). In a more general sense, this model of bladder tumor enhancement has been criticized as being inappropriate for the assessment of tumor enhancement of human dietary constituents (NCI Temporary Committee, 1976). Two additional studies in mice in which cyclamate was given in combination with 2-acetylaminofluorene or following X-irradiation produced negative results.

Rat Studies with Cyclamate

The initial study said to demonstrate the tumor–promoting action of orally administered cyclamate in rats is that of Hicks et al. (1975). In this study, groups of weanling female rats were given a single dose of MNU instilled into the urinary bladder (Hicks et al., 1975; Hicks and Chowaniec, 1977). The animals were then fed sodium cyclamate via the diet for 2 years. No bladder tumors were reported to have occurred in rats given MNU alone; however, approximately 50% of rats treated with MNU plus cyclamate developed bladder tumors. While this study appears to have been well conducted and sufficient numbers of animals survived the treatment period, it now appears that the dose of MNU used by Hicks and colleagues was uncertain and attempts to repeat this study have failed. For example, Mohr et al. (1979) administered the nominal dose of 2 mg MNU used by Hicks et al (1975) to female rats and followed this with a diet containing sodium cyclamate for lifetime. They found that 2 mg MNU, the nominal dose used by Hicks, produced a 57% incidence of bladder tumors, while MNU plus cyclamate produced a 70% incidence of tumors, a result not significantly different from the incidence found in MNU-treated rats. No further attempts have been undertaken to resolve this conflict.

In another promotion-type study, Ito et al. (1983) administered the bladder carcinogen N-butyl-N-(4-hydroxybutyl) nitrosamine (BBN) in the drinking water of weanling male rats for 4 wk and followed this with a diet containing 2.5 g/kg sodium cyclamate for an additional 32 wk, at which time the animals were killed. The incidence of papillary and nodular hyperplasia was similar in BBN-treated and BBN/cyclamate-treated rats, indicating cyclamate did not demonstrate promotion in this model. Investigators in Ito's laboratory have used this model in many other experiments both with cyclamate and saccharin. It should be noted that the end-point selected here is not tumors but a bladder epithelial lesion described by Ito et al (1983) as papillary and nodular hyperplasia, which is claimed to be a precursor to tumor development. It should be pointed out that the Ito model differs from the classical model of tumor promotion in that respect. Moreover, care must be taken in interpreting the results of work using this model since papillary and nodular hyperplasia is a very reversible bladder lesion.

In a cocarcinogenesis experiment, Schmahl and Kruger (1972) gave groups of rats either BBN in drinking water or BBN combined with sodium cyclamate in the diet for approximately 2 yr. Since all the rats given BBN alone developed bladder tumors, the value of this study is questionable; however, there was no evidence that cyclamate reduced the latent period for BBN-induced bladder carcinogenesis in this study.

Taken together, the available studies on promotion and cocarcinogenesis involving cyclamate provide little convincing experimental evidence that this sweetener, when administered by appropriate routes of exposure, possesses tumor-enhancing properties. The only suggestive evidence for promotion comes from the studies of Hicks et al. (1975), which have not been substantiated by further investigations. Since the actual dose of active MNU used by Hicks is unknown, it is unlikely that this study can be successfully reproduced.

Mouse Studies with Saccharin

Few studies are available in which the bladder tumor–promoting or cocarcinogenic action of saccharin has been studied in mice. Allen et al. (1957) conducted a study in which saccharin was mixed with four times its weight of cholesterol and implanted as a pellet into the bladder lumina of mice. Mice that received cholesterol implants alone served as controls. After 52 wk, 4% of control mice and 30% of saccharin-treated mice developed bladder tumors. In an extension of this work, Bryan et al. (1970) implanted cholesterol pellets containing sodium saccharin or cholesterol pellets alone into the bladders of Swiss mice. After 56 wk of treatment, 50% of saccharin-treated mice and 12% of mice exposed only to cholesterol developed tumors, a result which was reported by the authors to be statistically significant. The significance of these studies involving bladder implantation is uncertain for the reasons stated previously for cyclamate.

Rat Studies with Saccharin

Numerous studies have been conducted to evaluate the possible promoting effects of sodium saccharin on the urinary bladder of rats initiated with a variety of agents. As with cyclamate, the initial study said to demonstrate saccharin–promoting action was that of Hicks et al. (1975), in which rats were given 2 mg MNU by bladder instillation followed by a diet providing sodium saccharin for 2 yr. In this study it was reported (Hicks and Chowaniec, 1977) that MNU alone induced no tumors in 124 rats, while approximately 50% of rats given sodium saccharin plus MNU, respectively, developed bladder tumors. Mohr et al. (1979) were unable to repeat these experiments. They found a 57% incidence of bladder tumors in female rats given 2 mg MNU alone, while treatment with a saccharin-containing diet plus MNU led to a 65% bladder tumor incidence. Indeed, Hicks and colleagues failed to repeat their original studies involving MNU/saccharin combinations since a subsequent study by Hooson et al. (1980) found the bladder tumor incidence was 25% in rats given MNU alone and 24% in rats given MNU plus saccharin. In a more recent study, West et al. (1986), using the Hicks/Mohr protocol, reported that tumor promotion was observed at a dietary sodium saccharin concentration of 2.5% but not at lower doses (0.1, 0.5, or 1.0%) or at a dietary concentration of 5%. They also reported a dose-dependent decrease in latent period over the range of doses studied with the exception of the 5% dose level. This conclusion is difficult to justify, however, since no interim sacrifices were conducted to assess time-to-tumor formation. No satisfactory explanation was given for the failure to find an increased incidence of tumors at the 5% level. Overall, this study, like those of Mohr et al. (1979) and Hoosen et al. (1980), provides little convincing evidence that sodium saccharin acts as a promoter in MNU-initiated rats.

Studies involving use of the experimental bladder carcinogen N-[4-(5-nitro-2-furyl)-2-thiazoly] formamide (FANFT) conducted by Cohen et al. (1982) and Fukushima et al. (1981), in which this compound was fed in the diet of rats for periods of 4 to 6 wk and followed thereafter by a diet containing 5% saccharin, have demonstrated the promoting action of this sweetener in this promotion-type model. The cocarcinogenicity of saccharin also has been demonstrated using the FANFT model (Murasaki and Cohen, 1983). Other studies demonstrating the promoting effects of sodium saccharin on the urinary bladder include the work of Ito et al. (1983), who initiated rats using the bladder carcinogen BBN in the drinking water for 4 wk followed by a diet containing 5% sodium saccharin. Promotion of rat urinary bladder carcinogenesis by dietary sodium saccharin also has been reported after injection of subcarcinogenic doses of cyclophosphamide and the use of freeze ulceration (Cohen et al., 1982; Hasegawa et al., 1985). The latter studies suggest that nonspecific stimuli, which induce reparative regeneration and hyperplasia, are sufficient to act as the nidus for tumor development following long-term saccharin administration. The induction of hyperplasia and papillary carcinoma also has been reported to occur following repeated instillation of saline or sterile water into the urinary bladder (Akaza et al., 1984), and recently Murphy et al. (1986) have shown that maintenance of an indwelling catheter in the bladder of rats for 1 yr, without infusion, leads to the development of bladder tumors. These studies suggest that rats may develop bladder tumors in response to a variety of nonspecific stimuli similar to that reported for mice (Ball et al., 1964; Clayson, 1974).

Numerous studies have been conducted in an attempt to determine possible mechanisms by which sodium saccharin could induce tumors or promote the development of bladder tumors in rats. Since sodium saccharin is not considered to be mutagenic (Ashby, 1985), is not metabolized (IARC, 1980), and does not bind to cellular macromolecules (Lutz and Schlatter, 1977), studies aimed at identifying its mechanisms of action have concentrated on its possible physical and physiological actions on rat bladder epithelium. Several studies have repeatedly demonstrated that administration of 5% dietary sodium to rats leads to marked changes in urine composition (Schoening and Anderson, 1985). These changes include increased urinary pH and sodium ion concentration, decreased urine osmolality, and an increase in magnesium ammonium phosphate crystals in the urine. These extensive urinary electrolyte changes were not observed following administration of equimolar amounts of saccharin-free acid (Fukushima et al., 1986a). Following the hypothesis that sodium ion, rather than saccharin per se, is responsible for the development of bladder tumors in rats given sodium saccharin, several investigators have studied the promoting action of the sodium salts of other low molecular weight organic acids. Fukushima et al. (1983a,b, 1984) found that sodium ascorbate but not ascorbic acid promoted tumor development in rats pretreated with BBN. These authors noted that while sodium ascorbate produced the same changes in urine composition as did sodium saccharin, ascorbic acid did not. In subsequent studies, Fukushima et al (1986b,c) found that sodium bicarbonate and sodium citrate also promoted the development of carcinomas in BBN-initiated rats. These results add further evidence that the urinary compositional changes induced by sodium salts may be related to tumor enhancement. This view is supported by the fact that Hasegawa and Cohen (1986) reported that 5% dietary sodium saccharin, but not the calcium salt or free acid, induced significant urinary bladder epithelial proliferation, as measured by [H³]-thymidine incorporation. The degree of thymidine incorporation correlated with the extent of changes in urine composition.

Interpretation of Promotion/Cocarcinogenesis Studies

The available studies on sodium cyclamate, taken as a whole, do not provide convincing evidence that cyclamate has promoting effects in rodents when administered by routes relevant to human risk assessment. However, it must be pointed out that this sweetener has not been as thoroughly tested for promotion in classical systems as has sodium saccharin. If this testing were done, it would be important to investigate the role of excess dietary sodium from sodium cyclamate on any observed enhancing effect since cyclamate, like saccharin, possesses no convincing evidence of genotoxicity (NAS, 1985). In addition, unlike saccharin, sodium cyclamate has not demonstrated any evidence of carcinogenicity in long-term animals bioassays (NAS, 1985).

The research on saccharin provides a reasonably convincing case that excess sodium ion, increased urinary pH, and the other urinary changes produced by sodium saccharin play a major role in tumor promotion in rats administered saccharin at 5% of the diet in lifetime studies. In 32-week promotion studies, Nakanishi et al. (1980) demonstrated a dose-response relationship for papillary-nodular hyperplasia and simple hyperplasia in rats initiated with BBN and given diets containing graded doses of sodium saccharin. Statistically significant effects were noted only at 1 and 5% saccharin, suggesting a threshold for this response. Furthermore, Fukushima et al. (1986b) found that administration of ammonium chloride, which reduces the urinary pH, reduced the tumor–promoting action of sodium ascorbate in BBN-initiated rats. Increased urinary pH is apparently an important component among the factors responsible for promotion observed with sodium saccharin, since a diet of 5% sodium hippurate, which does not increase urinary pH, did not lead to papillary nodular hyperplasia or papillomas in BBN-initiated rats (Fukushima et al. 1986a). In addition Shibata et al. (1986) could find no convincing evidence for a promoting effect of 5 or 10% dietary sodium chloride in BBN-initiated rats. In this study urinary pH was not significantly different from controls fed a basal diet.

The existing data on sodium saccharin appear to suggest a relationship between high dietary levels of this sweetener and marked alterations in urine composition. Evidence to date suggests that these changes are associated in some way with the promoting action of saccharin on the urinary bladder of rats. These mechanistic studies are of importance in continuing efforts to unravel the etiological events associated with sodium saccharin–induced bladder tumorigenesis.

CONCLUSIONS

The toxicological studies on cyclamate and saccharin demonstrate that these substances are unlikely to pose a risk of human cancer at usual exposure levels. Based on carcinogenicity studies in animals, there is no convincing evidence that cyclamate or its major metabolite cyclohexylamine are carcinogenic. Studies on saccharin unequivocally indicate that this substance produces bladder cancer in rats but only under special test conditions involving high dose in utero exposure or exposure very early in life followed by continuous treatment over lifetime.

Mechanistic studies involving promotion and cocarcinogenesis bioassays have not produced convincing evidence that cyclamate promotes bladder cancer development, but it has not been as thoroughly tested in these models as saccharin. Saccharin, on the other hand, clearly promotes bladder tumor development in a variety of initiation-promotion models, employing several different physical and chemical initiating agents. Additional mechanistic studies appear to demonstrate that it is sodium saccharin and not saccharin per se that promotes bladder tumor development. The marked physiological changes induced in urine composition by high dose sodium saccharin administration appear to be closely associated with tumor formation.

The relevance to humans of experimental initiation-promotion models of carcinogenesis is uncertain. The unique conditions under which sodium saccharin promotes tumor development are unlikely to occur in humans since humans would not be exposed to sufficiently high doses of sodium saccharin to induce the marked physiological changes which appear to be a prerequisite for tumor development. Similarly, the risk of human cancer from saccharin based upon extrapolation of results from two-generation studies in rats seems unlikely for similar reasons.

In a more general sense, it can safely be stated that few substances have received the degree of regulatory attention that cyclamate and saccharin have. Many of the accepted principles of modern toxicology testing and the evaluation of test results can be traced to experience with these substances. Very often studies on saccharin and cyclamate were flawed because of poor experimental design, poor animal health, and misinterpretation of toxicological findings and their significance. The testing on these substances leads to the clear conclusion that great care must be taken in the design and interpretation of chronic studies and studies involving initiation-promotion protocols. As pointed out by the National Academy of Sciences (1985), a great deal more generic research is required in order to assess the significance to humans of promotion studies conducted in laboratory animals.

REFERENCES

Akaza, H., Murphy, W.M., and Soloway M.S. 1984. Bladder cancer induced by noncarcinogenic substances. *J. Urol.* 131: 152.

Allen, M. J., Boyland, E., Dukes, C. E., Horning, E. S., and Watson, J.G. 1957. Cancer of the urinary bladder induced in mice with metabolites of aromatic amines and tryptophan. *Br. J. of Cancer* 11: 212.

Arnold, D. L., Moodie, C. A., Grice, H. C., Charbonneau, S. M., Stavric, B., Collins, B. T., McGuire P. F., Zawidzka, Z.Z., and Munro, I.C. 1980. Long-term toxicity of ortho-toluenesulfonamide and sodium saccharin in the rat. *Toxic. Appl. Pharmacol.* 52: 113.

Ashby, J. 1985. The genotoxicity of sodium saccharin and sodium chloride in relation to their cancer-promoting properties. *Food Chem. Toxicol.* 23: 507.

Ball, J. K., Field, W. E. H., Roe, F. J.C., and Walters, M. 1964. The carcinogenic and co-carcinogenic effects of paraffin wax pellets and glass beads in the mouse bladder. *Br. J. Urol.* 36: 225.

Bar, F. and Griepentrog, F. 1974. Fehlen einer cancerogenen Wirkung bei Saccharin and Sacchrinnatrium Cyclamaten, ihrem moglichen Stoffwechselmetaboliten Cyclohexylamin sowie einer Mischung aus 10 Teilen Natriumcyclamat und einem Teil Saccharinnatrium. Teil III Cyclamate. *Dtsch. Apoth.* 2: 66.

Brantom, P. G., Gaunt, I. F., and Grasso, P. 1973. Long-term toxicity of sodium cyclamate in mice. *Food Cosmet. Toxicol.* 22: 735.

Bryan, G. T. and Ertürk, E, 1970. Production of mouse urinary bladder carcinomas by sodium cyclamate. *Science* 167: 996.

Bryan, G. T., Ertürk, E., and Yoshida, O. 1970. Production of urinary bladder carcinomas in mice by sodium saccharin. *Science* 168: 1238.

Carson, S. and Vogin, E. E. 1972. *Toxicological, Reproductive and Mutagenic Studies with Cyclohexylamine in Rats.* Food and Drug Research Laboratories, Maspeth, New York.

Clayson, D. B. 1974. Bladder carcinogenesis in rats and mice: Possibility of artifacts. *J. Nat. Cancer Inst.* 52: 1685.

Cohen, S.M., Murasaki, G., Fukushima, S., and Greenfield, R. E. 1982. Effect of regenerative hyperplasia on the urinary bladder: Carcinogenicity of sodium saccharin and N-[4-5-nitro-2-furyl)-2-thiazoly]formamide. *Cancer Res.* 42: 65.

Fitzhugh, O. G., Nelson, A. A., and Frawley, J. P. 1951. A comparison of the chronic toxicities of synthetic sweetening agents. *J. Am. Pharm. Assoc.* 40: 583.

Freidman, L., Richardson, H. L., Richardson, M.E., Lethco, E. J., Wallace, W. C., and Sauro, F. M. 1972. Toxic response of rats to cyclamates in chow and semisynthetic diets. *J. Natl. Cancer Inst.* 49: 751.

Fukushima, S., Friedell, G. H., Jacobs, J. B., and Cohen, S. M. 1981. Effect of L-tryptophan and sodium saccharin on urinary tract carcinogenesis initiated by N-(4-(5-nitro-2-furyl)-2-thiazoly)formamide. *Cancer Res.* 41: 3100.

Fukushima, S., Hagiwara, A., Ogiso, T., Shibata, M., and Ito N. 1983a. Promoting effect of various chemicals in rat urinary bladder carcinogenesis initiated by N-nitroso-n-butyl(4-hydroxybutyl)amine. *Food Chem. Toxicol.* 21: 59.

Fukushima, S., Imaida, K., Sakata, T., Okamura, T., Shibata, M., and Ito, N. 1983b. Promoting effects of sodium L-ascorbate on two stage urinary bladder carcinogenesis in rats. *Cancer Letters* 23: 29.

Fukushima, S., Shibata, M., Kurata, Y., Tamano, S., and Masui, T. 1986a. Changes in the urine and scanning electron microscopically observed appearance of the rat bladder following treatment with tumour promoters. *Jap. J. Cancer Res.* (GANN) 77: 1074.

Fukushima, S., Shibata, M. Kurata, Y., Tamano, S., and Masui, T. 1986a. Changes in the urine and scanning electron microscopically observed appearance of the rat bladder following treatment with tumour promoters. *Jap. J. Cancer Res.* (GANN) 77: 1074.

Fukushima, S., Shibata, M., Shirai, T., Tamano, S., and Ito, N. 1986b. Roles of urinary sodium ion concentration and pH in promotion by ascorbic acid of urinary bladder carcinogenesis in rats. *Cancer Res.* 46: 1623.

Fukushima, S., Thamavit, W., Kurata, Y., and Ito, N. 1986c. Sodium citrate: a promoter of bladder carcinogenesis, *Jap J. Cancer Res.* (GANN) 77: 2.

Gaunt, I. F., Hardy, J., Grasso, P., Gangolli, S. D., and Butterworth, K. R. 1974a. *The Long-Term Toxicity of Cyclohexylamine Hydrochloride in the Rat.* The British Industrial Biological Research Association, Surrey, England.

Gaunt, I. F., Hardy, J., Grasso, P., Gangolli, S. D., and Butterworh, K.R. 1974b. The long-term toxicity of cyclohexylamine hydrochloride in the rat. *Food Cosmet. Toxicol.* 14: 255.

Hardy, J., Gunt, I. F., Hooson, J., Hendry, R. J., and Butterworth, K. R. 1974. *Long Term Toxicity of Cyclohexylamine hydrochloride in mice.* The British Industrial Biological Research Association, Surrey, England.

Hardy, J., Gaunt, I.F., Hooson, J., Hendry, R. J., and Butterworthy, K.R. 1976. Long-term toxicity of cyclohexylamine hydrochloride in mice. *Food Cosmet. Toxicol.* 14: 269.

Hasegawa, R. and Cohen, S.M. 1986. The effect of different salts of saccharin on the rat urinary bladder. *Cancer Letters* 30: 261.

Hasegawa, R., Greenfield, R. E., Murasaki, G., Suzuki, T., and Cohen, S. M. 1985. Initiation of urinary bladder carcinogenesis in rats by freeze ulceration with sodium saccharin promotion. *Cancer Res.* 45: 1469.

Hicks, R. M. and Chowaniec, J. 1977. The important of synergy between weak carcinogens in the induction of bladder cancer in experimental animals and humans. *Cancer Res.* 37: 2943.

Hicks, R.M., Wakefield, J. St. J., and Chowaniec, J. 1975. Evaluation of a new model to detect bladder carcinogens or co-carcinogens: Results obtained with saccharin, cyclamate and cyclophosphamide. *Chem.-Biol. Interact.* 11: 225.

Homburger, F., Russfield, A. B., Weisburger, E. K., and Weisburger J. H. 1973. Final Report: Studies on Saccharin and Cyclamate. Bio-Research Consultants, Cambridge, MA.

Hoosen, J., Hicks, R. M., Grasso, P., and Chowaniec, J. 1980. Ortho-Toluene sulphonamide and saccharin in the promotion of bladder cancer in the rat. *Br. J. Cancer* 42: 129.

IARC. 1980. IARC *Monographs on the Evaluation of the Carcinogenic Risk of Chemicals to Humans: Some Non-Nutritive Sweetening Agents.* Vol. 22. Intl. Agency for Research on Cancer, Lyon, France.

Ikeda, Y., Horiuchi, S., Furuya, T., Kawamata, K., Kaneko, T., and Uchida, O. 1975. *Long-term Toxicity Study of Sodium Cyclamate and Saccharin Sodium in Rats.* Department of Toxicology, National Institute of Hygienic Sciences, Tokyo, Japan.

Ito, N., Fukushima, S., Shirai, T., and Nakanishi, K. 1983. Effects of promoters on N-butyl-N-(4-hydroxybutyl) nitrosamine-induced urinary bladder carcinogenesis in the rat. *Environmental Health Perspectives* 50: 61.

Kroes, R., Berkvens, J. M., Peters, P. W. J., Verschuuren, H.G., de Vries, T., and van Esch. G. J. 1975. *Long Term Toxicity and Reproduction Study (In-*

cluding a Teratogenicity Study) with Cyclamate, Saccharine and Cyclohex-ylamine. National Institute of Public Health, Bilthoven, the Netherlands.

Kroes, R., Peters, P. W. J., Berkvens, J. M., Verschuuren, H.G., de Vries, T., and van Esch, G. J. 1977. Long term toxicity and reproduction study (including a teratogenicity study) with cyclamate, saccharin and cyclohex-ylamine. *Toxicology* 8: 285.

Lutz, W. K. and Schlatter, C. 1977. Saccharin does not bind to DNA of liver or bladder in the rat. *Chem. Biol. Interactions* 19: 253.

Mohr, U., Green, U., Althoff, J., and Schneider, P. 1979. Syncarcinogenic action of saccharin and sodium cyclamate in the induction of bladder tumors in MNU-pretreated rats. *Health and Sugar Substitutes. Proceedings of the ERGOB Conference on Sugar Substitutes* Geneva, Switzerland, (Ed.) Goggenheim, B., p. 64. S. Karger, Basel, Switzerland.

Muranyi-Kovacs, I., Rudali, G., and Aussepe, L. 1975. *The Carcinogenicity of Sodium Cyclamate in Combination with Other Oncogenic Agents.* Labaratoire de Genetique, Fondation Curie, Institut de Radium, Paris.

Murasaki, G. and Cohen, S. M. 1983. Co-carcinogenicity of sodium saccharin and N-4-(5-nitro-2-furyl)-2-thiazolyl formamide for the urinary bladder. *Carcinogenesis* 4: 97.

Murphy, W. M., Blatnik, A. F., Shelton, T. B., and Soloway, M. S. 1986. Carcinogenesis in mammalian urothelium: Changes induced by non-carcinogenic substances and chronic indwelling catheters. *J. Urol.* 135: 840.

NAS. 1985. *Evaluation of Cyclamate for Carcinogenicity.* National Academy Press. Washington, DC.

Nakanishi, K., Hagiwara, A., Shibata, M., Imaida, K., Tatematsu, M., and Ito, N. 1980. Dose response of saccharin in induction of urinary bladder hyperplasia in Fischer 344 rats treated with N-butyl-N-(4-hydroxybutyl) nitrosamine. *J. Nat. Cancer Inst.* 65: 1005.

NCI (National Cancer Institute). 1976. *Report of the Temporary Committee for the Review of Data on Carcinogenicity of Cyclamate.* Division of Cancer Cause and Prevention, National Cancer Institute, Bethesda, MD.

NRC (National Research Council). 1969. *Report of the Ad Hoc Committee on Nonnutritive Sweeteners.* National Academy of Sciences, Washington, DC.

Oser, B. L. 1985. Highlights in the history of saccharin toxicology. *Food Chem. Toxicol* 23: 4/5 535.

Oser, B. L., Carson, S., Cox, G. E., Vogin, E. E., and Sternbert, S.S. 1976.

Long-term and multigeneration toxicity studies with cyclohexylamine hydrochloride. *Toxicology* 6: 47.

Plank, J. 1970. *Two-Year Chronic Oral Toxicity of Cyclohexylamine Sulfate—Albino Rats.* Report to Abbott Laboratories. IBT No. B5249. Industrial Bio-Test Laboratories, Northbrook, Illinois.

Pliss, G.V. 1958. Carcinogenic activity of dicyclohexylamine and its nitrite salts. *Vopr. Onkol.* 4: 659.

Report of an Expert Panel. 1985. Saccharin—Current status. *Food Chem. Toxicol.* 23(4/5): 543.

Roe, F. J. C., Levy, L. S., and Carter, R. L. 1970. Feeding studies on sodium cyclamate, saccharin and sucrose for carcinogenic and tumor–promoting activity. *Food Cosmet. Toxicol.* 8: 135.

Rudali, G., Coezy, E., and Muranyi-Kovacs, I. 1969. Investigations on the carcinogenic activity of sodium cyclamate in mice. *C.R. Acad. Sci. Paris.* 269: 1910.

Schoenig, G. P. and Anderson, R. L. 1985. The effects of high dietary levels of sodium saccharin on mineral and water balance and related parameters in rats. *Food Chem. Toxicol.* 23(4/5): 465.

Schoenig, G. P., Goldenthal, E.I., Geil, R. G., Frith, C. H., Richter, W.R., and Carlborg, F.W. 1985. Evaluation of the dose response and in utero exposure to saccharin in the rat. *Food Chem. Toxicol.* 23(4/5): 475.

Schmahl, D. 1973. Absence of carcinogenic activity of cyclamate, cyclohexylamine and saccharin in rats. *Arneim. Forsch.* 23: 1466.

Schmahl, D. and Habs, M. 1980. Absence of carcinogenic response to cyclamate and saccharin in Sprague-Dawley rats after transplacental application. *Arzneim.-Forsch.* 30: 1905.

Schmahl, D. and Kruger, F.W. 1972. Lack of syncarcinogenic action of cyclamate in the induction of bladder cancer by butyl-butanol-nitrosamine in rats. *Arzneim-Forsch.* 22: 999.

Shibata, M. A., Nakanishi, K., Shibata, M., Masui, T., and Ito, N. 1986. Promoting effect of sodium chloride in 2-stage urinary bladder carcinogenesis in rats initiated in N-butyl-N-(4-hydroxybutyl)-nitrosamine. *Urol. Res.* 14: 201.

Taylor, J. M., Weinberger, M. A., and Friedman, L. 1980. Chronic toxicity and carcinogenicity to the urinary bladder of sodium saccharin in the *in utero*-exposed rat. *Toxicol. Appl. Pharmacol.* 54: 57.

Tisdel, M. O., Nees, P. O., Harris, D. L., and Derse, P. H. 1974. Long term feeding of saccharin in rats. In Symposium *Sweeteners.* (Ed.) Inglett, G. E., p. 145. Avi Publishing Co., Westport, CT.

West, R. W., Sheldon, W. G., Gaylor, D. W., Haskin, M. G., Delongchamp, R. R., and Kadlubar, S. F. 1986. The effects of saccharin on the development of neoplastic lesions initiated with n-methyl-n-nitroso-urea in the rat urothelium. *Fund. Appl. Toxicol.* 7: 585.

7

Glutathione and Vitamin E in Protection Against Mutagens and Carcinogens

Donald J. Reed
Oregon State University
Corvallis, Oregon

INTRODUCTION

The pioneering work of the Millers (1966) demonstrated the metabolic activation of foreign chemicals to reactive intermediates capable of modification of macromolecules. Evidence supports the view that metabolism of chemical carcinogens has an important role in chemical carcinogenesis. The roles of cytochrome P-450 enzymes in such metabolism appear to indicate that the composition of these enzymes can affect in vitro and in vivo metabolism of chemicals in both animal models and humans (for a review see Guengerich, 1988). The tenet that bioactivation of foreign compounds yields reactive intermediates and metabolites capable of cellular interactions is well established for many different classes of chemical compounds (Anders, 1985). Whereas these interactions may be enzymatic or nonenzymatic in nature, formation of electrophiles and free radicals by such bioactivation processes is well documented. Moreover, the significance of various protective enzymes in the control of reactive metabolites is becoming more evident. These enzymes are thought to control the concentration of chemical intermediates which are the ultimate carcinogenic species of carcinogens. It has been concluded that these enzymes in general make an important contribution to species differences in susceptibilities to chemical carcinogens (Oesch, 1987). The enzymatic detoxification enzymes, which act as protective enzymes, and their metabolic pathways, which describe the reactions they catalyze, now represent well-defined processes for mutagen and carcinogen detoxification. However, the dynamics of these processes, such as competitive detoxitication pathways, determination of pool sizes of intermediates, lifetimes of these intermediates, rates of turnover of precursors of conjugate formation, and macromolecular adducts are not so well delineated.

The free-radical oxidant species of oxygen and hydrogen peroxide are being increasingly implicated as a major contributor to cellular injury in human disease. Such processes are dependent on the types of free radicals, and the interrelationship of oxidant-damaging mechanisms are complex. The features of radical processes and their implications in human disease have been reviewed recently (Sies, 1985; Halliwell, 1987).

When genetic and somatic alterations of cellular constituents by reactive metabolites occur, the extent of these alterations is determined by the status of the cellular defense systems that protect cellular constituents. This chapter will examine the general nature of reactive metabolites of mutagens and carcinogens in foods, their secondary reactive products, and the types of events involved in cellular protection. Pertinent to "built-in" protection at the cellular level during chemical exposure is the status of naturally occurring substances that modify mutagenic and carcinogenic effects. Additionally, compartmentalization of cellular protective systems must be considered since its role is beginning to be understood relative to cell injury during chemical exposure.

Cell protection is dependent upon the various inherent features of the cellular defense systems. The protection of vital cellular constituents appear dependent upon the structural integrity of the cell, the compartmentalization of both functions and constituents, and the presence of certain enzymes. These enzymes include glutathione S-transferases (GSTs), epoxide hydrolases, superoxide dismutases, catalase, glutathione peroxidases, and glutathione reductase. Essential low molecular weight constituents include water, thiol compounds (particularly glutathione), vitamins C and E, and the vitamin A precursor β-carotene, although an absolute requirement of any one of these agents for cellular protection has not been ascertained.

GENERAL CONCEPTS OF PROTECTION

Protection Against Electrophiles

Cellular defense against reactive intermediates of mutagens and carcinogens can be defined or expressed on the basis that reactive intermediates are organic reagents that possess a low electron density. These agents attack the cellular constituents at positions of high electron density and are therefore referred to as electrophilic reagents or electrophiles. Such reactive electrophiles with their electron-deficient centers are subject to attack by anions (negatively charged) such as hydroxide, or by an electron-rich center such as the nitrogen atom in amines. These electron-rich entities are referred to as nucleophilic reagents or nucleophiles. This electrophile/nucleophile dichotomy has been described as a unique case of the acid/base concept (Sykes, 1975). A Lewis acid becomes an electrophile by accepting electrons, and a Lewis base becomes a nucleophile by providing the electrons. Hard and soft electrophiles and nucleophiles can also show a relationship with oxidizing and reducing agents even when covalent bonding is not accompaying changes in electron states between two such reagents.

Swain and Scott (1953) described a linear free-energy relationship for nucleophilic substitution reactions that has been extremely useful to define nucleic acid alkylation. The relative nucleophilic strength of a nucleophile site is correlated with the ratio of the alkylation reaction rate of that nucleophilic site to the rate with water. The nucleophilic strength approximates the propensity of electrons at the reaction site to participate in covalent bond-forming activities (Jensen, 1978). Analysis of alkylation reactions with a variety of reaction sites over a range of nucleophilic strengths can indicate the sensitivity of the alkylating agent (electrophile) towards differences in nucleophilic strength, which is designated as n for such reagents (Table 7.1) (Koskikallio, 1969a, b). A greater selectivity of an alkylating agent is indicated by a higher substrate s-value, which can be related to the degree of S_N2 character of the reaction. Methyl bromide was chosen as a standard substrate for which $s = 1.00$ (Swain and Scott, 1953). The substrate s-values for N-methyl-N-nitrosoureas (MNU) and N-ethyl-N-nitrosourea (ENU) have estimated to be 0.42 and 0.26, respectively (Veleminsky et al., 1970). The larger the s-value, the greater the selectivity due to a greater tendency to react in a concerted fashion rather than the parent molecule decomposing to yield an alkylating species with less selectivity of target molecules for alkylation. Thus MNU reacts more selectively than ENU, and that behavior indicates that the reactive entity is not a carbonium ion but rather an intermediate occurring prior to the reaction chain (Veleminsky et al., 1970).

With target molecules, as a general rule, the higher the nucleophilic constant, the greater the effectiveness as the nucleophile functions as an electrophile scavenger. The ability of thiols to protect by being alkylated in lieu of cellular macromolecules depends greatly on the percentage of the thiol group present as an anion. Cysteine has a sixfold greater ionization than glutathione at pH 7.5 (Table 7.2), but the relative concentration

TABLE 7.1   Nucleophilic Constants[a]

Nucleophile	Nucleophilicity constant (n)
H_2O	0.01
SO_4^{2-}	2.5
CH_3OO^-	2.76
Cl^-	2.99
HPO_4^{2-}	3.52
HCO_3^{2-}	3.8
Br^-	4.02
$(NH_2)_2CS$	4.1
$C_6H_5NH_2$	4.35[b]
SCN^-	4.80
I^-	4.93
SO_3^{2-}	5.1
CN^-	5.1
$S_2O_3^{2-}$	6.35

[a]*Koskikallio (1969a).*
[b]*Koskikallio (1969b).*

TABLE 7.2   Thiol Groups in Cysteinyl Derivatives[a]

Compound	Percentage in the thiolate form at pH 7.5
L-Cysteinyl ester	16
L-Cysteinyl glycine	11
L-Cysteine	6
Glutathione	1

[a]*Source: Benesch and Benesch (1955).*

of glutathione (GSH) to cysteine (in liver it is about 50 to 1) gives an overall total reactivity that is greater with GSH due to its high concentration in most tissues.

Protection Against Free Radicals

Radicals are involved in the bioactivation of many mutagens and carcinogens. As chemical reactants they are less susceptible to variations in electron density than the substrate being attacked. Reactions of this type are highly susceptible to the presence of agents that either liberate or scavenge radicals (Sykes, 1975). Oxygen bioactivation can produce superoxide anion radical, hydrogen peroxide, and hydroxyl free radical. These reduced species of dioxygen (molecular oxygen) are endogenous to cells and tissues. Certain foreign chemicals cause an increase in the cellular content of these reactive intermediates in oxygen metabolism and are termed redox cycling agents (Kappus and Sies, 1981).

Cellular constituents that protect against free radical–mediated cellular damage reside in the various subcellular organelle compartments. These compartments are important, but attention must be paid to the distribution of both the prooxidants and antioxidants between the aqueous and the lipid phases. Additionally, oxidation-reduction (redox) potentials vary with the degree of complexation with metal ions, macromolecules, and so on. Thus, the general nature of the protective systems and their reactions are influenced by the particular milieu of the cellular interior.

The specific enzymes which have a major responsibility for cellular protection against oxygen-mediated toxicity include the glutathione peroxidase/reductase redox cycle enzymes, catalase (Cat), and superoxide dismutases (SOD). These enzymes catalyze reactions that cause rapid decreases in the concentration of reduced oxygen intermediates (Fig. 7.1) (Sies et al., 1983). Glutathione is a substrate for the glutathione peroxidase/reductase redox system (an enzyme reaction), but in nonenzymic reactions the cell primarily utilizes β-carotene, α-tocopherol, ascorbic acid, and certain extracellular agents including uric acid, bilirubin, and carnosine may be important cellular protective agents (Ames, 1987).

Correlation of cellular damage by reduced oxygen species with mutagenic and carcinogenic processes, particularly promotion, is a major thrust of current carcinogenesis research as described by Bailey *et al.* (1988).

TYPES OF PROTECTION

Water

Water at intracellular concentrations up to 55M participates in cellular protection against reactive intermediates by providing a low concentration of hydroxide ion as a nucleophile at physiological pH. The formation of corresponding alcohols of carbon electrophiles including the 2-chloroethyl carbonium ion (Reed et al., 1975) is evidence of such protection. Nonenzymatic competitive reactions with halide anions, oxygen-, nitrogen-, or sulfur-containing anions in proportion to their nucleophilicity and reaction rate constants are described in the early work of Swain and Scott (1953).

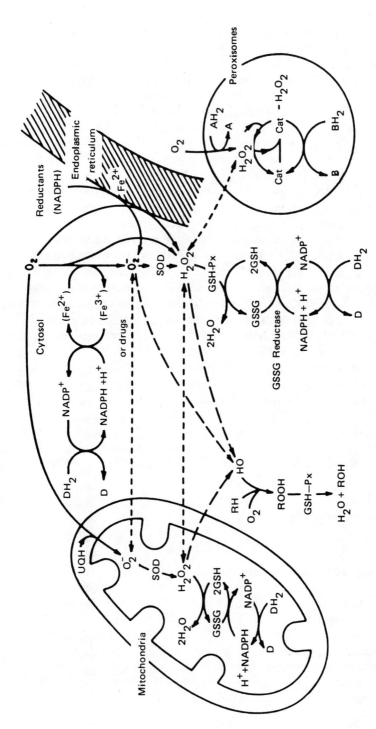

FIG. 7.1 Schematic diagram of cellular protection against oxygen-mediated toxicity. UQH: semiquinone of ubiquinone. D, DH AH₂, BH₂; various cellular substrates involved in enzymatic redox reactions. (*Modified from Sies et al., 1983.*)

Water has a vital role in cellular protection as a substrate for epoxide hydrolases, which convert epoxides to the corresponding diols. Although this role for water can be generally thought of as a protection mechanism, the conversion of certain arene oxides to the corresponding *trans*-dihydrodiols is a bioactivation step. For example, the 7,8-epoxide of benzo[a]pyrene, upon conversion to 7,8-*trans*-dihydrodiol, serves as the precursor of 7,8-*trans*-dihydrodiol 9,10-epoxide of benzo[a]pyrene, which is a potent mutagen and carcinogen (Jerina, 1983). Thus, polycyclic aromatic hydrocarbon epoxides present a most interesting challenge to the cellular protection systems.

The initial 7,8-epoxide undergoes "detoxification" with water to form the corresponding *trans*-dihydrodiol. Failure of an adequate cellular elimination of this product can result in formation of the "ultimate carcinogen" from the "proximate" form with a 9,10-epoxide ring, which is in the bay region of benzo[a]pyrene. The four possible metabolites are optically active isomers of the 7,8-diol-9,10-epoxide. The (+)-(7R,8S)-diol-(9S,10R)-epoxide (Fig. 7.2) is the isomer responsible for nearly all of the tumorigenic activity attributed to benzo[a]pyrene (Buening et al., 1978).

But why is one isomer much more carcinogenic than the other three isomers? One can suggest several important factors. The active isomer has an epoxide group that forms part of a bay region of the hydrocarbon. Although this isomer is predicted to have high chemical reactivity (Jerina, 1983), it shares the common features of all four isomers, that is, it is a part of the bay region and has a sterically hampered enzymatic detoxification of the epoxide function (Harvey, 1981).

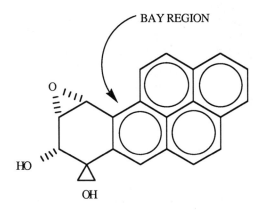

FIG. 7.2 Structure of the first ultimate carcinogen identified for any member of the polycyclic hydrocarbon class: (+)-(7R,8S)-dihydroxy-(9S,10R)-epoxy-7,8,9,10-tetrahydrobenzo(a)pyrene.

Many polycyclic aromatic hydrocarbons have been examined as candidates for proximate and ultimate carcinogens, and all the reactive intermediates found conformed to the bay region theory (for a review see Conney, 1982).

Protection by epoxide hydrolase activity can vary markedly as a result of differences in the efficiency of catalysis with different substrates. Microsomal epoxide hydrolase catalysis of the hydration of epoxides is thought to occur via a general base mechanism with the nucleophilic attack of water or hydroxide ion on the oxirane carbon (Hanzlik et al., 1976; Dansette et al., 1978; Armstrong et al., 1980). Efficiency of catalysis is illustrated with the hydration of phenanthrene 9,10-oxide. The enzyme rate over that of hydroxide ion (10^8) and spontaneous water reactions (10^{11}) is 10^3 times more efficient than hydronium ion catalysis (Armstrong et al., 1980).

Strong support for the concept of hampered detoxication rates for the ultimate carcinogens comes from a study of compounds that can cause destruction of the reactive epoxide group. A naturally occurring plant phenol with a high affinity for the diol epoxide through π-π interactions (between the aromatic regions of the diol epoxide and the blocking agent) was found that also had acidic and nucleophilic groups that are able to participate in the destruction of the epoxide group. This compound, elagic acid, reacts rapidly with benzo[a]pyrene-7,8-diol 9,10-epoxide to form a *cis* adduct that markedly inhibits mutagenicity in vitro (Sayer et al., 1982; Wood et al., 1982). Catalysis rates of epoxide hydrolases and glutathione *S*-transferases vary widely due to the nature of the polycyclic aromatic hydrocarbon epoxide isomers (see review Hernandez and Bend, 1982). Therefore, it was not too surprising that glutathione was shown to conjugate with (±)-benzo[a]pyrene-7,8-dihydrodiol and (±)-benzo[a]pyrene-7,8-diol 9,10 epoxide when Jernström et al. (1982) used isolated hepatocytes prepared from 3-methylchloranthrene–treated rats. More importantly, the intracellular level of glutathione must be maintained to prevent the reactive intermediates from interacting with the DNA in intact hepatocytes (Jernström et al., 1982).

Thiols

Glutathione (L-γ-glutamyl-L-cysteinylglycine) accounts for about 90% of the intracellular nonprotein thiol content. In the hepatocyte, the major subcellular compartments of glutathione appear to be the cytoplasm (85–90%) and the mitochondrial matrix (10–15%). The glutathione concentration of the matrix appears to be as high or higher than that in the cytoplasm (Meredith and Reed, 1982). GSH is resistant to typical proteases by virtue of the γ-glutamyl linkage. Hydrolytic degradation of GSH and its conjugates is mainly an extracellular process catalyzed by a specific enzyme known as γ-glutamyltransferase. Thus, GSH is an ideal cellular constituent for cellular protection systems.

The intracellular presence of a foreign chemical often requires that GSH function in a dual role for maintenance of cellular protection. Formation of GSH conjugates has been shown with many carcinogens (for reviews, see Boyland and Chasseaud, 1968; Chasseaud, 1979). The role of GSH as the main intracellular interceptor of reactive, electrophilic compounds is becoming well established. Early studies that demonstrated liver necrosis as a result of giving bromobenzene or acetaminophen led investigators to the determination that reactive intermediates can react enzymatically and nonenzymatically with GSH at rates sufficient to deplete the pool of glutathione in the liver. Because the hepatotoxicity of these and other similar foreign chemicals can be mitigated by prior treatment with cysteine, acetylcysteine, or methionine, it follows that GSH biosynthesis, rather than direct interaction of these thiols, provides the majority of the protective effects.

Protection provided by GSH against chemical damage is altered by various factors. The liver GSH content is altered by diurnal or circadian variations as well as by fasting. Fasting of rats for 1 or 2 days decreases the level of liver GSH to about 50 to 70% of the level in fed animals (Leaf and Neuberger, 1947; Maruyama et al., 1968; Tateishi et al., 1974). Diurnal variation of liver GSH content results in higher GSH concentrations at night and early morning and lower concentrations in the late afternoon, with maximum variation of 25 to 30% (Beck et al., 1958; Calcutt and Ting, 1969; Boyd et al., 1979).

Maintenance of intracellular GSH appears totally dependent on in situ biosynthesis of GSH. For example, rapid GSH depletion and resynthesis, after 2-chloroethanol treatment of rats, requires rapid replacement of the cysteine pool by either influx of cysteine or cystine or a conversion of methionine and serine to cysteine via the cystathione pathway (White, 1976). Thus far, however, it is only the hepatocyte and no other cell type that has been demonstrated to utilize the cystathionine pathway to an appreciable extent during GSH depletion and resynthesis (Reed, 1983).

In the liver, methionine metabolism is a dynamic cycle with a continual flow between methionine and homocysteine, in which the only outlet for the intermediates is the irreversible utilization of homocysteine to form cystathionine (Finkelstein, 1974). In fed rats, hepatic methionine sulfur has a half-life of about 5 minutes, and 40–60% of the tissue homocysteine is diverted to cystathionine formation at each pass through the cycle. During dietary protein restriction the half-life of methionine sulfur increases and the proportion of homocysteine diverted to cystathionine decreases, thereby conserving the tissue methionine content (Finkelstein, 1974). The interplay between dietary cystine and methionine for the maintenance of liver cysteine, and in turn GSH, is an important aspect of dietary influence on carcinogenesis.

Glutathione S-Transferases

The suggested nomenclature of the glutathione S-transferases (GSTs) is based on subunit structure of the isozymes (Jakoby et al., 1984). In addition, these enzymes have been divided into three classes based on structural and functional similarities (Mannervik et al., 1985). These three classes are by isolectric point (pI) and distinguishing substrates. The classes are α, μ, and π with pIs of alkaline (>8.0), neutral (7–8), and acidic (<7.0) nature, respectively. The substrates used for classification are organic hydroperoxides, epoxides, and ethacrynic acid, respectively. An important aspect of the GSTs is their induction and variable expression which has been reviewed recently (Boyer, 1988).

GSTs have a high specificity for glutathione, which is bound with a high affinity (approx. 0.3 mM) to provide an enzyme-bound glutathione thiolate anion (GS^-) at an estimated intracellular concentration in the liver ranging up to about 0.1 mM. The combined effects of substrate affinities and high concentration of substrate-bound nucleophilic anions provide a very effective conjugate formation. Reactive chemicals, particularly those which can be classed as hydrophilic electrophiles, are effectively sequestered by GSTs. These transferases are present in liver in higher concentrations; approximately 10% of the rat hepatic cystosolic protein is GSTs (Jakoby, 1978).

Because many oxygen-containing compound exist in cells, one might think that compounds, such as a sulfur compound like glutathione, are not needed to react with electrophiles. However, as a general rule, sulfur compounds have been assumed to be about 1000 times better nucleophiles than oxygen compounds (Janssen, 1972). Ketterer et al. (1983) have characterized GSH and its thiolate anion (GS^-) as strong nucleophiles which react best with "soft" electrophilic centers. When the electrophilic center is soft, the nucleophile causes polarization of the electrophile, and a rapid reaction ensues. In contrast, a "hard" electrophilic center polarizes a weak nucleophile so that there is much less dependency on the nucleophile, and often competing reactions with water or other compounds result. The efficacy of glutathione against most carbon-centered electrophiles, which have hard electrophilic centers, is not understood.

An interesting comparison of reactivity towards acrylontrile has been made between $HS\text{-}CH_2CH_2COOH$ (β-mercaptopropionic acid) and $NH_2\text{-}CH_2CH_2COOH$ (β-alanine) since the thiol and amino groups of these compounds have identical pK_a values (10.05–10.06) (Friedman et al., 1965). Steric environments for these compounds are also comparable. Therefore, the 280-fold greater reactivity of the sulfur group compared to the amino group must be explained on the basis of differences in reactivities, which depend on polarizabilities of nonbonded electrons on nitrogen and sulfur, charge distributions in ground and transition states, and solvation factors (Friedman et al., 1965). The thiol group of GSH has a pK_a of 8.56, and the ratio of rate constants was 3×10^3 when the reaction of GSH with acrylonitrile was determined at pH 10.5 (GS^- only).

At physiological pH, 99% of the glutathione exists as glutathione and 1% as the anion, GS^-. Because the reactive rate with electrophiles is about three orders of magnitude greater for the anion, it is not surprising that GSTs catalyze GSH conjugation reactions by binding GSH, promoting the formation of the anion, as well as by binding lipophilic electrophiles.

Thiols and Radicals

Protection by thiols against free radicals can be described by either a hydrogen donation reaction:

$$R\cdot + R'SH \rightarrow RH + R'S\cdot$$

or a charge transfer reaction:

$$R^{\overset{+}{\cdot}} + R'SH \rightarrow R + R'S\cdot + H^+$$

The thiol radical $RS\cdot$ is probably the most prominent sulfur-centered radical within cells and is formed either by hydrogen atom abstraction from thiols by other radicals ($R\cdot + R'SH \rightarrow RH + R'S\cdot$), by reduction ($RSSR + R'_{aq} \rightarrow RS\cdot + RS^- + R'_{aq}$), or displacement reactions of disulfides ($RSSR + PO_3\cdot^{2-} \rightarrow RS\cdot + RSPO_3^{2-}$). Sulfur-centered radical anion formation results from the stabilization of the thiol radical ($RS\cdot + RS^- \rightarrow RSSR^-$). The thiol radical may interact with oxygen to form peroxysulfenyl radicals such as the glutathione peroxysulfenyl radical ($GSO\cdot0$). The reaction of these radicals has been reviewed (Ross, 1988). Radical cation formation can occur with disulfides by a one-electron oxidation to yield RSSR$^{+\cdot}$. Because sulfur-centered radicals undergo many types of radical reactions, including rearrangement, displacement, fragmentation, addition, abstraction, and redox reactions, the potential for multiple cellular effects is obvious.

Formation of xenobiotic radicals may lead to the formation of radicals including the glutathionyl radical of GSH. The majority of thiol radicals generated in biological systems undergo reactions leading to superoxide anion radical generation from O_2 (Subrahmanyam and O'Brien, 1985; Ross, 1988).

An important aspect of oxidative challenge by exogenous thiols such as cysteamine is the effect of thiol-disulfide interchange reactions. Rate constants and equilibrium constants for thiol-disulfide interchange reactions involving glutathione disulfide have been reported for a variety of reducing thiols (Szajewski and Whitesides, 1980). The rate of reduction follows an expression derived from the relative pK_a values of the reducing thiols and the thiols derived from the disulfide. Interestingly, the rate of reduction does not necessarily correlate with the equilibrium constant for the reduction of a disulfide by a thiol (Szajewski and Whitesides, 1980). A S_N2 displacement reaction characterizes such thiolate-disulfide interchanges.

$$RSH \rightleftharpoons RS^- + H^+$$

$$RS^- + GSSG \rightleftharpoons GSSR + GS^-$$

$$RS^- + GSSR \rightleftharpoons RSSR + GS^-$$

$$GS^- + H^+ \rightleftharpoons GSH$$

The susceptibility of strong reducing thiols to autoxidation, including protein thiols,

$$2\ RSH + O_2 \rightarrow RSSR + H_2O_2$$

$$RSSR + GS^- \rightleftharpoons RSSG + RS^-$$

$$RSSG + GS^- \rightleftharpoons RSH + GSSG$$

and hydrogen peroxide production means that protection of intracellular thiols is a complex process. GSH is thought to be important in limiting the interaction of reactive thiols with molecular oxygen. Thus, thiols are generally given a protective role in the prevention of lipid peroxide formation. However, thiols may promote lipid peroxidation under certain in vitro conditions. Recent studies have suggested that certain thiols may reduce iron (Fe^{3+}) directly, and, in turn, iron may undergo autoxidation without an O_2^- intermediate:

$$2\ Fe^{2+} + O_2 + 2\ H^+ \rightarrow 2\ Fe^{3+} + H_2O_2$$

Therefore, a thiol-dependent lipid peroxidation may occur by a direct reduction of iron by thiols followed by initiation of

$$RS^- + Fe^{3+} \rightarrow Fe^{2+} + RS \cdot$$

lipid peroxidation by the thiol radical that is independent of superoxide anion radical (Tien et al., 1982). Such reactions may have important contributions to the promotion of carcinogenesis (Cerutti, 1985).

Vitamin E

Vitamin E (Fig. 7.3) is an efficient inhibitor of lipid peroxidatioin in vivo (for review see Tappel, 1979). Autoxidation, in simple terms, is a chain reaction and is in the following reaction scheme of Burton and Ingold (1981). RH represents the organic substrate:

Initiation:	$RH \rightarrow R \cdot$ or $ROO \cdot$	(1)
Propagation:	$R \cdot + O_2 \rightarrow ROO \cdot$	(2)
	$ROO \cdot + HR' \rightarrow ROOH + R'$	(3a)
	$ROO \cdot + R'H \rightarrow ROOR' + H \cdot$	(3b)
Termination:	$ROO \cdot + ROO \cdot \rightarrow$ nonradical products	(4)

with $ROO \cdot$ the peroxy radical as the product.

Several individual tocopherols constitute vitamin E, and the relative and the absolute antioxidant effectiveness in vitro has only recently been clarified (Burton and Ingold, 1981). These chain-breaking phenolic antioxidants (ArOH) shorten the oxidation chain. Whereas chain termination by reaction (Veleminsky et al., 1970) is suppressed, termination may occur by reactions (Reed et al., 1975; Jerina, 1983), with n being the stoichiometric factor for the antioxidant.

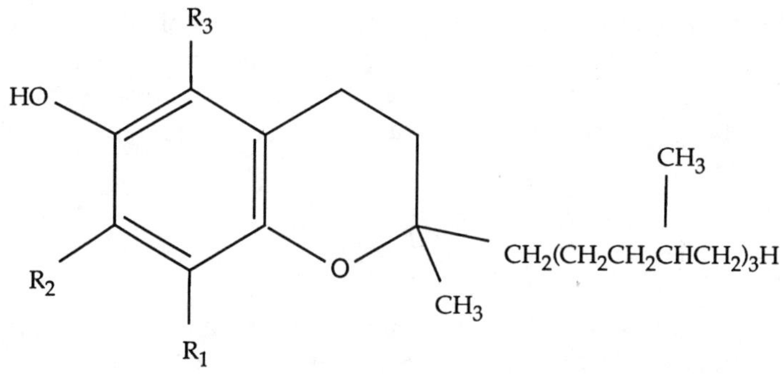

α-Tocopherol (α-T): $R_1 = R_2 = R_3 = CH_3$
β-Tocopherol (β-T): $R_1 = R_3 = CH_3$; $R_2 = H$
γ-Tocopherol (γ-T): $R_1 = R_2 = CH_3$; $R_3 = H$
δ-Tocopherol (δ-T): $R_1 = CH_3$; $R_2 = R_3 = H$

FIG. 7.3   Structure of vitamin E.

$$ROO \cdot + ArOH \rightarrow ROOH + ArO \cdot \qquad (5)$$

$$(n - 1) ROO \cdot + ArO \cdot \rightarrow \text{nonradical products} \qquad (6)$$

In an inhibited reaction in which all $ArO \cdot$ are destroyed by reaction (6), the rate of autoxidation has been described by the following equation:

$$\frac{-d[O_2]}{dt} = \frac{k_3[RH]R_i}{nk_5[ArOH]}$$

where R_i is the rate of chain initiation.

The abstraction of peroxyl radicals of the phenolic hydrogens from these tocopherols has been described as the rate constant k_5. The values of k_5 for α-, β-, γ-, and δ-tocopherols are 23.5, 16.6, 15.9, and 6.5×10^5 M^{-1} sec^{-1}, respectively, at 30°C (Burton and Ingold, 1981). Each tocopherol was found to react with exactly two peroxyl radicals, and all the tocopherols appear to be exceptionally good chain-breaking antioxidants in vitro. Further, the data of Burton and Ingold (1981) are in agreement with in vivo tests of the relative biological activities of these tocopherols(T): α-T > β-T > γ-T > δ-T (Century and Horwitt, 1965).

Covalent Binding of Reactive Intermediates

During the past two decades, it has become generally accepted that chemically inert foreign compounds can be transformed to chemically reactive intermediates that react covalently with cellular macromolecules as well as with low molecular weight nucleophiles.

The Millers pioneered in establishing the transformation processes of the endoplasmic reticulum, and they advanced our understanding of covalent interactions as related to specific chemical carcinogens (Miller and Miller, 1966).

Chemically reactive metabolites of chemicals have been shown to bind to cellular proteins including endoplasmic reticulum (Uehleke, 1974; Raha et al., 1976), nuclear (Ketterer, 1980; MacLeod et al., 1980; Stout et al., 1980) and cytosolic proteins (Jakoby and Keen, 1977;Ohmi et al., 1981; Reeve et al., 1981).

There is some evidence that protein binding may occur preferentially to certain proteins rather than as a random binding event. For example, ligandin is the preferred target protein in rat liver cytosol when either 3-methylcholanthrene or benzo[a]pyrene is administered in vivo, (Singer and Litwack, 1971; Ketterer et al., 1976; Jakoby and Keen, 1977;Ketterer, 1980; Schelin et al., 1983).

Protection against certain substrates containing olefinic bonds is afforded by cytochrome P-450 monooxygenases, especially the isozymes that are inducible by phenobarbital treatment. The protection results from the selective destruction of the enzyme prosthetic heme group and the formation of "green" porphyrin by N-alkylation (Ortiz de Montellano et al., 1980).

An important food antioxidant, 3,5-di-*tert*-butyl-4-hydroxytoluene (BHT), undergoes a cytochrome P-450 catalyzed conversion to a quinone methide (Nakagawa, et al., 1983). The specific binding to protein, but not to nucleic acids, has led to the detection of conjugate between the 4-methyl group and the sulfhydryl group of microsomal protein cysteine residues. Nakagawa and coworkers have concluded that in vivo, BHT can conjugate not only to glutathione and cysteine, but also to protein sulfhydryls, and that the latter reaction may produce BHT-mediated damage leading to the observed latent toxicity of this compound (Kehrer and Witschi, 1980).

Since covalent binding to DNA was described as a quantitative indicator for genotoxicity (Lutz, 1979), many advances have occurred to aid in the understanding of such covalent interactions. A potential mutagen or carcinogen has been defined as any chemical capable of forming covalent bonds with DNA of somatic and reproductive mammalian cells in vivo (Randerath et al., 1985). Conference reports clearly demonstrate the importance of DNA adducts in assessing the risk potential of carcinogens. Pertinent voluminous scientific literature includes characterizations of the formation of DNA adducts including an extensive review on DNA adducts as dosimeters to monitor humans exposed to environmental mutagens and carcinogens (Environmental Health Perspectives, 1985; Farmer et al., 1987).

CELLULAR ASPECTS OF PROTECTION

Compartmentation

The concentration and nature of nonprotein thiols and protein sulfhydryl groups has been a topic of long-standing interest. Vital cellular functions of protein sulfhydryls are numerous and cannot be enumerated here. The high concentration of protein sulfhydryl groups (15–20 mM in liver) exceeds the concentration of total nonprotein thiols (6–10 mM in liver). Protection of protein thiols from alterations (including the homeostasis oxidation state) involves the total cellular thiol:disulfide potential (Ziegler et al., 1980). Subcellular distribution and concentrations of both nonprotein thiols and protein sulfhydryls may relate closely to their respective functions. More than 90% of the total nonprotein thiols present in cells appears to be glutathione. The presence of a discrete mitochondrial pool of glutathione was proposed by Vignais and Vignais (1973). Others found that mitochondria retained GSH during experiments involving nonaqueous media (Jocelyn and Kamminga, 1974; Jocelyn, 1975) and that isolated rat mitochondria contain about 10% of the total hepatic glutathione with about 90% of it being present as reduced glutathione (Jocelyn and Kamminga, 1974). Wahlländer et al. 1979) reported the mitochondrial glutathione content to be 13% of total liver content by a nonaqueous extraction procedure. Meredith and Reed (1982) suggested that, based on compartment water space (Elbers et al., 1974; Wahlländer et al., 1979), the mitochondrion maintains a higher glutathione concentration than the cytoplasm, 10 mM versus 7 mM, respectively. The apparent impermeability of the inner membrane of the mitochondrion led to the speculation that mitochondria maintain intramitochondrial glutathione by in situ synthesis (Wahlländer et al., 1979). Higashi et al. (1977) have suggested that liver glutathione is a two-compartment physiological reservoir of L-cysteine. A labile compartment serves as a cysteine reservoir and as a more stable compartment, which is not readily available even during starvation. Cho et al. (1981) have provided confirmatory evidence in that fasted and refed rats maintain a constant level of plasma cystine.

Studies on glutathione biosynthesis demonstrate separate pools of glutathione in the cytosol and the mitochondria with the in vivo turnover half-lives being 2 and 30 hr, respectively (Meredith and Reed, 1982). Short-term starvation depleted the cytosol pool but not the mitochondrial pool. However, no evidence exists for synthesis of GSH in the mitochondria. The lack of loss of either GSG or GSSG from isolated mitochondria (Olafsdottir and Reed, 1988) continues to raise important questions about the mechanism for maintenance of glutathione homeostasis in mitochondria.

Induction of Protective Enzymes

Administration of certain "antioxidants" or "anticarcinogens" is an important aspect of cellular protection for the prevention of induction of experimental tumors by a variety of chemical carcinogens (for a review see Wattenberg, 1985). Wattenberg (1972a, b; 1974; Wattenberg et al., 1977) made an extensive study of this phenomenon followed by reports by Weisburger's laboratory (Grantham et al., 1973; Ulland et al., 1973; Weisburger et al., 1977).

Theories advanced to explain these effects of antioxidants or anticarcinogens have been discussed by Benson et al. (1978) and include (a) direct interaction of either the carcinogen or its activated metabolic products with the antioxidant; (b) enhanced activities of enzymes that inactivate the proximate or ultimate carcinogens, and thereby limit the damaging interactions with critical macromolecular components and also thereby prevent the initiation process of cellular transformation; (c) blockage or competition against specific metabolic activation processes required to convert procarcinogens to their reactive intermediates; and (d) increased efficiency in repair of damaged DNA.

Following in vivo exposure to a variety of chemicals including polycyclic hydrocarbons, phenobarbital, and antioxidants, the level of GSH in liver may be increased substantially (for a review see Boyer and Kenney, 1985).

Addition of either 2(3)-*tert*-butyl-4-hydroxyanisole (BHA) or 1,2-dihydro-6-ethoxy-2,2,4-trimethyl quinoline (ethoxyquin) to the diet greatly decreases the levels of mutagenic metabolites of benzo[a]pyrene in CD-1 mice (Batzinger et al., 1978). These observations have led to the finding that liver cytosol from BHA-fed mice and rats exhibits GST activities that are enhanced more than 10-fold (Benson et al., 1978). Increased enzyme protein included multiple GST species (Benson et al., 1978).

Studies by Nakagawa et al. (1983) show that butylated hydroxytoluene (BHT) given orally, increases the total GSH in rat liver and the activities of GST and GSSG reductase but has no effect on GSH peroxidase (Nakagawa et al., 1981). The isomers of BHA, 2-*tert*-butyl-4-hydroxy-anisole (2-BHA) and 3-*tert*-butyl-4-hydroxyanisole (3-BHA) have been compared in their induction properties in mouse liver, and both isomers were found to increase acid-soluble thiol content and to increase activities of GST and epoxide hydrolase (Lam et al., 1981). The 3-BHA induction was more than three times higher than that of 2-BHA in the liver. However, in the mouse forestomach the order of induction by the isomers was reversed (Lam et al., 1981).

Dietary administration of BHA to mice also enhances dicoumaryl-inhibited NADPH: quinone reductase [NADPH dehydrogenase (quinone); NADPH (quinone acceptor) oxidoreductase, EC 1.6.99.2] activity to 10 times control levels in the liver (Benson et al., 1980). Increases of severalfold were observed in kidney, lung, and mucosa of the upper small intestine. The protective effects of BHA may be a result of increased conversion of quinones to readily excreted conjugates (Benson et al., 1980).

There is a growing body of evidence that vicinal diol epoxides, the reactive intermediates of polycyclic hydrocarbon, are largely responsible for most of the mutagenic and carcinogenic effects induced by polycyclic hydrocarbons (Boyland and Sims, 1967; Sims et al., 1974; Flesher et al., 1976; Huberman et al., 1976; Newbold and Brookes, 1976; Slaga et al., 1976; Wislocki et al., 1976; Levin et al., 1977; Hecht et al., 1978; Bigger et al., 1980; Cooper et al., 1980; MacNicoll et al., 1981).

Experiments with *trans*-7,8-dihydro-7,8-dihydroxybenzo[*a*]pyrene and 7β,8α-dihydroxy-9α-epoxy-7,8,9,10-tetrahydrobenzo[*a*]pyrene indicate some inactivation is glutathione-dependent (Burke et al., 1977; Glatt and Oesch, 1977; Shen et al., 1980; Hesse et al., 1980; Guenthner et al., 1980; Ketterer, 1980; Glatt et al., 1981; Jernström et al., 1982) but not dependent on microsomal epoxide hydrolase (Wood et al., 1976, 1977; Bentley et al., 1977; Glatt et al., 1981).

Earlier studies on the induction of phase II enzymes by phenobarbital and 3-methylcholanthrene (including those of Hales and Neims, 1977; Baars et al., 1978; Clifton and Kaplowitz, 1978;) as well as TCDD (2,3,7,8-tetrachlorodibenzo-*p*-dioxin) (Baars et al., 1978) and 3,4-benzo(*a*) (Clifton and Kaplowitz, 1978) indicated less induction than by antioxidants such as BHA (Benson et al., 1978).

Phenobarbital induction followed by isolation of liver poly(A)$^+$RNA and translation experiments have led Pickett et al. (1981) to conclude that the level of translatable GST B mRNA is elevated about three- to fourfold by phenobarbital administration. Felton et al. (1980) have shown that induction of hepatic GST activity by polycyclic aromatic compounds does not correlate with the Ah receptor, which controls the inducible aryl hydrocarbon (benzo[a]pyrene) hydroxylase activity.

trans-Stilbene oxide appears to be a different type of inducing agent than those having properties of either phenobarbital or 3-methylcholanthrene (see reviews by Conney, 1967, 1982; Estabrook and Lindenlaub, 1979). Treatment of rats with trans-stilbene oxide increases the epoxide hydratase activity of liver microsomes to more than 700% of control values (Schmassman and Oesch, 1978, Guthenberg et al., 1980). Cytoplasmic GST activity increases 300 to 400%, leading to the conclusion that this agent induces phase II enzymes considerably more than the cytochrome P-450 system (which is about doubled) (Guthenberg et al., 1980). The structural requirements of stilbene oxide induction have been examined. A comparison of induction in rats by cis- and trans-stilbene, cis- and trans-stilbene oxide, benzoin and benzil led to the conclusion that trans-stilbene oxide is the actual inducing agent and that benzyl is more selective as an inducer of epoxide hydrolase than is trans-stilbene oxide (Seidegard et al., 1981).

The discovery that selenium (Se), as selenocysteine (Rotruck et al., 1973), is an essential element of glutathione peroxide has provided enormous insight to the role of selenium in oxidative processes. Glutathione peroxidase is the only identified selenium-containing mammalian enzyme (Stadtman, 1980). The structure and function of this enzyme has been reviewed (Flohé et al., 1979; Wendel, 1980; Sunde and Hoekstra, 1980).

Se-deficient rat liver has a non-Se-dependent GSH peroxidase activity that is associated with one or more of the GSTs (Prohaska and Ganther, 1977; Lawrence and Burk, 1978). Organic hydroperoxides such as cumene- and t-butyl hydroperoxide, but not hydrogen peroxide, are reduced by these enzymes.

Recently, a membrane-bound glutathione peroxidase–like activity has been described for mouse liver and cardiac mitochondrial membrane (Katki and Myers, 1980). This enzyme activity has been distinguished from the cytosol and mitochondrial matrix selenium-dependent glutathione peroxidases. Three features are important: (1) the enzyme activity is membrane-bound and is not affected by selenium deficiency, (2) it does not appear to be a GSH S-transferase (Katki and Myers, 1980), and (3) the enzyme appears to be located in mitochondrial intermembrane space.

The relationship between selenium and glutathione in cells is understood in terms of the essential role of selenium in the function of glutathione peroxidase (Rotruck et al., 1973). Recently, Hill and Burk (1982) reported that when selenium-deficient rats were used as a source of freshly isolated hepatocytes, those hepatocytes demonstrated an altered glutathione status on incubation. The glutathione concentration in selenium-deficient hepatocytes rose to 1.4 times that in control hepatocytes. The selenium-deficient cells released twice as much glutathione into the incubation medium as did the control cells. Plasma glutathione concentration in selenium-deficient rats was found to be twofold that in control rats, indicating that increased glutathione synthesis and release occurs in vivo during selenium deficiency (Hill and Burk, 1982).

A soluble, heat-labile factor, which is not glutathione peroxidase, can confer glutathione-dependent inhibition of lipid peroxidation to both microsomal and mitochondria preparations from rat liver (McCay et al., 1981). The relationship of this protection system to the protective functions of vitamin E are yet to be established.

Redox Cycling

A second role for GSH in a powerful protection system against oxidative damage is mediated largely by metabolites of molecular oxygen. Toxic chemical effects associated with oxygen metabolism and subsequent redox cycling and lipid peroxidation appear to be a part of aerobic life. The relationship of very important events to reactive intermediates of chemicals has been reviewed by Kappus and Sies (1981). We are just beginning to understand and assess the energy required by the consumption of reducing equivalents that result from redox cycling.

Since superoxide anion radicals can migrate across artificial lipid bilayer membranes at temperatures above the lipid phase-transition (Rumyantseva et al., 1979), they may traverse membranes in general. However, in erythrocytes (Lynch and Fridovich, 1978) and granulocytes (Gennaro and Romeo, 1979) the migration is thought to occur via anion channels. This point could be important since most quinones are in membrane and the concentration of O_2 in the lipid plasma membrane is eight times that in the aqueous medium (Pryor, 1973). Thus, superoxide anion radicals may be migrating in both directions across membrane from their site of formation. The rapid reaction of semiquinones with oxygen would indicate that semiquinones would not diffuse far in the presence of oxygen (Powis et al., 1981). Lack of protection by superoxide dismutase may indicate some superoxide anion production outside of cells (Powis et al., 1981).

Protection from reduced oxygen species therefore may occur in membrane by specific membrane-associated proteins that are capable of membrane protection and therefore can be shown to limit lipid peroxidation of membrane-associated polyunsaturated lipids.

An excellent example of the complexity of redox cycling has been discussed by Biaglow (1981) concerning the reduction of nitro compounds. Reduction of the nitro functional group to nitro radical anions is catalyzed by reductases including NADPH cytochrome P-450 reductase (A.Y.H. Lu, 1982, private communication). The fate of such radicals depends on many factors including O_2 concentration and GSH. Oxygen and GSH compete for the nitro radical anion electron and, in turn, form superoxide anion radical and $GS \cdot$, which then form GSSG. Decreasing the concentration of either oxygen or GSH appears to increase macromolecular damage.

Protection against quinones appears to involve several aspects of cellular function involving oxygen reduction. Quinones can undergo either two-electron reduction to corresponding hydroquinones or one-electron reduction to the corresponding semiquinone radicals (Iyanagi and Yamazaki, 1970). However, the main cytotoxic effects of quinones are thought to be mediated through one-electron reduction to the semiquinone radical (Bachur et al., 1978) (Fig. 7.4). This radical is known to be capable of formation of the superoxide anion radical by the one-electron reduction of molecular oxygen (Fridovich, 1976).

It has been suggested that, whereas the rate of NADPH formation is not limiting for monooxygenase activity, it may be rate-limiting for quinone-stimulated superoxide formation (Powis et al., 1981). Simple quinones stimulate the formation of O_2^- by isolated rat hepatocytes at rates up to 15 nmol/min per 10^6 cells. Destruction of O_2^- and water formation would require the consumption of 15 nmol/min per 10^6 cells of intracellular GSH or nearly a complete turnover of GSH to GSSG and reduction back to GSH in 2 minutes. An equal quantity (7.5 nmol) of NADPH must be furnished. However, Sies et al., Gerstenecker and Sies, 1980; Sies et al., 1982) have calculated the maximum rate of NADPH production to be equivalent to 15 nmol/min per 10^6 cells.

Sies et al. (1982) have reviewed the metabolism of organic hydroperoxides and concluded that enzymatic reduction of organic hydroperoxides is the result of the activities of two GSH-requiring enzymes, glutathione peroxidase [EC 1.11.1.9] and glutathione S-transferase [EC 2.5.1.18]. Additional protection against hydroperoxides is afforded by endogenous

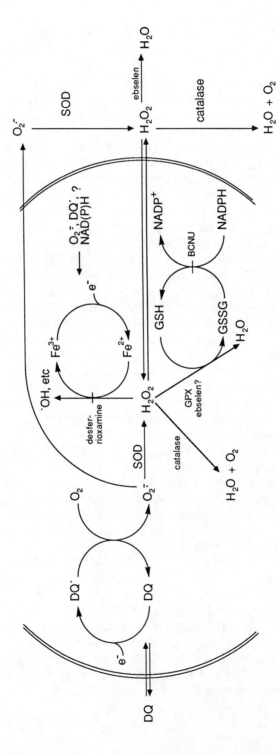

FIG. 7.4 Protective systems against quinone-generated reduction of oxygen.

"antioxidants" including α-tocopherol, ascorbic acid, and β-carotene. Synthetic antioxidants such as butylhydroxytoluene (BHT) are thought to act primarily as mimics of α-tocopherol in the termination of free radical reaction sequence.

The rate of cellular generation of NADPH from $NADP^+$ appears to be rate-limiting for monooxygenase reactions. In intact liver, cytochrome P-450–dependent drug metabolism is decreased when an organic hydroperoxide is being reduced to the corresponding alcohol by glutathione peroxidase, and, in turn, GSSG consumes NADPH reducing equivalents in the conversion of newly generated GSSG to GSH (Morehouse et al., 1983).

A serious question has been raised concerning the role that hydrogen peroxide may have in microsomal lipid peroxidation. Hydrogen peroxide reacts with reduced transition metals, especially ferrous iron, to generate the most oxidative of oxygen species, the highly reactive hydroxyl radical, · OH. This radical is thought to predominate in initiation of microsomal lipid peroxidation. However, Morehouse et al. (1983) have concluded that hydroxyl radical generated from hydrogen peroxide does not initiate microsomal lipid peroxidation.

NADPH-dependent lipid peroxidation, which is initiated by NADPH-cytochrome P-450 reductase, may occur either by hydroxyl radical formation through an iron-catalyzed, Haber-Weiss reaction (Tien et al., 1981), or it may arise also from the formation of a reactive ADP-Fe-oxygen complex (Bucher et al., 1982). Possible events include the reduction of perferryl ion to the ferryl ion for initiation of lipid peroxidation. Superoxide anion maybe the reductant:

$$ADP - Fe^{3+} + O_2^- \rightarrow ADP - Fe^{2+}O_2$$

followed by

$$ADP - Fe^{2+}O_2 \underset{2\,H^+}{\overset{2e^-}{\rightleftharpoons}} ADP-[FeO]^{2+} + H_2O$$

to yield the initiating species.

In contrast, NADPH-cytochrome P-450 reductase-dependent lipid peroxidation with EDTA-Fe may occur through a hydroxyl ion–dependent mechanism rather than an ADP ferrous ion–oxygen type of complex (Lötscher et al., 1979). These processes appear to be very important to radical damage to DNA (Imlay et al., 1988).

REFERENCES

Ames, B. N. 1987. Measuring oxidative damage in humans: Relation to cancer and aging. Presented at IARC Meeting on Detection Methods for DNA-Damaging Agents in Man, Espoo, Finland, September 2–4.

Anders, M. W. (Ed.). 1985. *Bioactivation of Foreign Compounds.* Academic Press, New York.

Armstrong, R. N., Levin, W., and Jerina, D. M. 1980. Hepatic microsomal epoxide hydrolase—Mechanistic studies of the hydration of K-region arene oxides. *J. Biol. Chem.* 255: 4698.

Baars, A. J., Jansen, M., and Breimer, D. D. 1978. The influence of phenobarbital, 3-methylcholanthrene and 2,3,7,8-tetrachlorodibenzo-*p*-dioxin on glutathione *S*-transferase activity of rat liver cytosol. *Biochem. Pharmacol.* 27: 2487–2494.

Bachur, N. R., Gordon, S. L., and Gee, M. V. 1978. A general mechanism for microsomal activation of quinone anticancer agents to free radicals. *Cancer Res.* 38: 1745–1750.

Bailey, G. S., Hendricks, J. D., and Williams, D. E. 1988. Presented at IFT-IUFoST Basic Symposium, New Orleans, LA, June 17-18.

Batzinger, R. P., Ou, S-Y. L., and Beuding, E. 1978. Anti-mutagenic effects of 2(3)-tert-butyl-4 hydroxyanisole and of antimicrobial agents. *Cancer Res.* 38: 4476.

Beck, L. V., Rieks, V. D., and Duncan, B. 1958. Diurnal variation in mouse and rat liver sulfhydryl. *Proc. Soc. Exp. Biol. Med.* 97: 229.

Benesch, R. E. and Benesch, R. 1955. The acid strength of the -SH group in cysteine and related compounds. *J. Am. Chem. Soc.* 77: 5877.

Benson, A. M., Batzinger, R. P., Ou, S. -Y. L., Bueding, E., Cha, Y. -N., and Talalay, P. 1978. Elevation of hepatic glutathione S-transferase activities and protection against mutagenic metabolites of benzo[*a*]pyrene by dietary antioxidants. *Cancer Res.* 38: 4486.

Benson, A. M., Hunkeler, M. J., and Talalay, P. 1980. Increase of NAD(P)H:quinone reductase by dietary antioxidants: Possible role in protection against carcinogenesis and toxicity. *Proc. Natl. Acad. Sci. U.S.A.* 77: 5216.

Bentley, P., Oesch, F., and Glatt, H. R. 1977. Dual role of epoxide hydratase in both activation and inactivation of benzo(*a*)pyrene. *Arch: Toxicol.* 39: 65.

Biaglow, J. E. 1981. Cellular electron transfer and radical mechanisms for drug metabolism, *Rad. Res.* 86: 212.

Bigger, C. A. H., Tomaszweski, J. E., and Dipple, A. 1980. Differences between products of binding of 7,12-dimethylbenz(a)anthracene to DNA in mouse skin and in a rat liver microsomal system. *Biochem. Biophys. Res. Commun.* 80: 229.

Boyd, S. C., Sasame, H. A., and Boyd, M. R. 1979. High concentrations of glutathione in glandular stomach—Possible implications for carcinogenesis. *Science* 205: 1010.

Boyer, T. D. 1988. The glutathione S-transferases. *Hepatology.* In press.

Boyer, T. D. and Kenney, W. C. 1985. Preparation, characterization and properties of glutathione S-transferases. In *Biochemical Pharmacology and Toxicology.* (Ed.) Zakim, D. and Vessey, D. A., Vol 1, p. 297. John Wiley and Sons, New York.

Boyland, E. and Chasseaud, L. F. 1969. Role of glutathione and glutathione S-transferases in mercapturic acid biosynthesis. *Adv. Enzymol.* 32: 173.

Boyland, E. and Sims, P. 1967. Carcinogenic activities in mice of compounds related to benz(a)anthracene. *Int. J. Canc.* 2: 500.

Bucher, J. R., Tien, M. Morehouse, L. A., and Aust, S. D. 1982. Redox cycling and lipid peroxidation: The central role of iron chelates. *Fund. Appl. Toxicol.* 3: 222.

Buening, M. K., Wislocki, P. G., Levin, W., Yagi, H., Thakker, D. R., Akagi, H., Koreeda, M., Jerina, D. M., and Conney, A. H. 1978. Tumorgenicity of the optical enantiomers of the diastereomeric benzo[a]pyrene-7,8-diol-9,10-epoxides in newborn mice: Exceptional activity of (+)-(7R, 8S) 8'-dihydroxy-(9S, 10R)-epoxy-7,8,9,10-tetrahydro-benzo[a]pyrene. *Proc. Natl. Acad. Sci. U.S.A.* 75: 5358.

Burke, M. D., Vadi, H., Jernström, B., and Orrenius, S. 1977. Metabolism of benzo(a)pyrene with isolated hepatocytes and the formation and degradation of DNA binding derivatives. *J. Biol. Chem.* 252: 6424–6436.

Burton, G. W. and Ingold, K. U. 1981. Autoxidation of biological molecules. I. The antioxidant activity of vitamin E and related chain-breaking phenolic antioxidants *in vitro*. *J. Am. Chem. Soc.* 103: 6472.

Calcutt, G. and Ting, M. 1969. Diurnal variations in rat tissue disulphide levels. *Naturwissenschraften* 56: 419.

Century, B. and Horwitt, M. 1965. Biological availability of various forms of vitamin E with respect to different indices of deficiency. *Fed. Proc., Fed. Am. Soc. Exp. Biol.* 24: 906.

Cerutti, P. A. 1985. Prooxidant states and tumor promotion. *Science* 227: 375.

Chasseaud, L. F. 1979. Role of glutathione and glutathione S-transferases in the metabolism of chemical carcinogens and other electrophilic agents. *Adv. Cancer Res.* 29: 175.

Cho, E. S., Sahyoun, N., and Stegink, L. D. 1981. Tissue glutathione as a cysteine reservoir during fasting and refeeding of rats. *J. Nutr.* 111: 914.

Clifton, G. and Kaplowitz, N. 1978. Effect of dietary phenobarbital, 3,4-benzo(a)pyrene and 3-methyl cholanthrene on hepatic, intestinal and renal glutathione S-transferase activities in the rat. *Biochem. Pharmacol.* 27: 1284.

Conney, A. H. 1982. Induction of microsomal enzymes by foreign chemicals and carcinogenesis by polycyclic aromatic hydrocarbons: G.H.A. Clowes Memorial Lecture. *Cancer Res.* 42: 4875.

Conney, A. H. 1967. Pharmacological implications of microsomal enzyme induction. *Pharmacol. Rev.* 19: 317.

Cooper C. S., MacNicoll, A. D., Ribeiro, O., Gervasi, P.G., Hewer, A., Walsh, C., Pal, K. Grover, P. L., and Sims, P. 1980. Involvement of a non-bay-region diol-epoxide in the metabolic activation of benz (a)anthracene in hamster-embryo cells. *Cancer Lett.* 9: 53.

Dansette, P. M., Makedonska, V. B., and Jerina, D. M. 1978. Mechanism for catalysis for the hydration of substituted styrene oxides by hepatic epoxide hydrase. *Arch. Biochem. Biophys.* 187: 290.

Elbers, R., Heldt, H. W., Schmucker, P., Soboll, S., and Wiese, H. 1974. Measurement of the ATP/ADP ratio in mitochondria and in the extramitochondrial compartment by fractionation of freeze-stopped liver tissue in non-aqueous media. *Hoppe-Seyler's Z. Physiol. Chem.* 355: 378.

Environmental Health Perspectives. 1985. Vol. 62 (Ed.) Lucier, G. W. and Hook, G. E. R., pp. 3–231. U. S. Department of Health and Human Services.

Estabrook, R. W. and Lindenlaub E. (Ed.) 1979. *The Induction of Drug Metabolism.* Symposium Ashford Castle, Ireland. May 24–27, 1978. p. 645. Verlag-Struttgart, New York.

Farmer, P. B., Neumann, H. -G., and Henschler, D. 1987. Estimation of exposure of man to substances reacting covalently with macromolecules. *Arch. Toxicol.* 60: 251.

Felton, J. F., Ketley, J. N., Jakoby, W. B., Aitio, A., Bend, J. R., and Nebert, D. W. 1980. Hepatic glutathione transferase (EC 2.5.1.18) activity induced by polycyclic aromatic compounds: Lack of correlation with the murine Ah locus. *Mol. Pharmacol.* 18: 559.

Finkelstein, J. D. 1974. 1. Methionine metabolism in mammals. Biochemical basis for homocystinuria. *Metabolism* 23: 387.

Flesher, J. W., Harvey, R. G., and Sydnor, K. L. 1976. Oncogenicity of K-region epoxides of benzo(*a*)pyrene and 7,12-dimethylbenz(*a*)anthracene. *Int. J. Cancer* 18: 351.

Flohé, L., Gönzler, W. A., and Loschen, G. 1979. The glutathione peroxidase reaction: A key to understand the selenium requirement of mammals. In *Trace Metals in Health and Disease.* (Ed.) Karasch, N. p. 263. Raven Press, New York.

Fridovich, I. 1976. Oxygen radicals, hydrogen peroxide, and oxygen toxicity. In *Free Radicals in Biology.* (Ed.) Pryor, W. A., Vol. 1. Academic Press, New York.

Friedman, M., Cavins, J.F., and Wall, J. S. 1965. Relative nucleophilic reactivities of amino groups and mercaptide ions in addition reactions with α,β-unsaturated compounds. *J. Amer. Chem. Soc.* 87: 3672.

Gennaro, R. and Romeo, D. 1979. The release of superoxide anion from granulocytes: Effect of inhibitors of anion permeability. *Biochem. Biophys. Res. Commun.* 88: 44–99.

Gerstenecker, C. and Sies, H. 1980. Restriction of hexobarbital metabolism by t-butyl hydroperoxide in perfused rat liver. *Biochem. Pharmacol.* 29: 3112–3113.

Glatt, H. R., Billings, R., Platt, K. L., and Oesch, F. 1981. Improvement of the correlation of bacterial mutagenicity with carcinogenicity of benzo(*a*)pyrene and four of its major metabolites by activation with intact liver cells instead of cell homogenate. *Cancer Res.* 41: 270–277.

Glatt, J. R. and Oesch F. 1977. Inactivation of electrophilic metabolites by glutathione *S*-transferase and limitation of the system due to subcellular localization. *Arch. Toxicol.* 39: 87.

Grantham, P. H., Weisburger, J. H., and Weisburger, E. K. 1973. Effect of the antioxidant butylated hydrotoxytoluene (BHT) on the metabolism of the carcinogens N-2 fluorenylacetamide and N-hydroxy-N-2-fluorenylacetamide. *Food Cosmet. Toxicol.* 11: 209.

Guengerich, F. P. 1988. Roles of cytochrome P-450 enzymes in chemical carcinogenesis and cancer chemotherapy. *Can. Res.* 48: 2946.

Guenthner, T. M., Jernström, B., and Orrenius, S. 1980. On the effect of cellular nucleophiles on the binding of metabolites of 7,8-dihydroxy-7,8-dihydrobenzo(*a*)pyrene and 9-hydroxybenzo(*a*)pyrene to nuclear DNA. *Carcinogenesis* 1: 407–418.

Guthenberg, C., Morgenstern, R., DePierre, J. W., and Mannervik, G. 1980. Induction of glutathione *S*-tranferase-A, *S*-transferase-B and *S*-

transferase-C in rat liver cytosol by *trans*-stilbene oxide. *Biochem. Biophys. Acta* 631: 1–10.

Hales, B. F. and Neims, A. H. 1977. Induction of rat hepatic glutathione S-transferase B by phenobarbital and 3-methylcholanthrene. *Biochem. Pharmacol.* 26: 555–556.

Halliwell, B. 1987. Oxidants and human disease: some new concepts. *FASEB J.* 1: 358.

Hanzlik, R. P., Edelman, M., Michaely, W. J., and Scott, G. 1976. Enzymatic hydration of epoxides [3-18] role of nucleophilic mechanisms. *J. Am. Chem. Soc.* 98: 1952.

Harvey, R. G. 1981. Activated metabolites of carcinogenic hydrocarbons. *Acc. Chem. Res.* 14: 218.

Hecht, S. S., LaVoie, E., Mazzarese, R., Amin, S., Bedenko, V., and Hoffman, D. 1978. 1,2-Dihydro 1,2-dihydroxy-5-methylchrysene, a major activated metabolite of the environmental carcinogen 5-methylchrysene. *Cancer Res.* 38: 2191–2194.

Hernandez, O. and Bend, J. J. 1982. Metabolism of epoxides. In *Metabolic Basis of Detoxication.* (Ed.) Jakoby, W. B., Bend, J. R. and Caldwell, J., p. 207. Academic Press, New York.

Hesse, S., Jernström, B., Martinez, M., Guenthner, O., and Orrenius, S. 1980. Inhibition of binding benzo[a]pyrene metabolites to nuclear DNA by glutathione and glutathione S-transferase B. *Biochem. Biophys. Res. Commun.* 94: 612.

Higashi, T., Tateishi, N., Naruse, A., and Sakamoto, Y. 1977. A novel physiological role of liver glutathione as a reservoir of L-cysteine. *J. Biochem.* 82: 117.

Hill, K. E. and Burk, R. F. 1982. Effect of selenium deficiency and vitamin E deficiency on glutathione metabolism in isolated rat hepatocytes. *J. Biol. Chem.* 257: 10668.

Huberman, E., Sachs, L., Yang, S. K., and Gelboin, H. V. 1976. Identification of mutagenic metabolites of benzo(a)pyrene in mammalian cells. *Proc. Natl. Acad. Sci. U.S.A.* 73: 607.

Imlay, J. A., Chin, S. M., and Linn, S. 1988. Toxic DNA damage by hydrogen peroxide through the fenton reaction *in vivo* and *in vitro*. *Science* 240: 640–642.

Iyanagi, T. and Yamazaki, I. 1970. One-electron transfer reaction in biochemical systems. V. Difference in the mechanism of quinone reduction by the NADH dehydrogenase and the NAD(P)H dehydrogenase (DT-diaphorase). *Biochim. Biophys. Acta* 216: 282.

Jakoby, W. B. and Keen, J. H. 1977. A triple-threat in detoxification: The glutathione S-transferases. *Trends Biochem. Sci.* 2: 229.

Jakoby, W. B., Ketterer, B., and Mannervik, B. 1984. Glutathione transferases: nomenclature. *Biochem. Pharmacol.* 33: 2539.

Jakoby, W. B. 1978. The glutathione *S*-transferases: A group of multifunctional detoxication proteins. *Adv. Enzymol.* 46: 383.

Janssen, M. J. 1972. Nucleophilicity of organic sulphur compounds. In *Sulfur in Organic and Inorganic Chemistry.* (Ed.) Senning, A., Vol. 3, p. 355. Marcel Dekker, New York.

Jensen, D. E. 1978. Reaction of DNA with alkylating agents. Differential alkylation of poly[dA-dT] by methylnitrosourea and ethylnitrosourea. *Biochemistry* 17: 5108.

Jerina, D. M. 1983. The 1982 Bernard B. Brodie Award Lecture. Metabolism of aromatic hydrocarbons by the cytochrome P-450 system and epoxide hydrolase. *Drug Metab. Drug. Dispos.* 11: 1.

Jernström, B., Babson, J. R., Moldéus, P., Holmgren, A., and Reed, D.J. 1982. Glutathione conjugation and DNA-binding of (+)-7β,8α-dihydroxy-9α,10α-epoxy-7,8,9,10-tetrahydrobenzo[*a*]pyrene in isolated rat hepatocytes. *Carcinogenesis* 3: 861.

Jocelyn, P. C. 1975. Some properties of mitochondrial glutathione. *Biochim. Biophys. Acta* 396: 427.

Jocelyn, P. C. and Kamminga, A. 1974. The non-protein thiol of rat liver mitochondria. *Biochim. Biophys. Acta* 343: 356.

Kappus, H. and Sies, J. 1981. Toxic drug effects associated with oxygen metabolism - redox cycling and lipid peroxidation. *Experientia* 37: 1233–1241.

Katki, A. G. and Myers, C. E. 1980. Membrane-bound glutathione peroxidase-like activity in mitochondria. *Biochem. Biophys. Res. Commun.* 96: 85–91.

Kehrer, J. P. and Witschi, H. 1980. Effects of drug metabolism inhibitors on butylated hydroxytoluene induced pulmonary toxicity in mice. *Toxicol. Appl. Pharmacol.* 53: 333.

Ketterer, B., Tipping, E., Beale, D., and Meuwissen, J. A. T. P. Ligandin, glutathione and carcinogen binding. In *Glutathione: Metabolism and Function.* (Ed.) Arias, I. M. and Jakoby, W. B., p. 243. Raven Press, New York.

Ketterer. B. 1980. Interactions between carcinogens and proteins. *Br. Med. Bull.* 36: 71.

Ketterer, B., Coles, B., and Meyer, D. J. 1983. The role of glutathione in detoxication. *Environ. Health Perspect.* 49: 56.

Koskikallio, J. 1969a. Nucleophilic reactivity. Part II. Kinetics of reactions of methyl perchlorate with nucleophiles in water. *Acta Chem. Scand.* 23: 1477.

Koskikallio, J. 1969b. Nucleophilic reactivity. Part III. Kinetics of methyl perchlorate with amines in water and methanol. *Acta Chem. Scand.* 23: 1490.

Lam, L. K., Sparnins, V. L., Hochalter, J. B., and Wattenberg, L. W. 1981. Effects of 2- and 3-*tert*-butyl-4-hydroxyanisole on glutathione *S*-transferase and epoxide hydrolase activities and sulfhydryl levels in liver and forestomach of mice. *Cancer Res.* 41: 3940.

Lawrence, R. A. and Burk, R. F. 1978. Species, tissue and subcellular distribution of non Se-dependent glutathione peroxidase activity. *J. Nutr.* 108: 211–215.

Leaf, G. and Neuberger, A. 1947. The effect of diet on the glutathione content of the liver. *Biochem. J.* 41: 280.

Levin, W., Wood, A. W., Lu, A. Y. H., Ryan, D., West S., Conney, A. H., Thakker, D. R., Yagi, H., and Jerina, D. M. 1977. Role of purified cytochrome P-448 and epoxide hydrase in the activation and detoxification of benzo(a)pyrene. In *Concepts in Drug Metabolism.* (Ed.) Jerina, D. M., pp. 99–126. American Chemical Society Symposium Series, Washington, DC.

Lötscher, H. R., Winterhalter, K. H., Carafoli, E., and Richter, C. 1979. Hydroperoxide can modulate the redox state of pyridine nucleotides and the calcium balance in rat liver mitochondria. *Proc. Natl. Acad. Sci. U.S.A.* 76: 4340.

Lutz, W. K. 1979. *In vivo* covalent binding of organic chemicals to DNA as a quantitative indicator in the process of chemical carcinogenesis. *Mutat. Res.* 65: 289.

Lynch, R. E. and Fridovich, I. 1978. Permeation of erythrocyte stroma by superoxide radical. *J. Biol. Chem.* 253: 4697–4699.

MacLeod, M. C., Kootstra, A. Mansfield, B. K., Slaga, T. J., and Selkirk, J. K. 1980. Specificity in interaction of benzo[a]pyrene with nuclear macromolecules: Implication of derivatives of two dihydrodiols in protein binding. *Proc. Nat. Acad. Sci. U.S.A.-Biol. Sci.* 77: 6396.

MacNicoll, A. D., Cooper, C. S., Ribeiro, O., Pal, K., Hewer, A., Grover, P. L., and Sims, P. 1981. The metabolic activation of benz(a)anthracene in 3 biological systems. *Cancer Lett.* 11: 243–249.

Mannervik, B., Alin, P., Guthenberg, C. Jensson, H., Tahir, M. K., Warholm, M., and Jörnvall, H. 1985. Identification of three classes of cytosolic glutathione transferase common to several mammalian species: Correlation between structural data and enzymatic properties. *Proc. Natl. Acad. Sci. U.S.A.* 82: 7202.

Maruyama, E., Kojima, J., Higashi, T. and Sakamoto, Y. 1968. Effect of diet on liver glutathione and glutathione reductase. *J. Biochem.* 63: 398.

McCay, P. B., Gibson, D. D., and Hornbrook, K. R. 1981. Glutathione-dependent inhibition of lipid peroxidation by a soluble, heat-labile factor not glutathione peroxidase. *Fed. Proc.* 40: 199–205.

Meredith, M. J. and Reed, D. J. 1982. Status of the mitochondrial pool of glutathione in the isolated hepatocyte. *J. Biol. Chem.* 257: 3447.

Miller, E. C. and Miller, J. A. 1966. Mechanisms of chemical carcinogenesis: Nature of proximate carcinogens and interactions with macromolecules. *Pharmacol. Rev.* 18: 805.

Morehouse, L. A., Tien, M., Bucher, J. R., and Aust., S. D. 1983. Effect of hydrogen peroxide on the initiation of microsomal lipid peroxidation. *Biochem. Pharm.* 32: 123–127.

Nakagawa, Y., Hiraga, K., and Suga. T. 1983. On the mechanism of covalent binding of butylated hydroxytoluene to microsomal protein. *Biochem. Pharmacol.* 32: 1417.

Nakagawa, Y., Hiraga, K., and Suga. T. 1981. Effects of butylated hydroxytoluene (BHT) on the level of glutathione and the activity of glutathione *S*-transferase in rat liver. *J. Pharmacobio-Dyn.* 4: 823.

Newbold, R. F. and Brookes, P. 1976. Exceptional mutagenicity of a benzo(*a*)pyrene diol epoxide in cultured mammalian cells. *Nature* 261: 52.

Oesch, F. 1987. Significance of various enzymes in the control of reactive metabolites. *Arch. Toxicol.* 60: 174.

Ohmi, N., Bhargava, M., and Arias, I. M. 1981. Binding of 3'-methyl-N,N-dimethyl-4-aminoazobenzene metabolites to rat liver cytosol proteins and ligandin subunits. *Cancer Res.* 41: 3461.

Olafsdottir, K. A. and Reed, D. J. 1988. Retention of oxidized glutathione by isolated rat liver mitochondria during hydroperoxide treatment. *Biochim. Biophys. Acta.* 964: 377–382.

Ortiz de Montellano, P. R., Kunza, K. L., and Mico, B. A. 1980. Destruction of cytochrome P-450 by olefins. N-alkylation of prosthetic heme. *Mole. Pharmacol.* 18: 602.

Pickett, C. B., Wells, W., Lu, A. Y. H., and Hales, B. F. 1981. Induction of translationally active rat liver glutathione *S*-transferase B messenger RNA by phenobarbital. *Biochem. Biophys. Res. Commun.* 99: 1002–1010.

Powis, G., Svingen, B. A., and Appel, P. 1981. Quinone-stimulated superoxide formation by subcellular fractions, isolated hepatocytes, and other cells. *Molec. Pharmacol.* 20: 387–394.

Prohaska, J. R. and Ganther, H. E. 1977. Glutathione peroxidase activity of glutathione S-transferases purified from rat liver. *Biochem. Biophys. Res. Commun.* 76: 437–445.

Pryor, W. A. 1973. Free radical reactions and their importance in biochemical systems. *Fed. Proc.* 32: 1862–1868.

Raha, C. R., Gallagher, C. H., Shubik, P., and Peratt, S. 1976. Covalent binding to protein of the K-region oxide of benzo[a]pyrene formed by microsome incubation. *J. Nat. Cancer. Ins.* 57: 33.

Randerath, K., Randerath, E., Agrawal, H. P., Gupta, R. C., Schurdak, M. E., and Reddy, M. V. 1985. Postlabeling methods for carcinogen-DNA adduct analysis. *Environ. Health Perspect.* 62: 57.

Reed, D. J., May, H. E., Boose, R. B., Gregory, K. M., and Beilstein, M. A. 1975. 2-Chloroethanol formation as evidence for a 2-chloroethyl alkylating intermediate during chemical degradation of 1-(2-chloroethyl)-3-cyclohexyl-1-nitrosourea and 1-(2-chloroethyl)-3-(trans-4-methylcyclohexyl)-1-nitrosourea. *Cancer Res.* 35: 568.

Reed, D. J. 1983. Regulation and function of glutathione in cells. In *Radioprotectors and Anticarcinogens.* (Ed.) Nygaard, O. F. and Simic, M. G., p. 153. Academic Press, New York.

Reeve, V. E., Gallagher, C. H., and Raha, C. R. 1981. The water-soluble and protein-bound metabolites of benzo[a]pyrene formed by rat liver. *Biochem. Pharmacol.* 30: 749.

Ross, D. 1988. Glutathione, free radicals and chemotherapeutic agents. Mechanisms of free-radical induced toxicity and glutathione-dependent protection. *Pharmac. Ther.* 37: 231–249.

Rotruck, J. T., Pope, A. L., Ganther, H. E., Swanson, A. B., Hafeman, D. G., and Hoekstra, W. G. 1973. Selenium: Biochemical role as a component of glutathione peroxidase. *Science* 179: 588–591.

Rumyantseva, G. V., Weiner, L. M., Molin, Y. N., and Budker, V. G. 1979. Permeation of liposome membrane by superoxide radical. *F.E.B.S. Lett.* 108: 477–480.

Sayer, J. M., Yagi, H., Wood, A. W., Conney, A. H., and Jerina, D. M. 1982. Extremely facile reaction between the ultimate carcinogen benzo(a)pyrene-7,8-diol 9,10-epoxide and ellagic acid. *J. Am. Chem. Soc.* 104: 5562.

Schelin, C., Tunek, A., and Jergil, B. 1983. Covalent binding of benzo(a)pyrene to rat liver cytosolic proteins and its effect on the binding to microsomal proteins. *Biochem. Pharmacol.* 32: 1501.

Schmassman, H. U. and Oesch, H. 1978. *Trans*-silbene oxide: A selective inducer of rat liver epoxide hydratase. *Mol. Pharmacol.* 14: 834.

Seidegard, J., DePierre, J. W., Morgenstern, R., Pilotti, A., and Ernster, L. 1981. Induction of drug-metabolizing systems and related enzymes with metabolites and structural analogues of stilbene. *Biochim. Biophys. Acta* 672: 65.

Shen, A. L., Fahl, W. E., and Jefcoate, C. R. 1980. Metabolism of benzo(*a*)pyrene by isolated hepatocytes and factors covalent binding of benzo(*a*)pyrene metabolites to DNA in hepatocytes and microsomal systems. *Arch. Biochem. Biophys.* 204: 511.

Sies, H. (Ed.) 1985. *Oxidative Stress.* Academic Press, London.

Sies, H., Wefers, H., Graf, P., and Akerboom, T. P. M. 1983. Hepatic hydroperoxide metabolism: Studies on redox cycling and generation of H_2O_2. In *Isolation, Characterization, and Use of Hepatocytes.* (Ed.) Harris, R. A. and Cornell, N. W., p. 341. Am. Elsevier, New York..

Sies, H., Wendel, A., and Bors, W. 1982. Metabolism of organic hydroperoxides. Ch. 16. In *Metabolic Basis of Detoxication* (Ed.) Jakoby, W. B., Bend, J. R., and Caldwell, J., p. 307. Academic Press, New York.

Sims, P., Grover, P. L., Swaisland, A., Pal, K., and Hewer, A. 1974. Metabolic activation of benzo(a)pyrene proceeds by a diol-epoxide. *Nature* 252: 326.

Singer, S. and Litwack, G. 1971. Identity of corticosteroid binder 1 with the macromolecule binding 3-methylcholanthrene in liver cytosol *in vivo*. *Cancer Res.* 31: 1364.

Slaga, T. J., Viaje, A., Berry, D. L., Bracken, W. M., Buty, S. G., and Scribner, J. D. 1976. Skin tumor initiating ability of benzo(*a*)pyrene-4,5-epoxides, 7,8-epoxides and 7,8-diol-9,10-epoxides and 7,8-diols. *Cancer Lett.* 2: 115.

Stadtman, T. C. 1980. Selenium-dependent enzymes. *Annu. Rev. Biochem.* 49: 93.

Stout, D. L., Hemminki, K., and Becker, F. F. 1980. Covalent binding of 2-acetylaminofluorene, 2-amino fluorene and *N*-hydroxy-2-acetylaminofluorene to rat liver nuclear DNA and protein *in vivo* and *in vitro*. *Cancer Res.* 40: 3579.

Subrahmanyam, V. V. and O'Brien, P. J. 1985. Peroxidase catalyzed oxygen activation by arylamine carcinogens and phenol. *Chem. Biol. Interact.* 50: 185.

Sunde, R. A. and Hoekstra, W. G. 1980. Structure, synthesis and function of glutathione peroxidase. *Nutr. Rev.* 38: 265.

Swain, C. G. and Scott, C. B. 1953. Quantitative correlation of relation rates. Comparison of hydroxide ion with other nucleophilic reagents toward alkyl halides, esters, epoxides and acyl halides. *J. Am. Chem. Soc.* 75: 141.

Sykes, P. 1975. *A Guidebook to Mechanisms in Organic Chemistry,* Fourth edition. Halsted Press, a Division of John Wiley & Sons, Inc., New York.

Szajewski, R. P. and Whitesides, G. M. 1980. Rate constants and equilibrium constants for thiol-disulfide interchange reactions involving oxidized glutathione. *J. Am. Chem. Soc.* 102: 2010.

Tappel, A. L. 1979. Measure of and protection from vivo lipid peroxidation. In *Biochemical and Clinical Aspects of Oxygen.* (Ed.) Caughey, W. A., p. 679. Academic Press, New York.

Tateishi, N., Higashi, T., Shinya, S., Naruse, A., and Sakamoto, Y. 1974. Studies on the regulation of glutathione level in rat liver. *J. Biochem.* 75: 93.

Tien, M., Morehouse, L. A., Bucher, J. R., and Aust, S. 1982. The multiple effects of ethylenediaminetetraacetate in several model lipid peroxidation systems. *Arch. Biochem. Biophys.* 218: 450.

Tien, M., Svingen, B. A., and Aust, S. D. 1981. Superoxide-dependent lipid peroxidation. *Fed. Proc.* 40: 179–182.

Uehleke, H. 1974. The model system of microsomal drug activation and covalent binding to endoplasmic proteins. *Proc. Eur. Soc. Study Drug Toxic.* 15: 119.

Ulland, B. M., Weisburger, J. H., Yamamoto, R. S., and Weisburger, E. K. 1973. Antioxidants and carcinogenesis: Butylated hydroxytoluene, but not diphenyl p-phenylenediamine, inhibits cancer induction by N-2-fluorenylacetamide and by N-hydroxy-N-2-fluorenylacetamide in rats. *Food Cosmet. Toxicol.* 11: 199.

Veleminsky, J., Osterman-Golkar, S., and Ehrenberg, L. 1970. Reaction rates and biological action of N-methyl- and N-ethyl-N-nitrosourea. *Mutat. Res.* 10: 169.

Vignais, P. M. and Vignais, P. V. 1973. Fuscin, an inhibitor of mitochondrial SH-dependent transport linked functions: *Biochim. Biophys. Acta* 325: 357.

Wahlländer, A., Soboll, S., Sies, H., Linke, I., and Muller, M. 1979. Hepatic mitochondrial and cytosolic glutathione content and the subcellular distribution of GSH S-transferases. *F.E.B.S. Lett.* 97: 138.

Wattenberg, L. W., Lam, L. K. T., Speier, J. L., Loub, W. D., and Borchert, P. 1977. Inhibitors of chemical carcinogenesis. In *Origins of Human Can-*

cer, Book B, (Ed.) Hiatt, H. H., Watson, J. D., and Winsten, J. A., p. 785. Cold Spring Harbor, New York.

Wattenberg, L. W. 1974. Inhibition of carcinogenic and toxic effects of polycyclic hydrocarbons by several sulfur-containing compounds. *J. Natl. Cancer Inst.* 52: 1583.

Wattenberg, L. W. 1972a. Inhibition of carcinogenic effects of diethyl-nitrosamine and 4-nitroquinoline-*N* oxide by antioxidants. *Fed. Proc.* 31: 633.

Wattenberg, L. W. 1972b. Inhibition of carcinogenic and toxic effects of polycyclic hydrocarbons by phenolic antioxidants and ethoxyquin. *J. Natl. Cancer Inst.* 48: 1425.

Wattenberg, L. W. 1985. Chemoprevention of cancer. *Cancer Res.* 45: 1–8.

Weisburger, E. K., Evarts, R. P., and Wenk, M. L. 1977. Inhibitory effect of butylated hydroxytoluene (BHT) on intestinal carcinogenesis in rats by azoxymethane. *Food Cosmet. Toxicol.* 15: 139.

Wendel, A. 1980. Glutathione peroxidase. In *Enzymatic Basis of Detox-ication.* (Ed.) Jakoby, W. B., Vol. 1, p. 333. Academic Press, New York.

White, I., N., H. 1976. The role of liver glutathione in the acute toxicity of retroresine to rats. *Chem. Biol. Interact.* 13: 333.

Wislocki, P. G., Wood, A. W., Chang, R. L., Levin, W., Yagi, H., Hernandez, O., Jerina, D. M., and Conney A. H. 1976. Toxicity of a diol epoxide derived from benzo(a)pyrene. *Biochem. Biophys. Res. Commun.* 68: 1006.

Wood, A. W., Chang, R. L., Levin, W., Lehr, R. E., Schaefer-Ridder, M., Karle, J. M., Jerina, D. M., and Conney, A. H. 1977. Mutagenicity and cytotoxicity of benz(a)anthracene diol epoxides and tetrahydro epox-ides; experimental activity of the bay regions 1,2-epoxides. *Proc. Natl. Acad. Sci. U.S.A.* 74: 2746.

Wood, A. W., Levin, W., Lu, A. Y. H., Yagi, H., Hernandez, O., Jerina, D. M., and Conney, A. H. 1976. Metabolism of benzo(*a*)pyrene and benzo(*a*)pyrene derivatives to mutagenic products by highly purified hepatic microsomal enzymes. *J. Biol. Chem.* 251: 4882.

Wood, A. W., Huang, M. -T., Chang, R. L., Newmark, H. L., Lehr, R. E., Yagi, H., Sayer, J. M., Jerina, D. M., and Conney, A. H. 1982. Inhibition of the mutagenicity of bay-region diol epoxides of polycyclic aromatic hydrocarbons by naturally occurring plant phenols—Exceptional ac-tivity of ellagic acid. *Proc. Natl. Acad. Sci. U.S.A.* 79: 5513.

Ziegler, D. M., Duffel, M. W., and Poulsen, L. L. 1980. Studies on the na-ture and regulation of the cellular thiol: disulphide potential. Ciba Foundation Symposium 72, *Sulfur in Biology,* p. 191.

8

Comparison of the Carcinogenic Risks of Naturally Occurring and Adventitious Substances in Food

Richard L. Hall and Bob J. Dull

McCormick & Company, Inc.
Hunt Valley, Maryland

Sara Hale Henry, Robert J. Schleuplein, and Alan M. Rulis

Food and Drug Administration
Washington, D.C.

INTRODUCTION

During the past 50 years, improvements in public health measures and the development of chemotherapeutic agents and vaccines have drastically diminished the threat of the communicable diseases—chiefly pneumonia, influenza, and tuberculosis—that were once the principal causes of death. The reduction of this category of threat has left open the way for the rise of the chronic diseases—those one must live long enough to develop. Of these, by far the most feared is cancer. Doll and Peto (1981), using the sketchy data available, present what is probably the most balanced and by now well-known synthesis of data and estimates of the causes of cancer (Table 8.1).

Cigarette smoking is the cause of approximately 88,000 deaths from lung cancer per year in the United States. A much smaller number of other

TABLE 8.1 Proportions of Cancer Deaths Attributed to Various different Factors

	Percent of all cancer deaths	
Factor or class of factors	Best estimate	Range of acceptable estimates
Tobacco	30	25–40
Alcohol	3	2–4
Diet	35	10–70
Food additives	1	−5–2
Reproductive and sexual behavior	7	1–13
Occupation	4	2–8
Pollution	2	1–5
Industrial products	1	1–2
Medicines and medical procedures	1	0.5–3
Geophysical factors	3	2–4
Infection	10?	1–?
Unknown	?	?

Source: Doll and Peto (1981).

fatal cancers are known to be attributable to specific occupational or industrial exposures. Together, as shown in Table 8.1, these account for approximately a third of all deaths from cancer. Beyond these are risk factors which show a strong association with cancer, a history of hepatitis and excessive alcohol consumption among them. As one attempts to reach for still other causative factors, the associations become weaker and more speculative. The breadth of the "range of acceptable estimates" in Table 8.1 underscores this increasing uncertainty. Thus, Doll and Peto estimate that alcohol accounts for 2 to 4 percent of cancer deaths, tobacco 25 to 40 percent, and diet 10 to 70 percent. It is virtually impossible at this point, given our limited knowledge of cancer causation and mechanisms and the current level of progress in epidemiology, to assign the causes of most human cancers with any great degree of accuracy.

Our knowledge of the mechanisms by which tumors form and progress is even less satisfactory. Through patient and skillful research, we have begun to gain, in a few limited instances, some knowledge of the initiation of chemical carcinogenesis by, for example, the nitrosamines (Pegg, 1977) or the *para*-alkoxy allylbenzenes (Miller et al., 1983). We do not know if these are significant or trivial in overall cancer incidence.

We have only just begun to appreciate the role of oncogenes (Land et al., 1983). The importance of cancer "promoters" and "promotion" is widely recognized and not at all well understood. Overall, our knowledge is fragmentary.

Because we fear what we do not understand, ignorance adds to fear. We typically discount the adverse consequences of our own actions, particularly when those actions bring us pleasure—as with smoking or alcohol consumption. We prefer to focus on external causes of involuntary risks. Because we do not know specifically where to look for the major causes of cancer other than tobacco and alcohol, we tend to focus on involuntary risks we think we can "see"—pollution, pesticide residues, and food additives (Efron, 1984).

In contrast to this emotional, subjective, and sometimes political approach, one should note, again referring to Table 8.1, that Doll and Peto (1981) consider pollution a minor contributor to overall cancer mortality. They do not mention pesticide residues, and they treat food additives as perhaps more a net benefit than a net risk. Unfortunately, given our ignorance and our fear of cancer, the rational analysis and informed speculation of Doll and Peto have had little impact on public perceptions or on the ways in which risks are often estimated and regulated in response to those perceptions.

Public attention fixes instead on the results of carcinogenicity tests in animals, perhaps because they appear to provide "hard numbers," seem intuitively easier to understand, and deal with the external, "involuntary" risks—the chemical carcinogens. In fact, the results of animal tests are rarely precise as this paper repeatedly stresses; an understanding of the cause and extent of their uncertainties should be an essential part of any risk analysis. Nor is the relevance of animal test results to human safety necessarily obvious. Determination of relevance requires that expert judgment consider all of the evidence in each case, and even that is often not enough to settle the issue. Nevertheless, the extreme fear of cancer further enhances public concern with experimental results in animals. This in turn has led to exceedingly conservative methods of risk estimation. It is the application of the process of risk estimation—Quantitative Risk Assessment (QRA)—to compare the risks of various chemicals and categories of foodborne chemicals that is the focus of this paper. Despite its limitations and inadequacies, QRA applied in this way can, we hope, yield useful comparisons of relative risks.

RISK COMPARISONS

Risk comparison is by no means new. There have been numerous books and articles dealing with natural toxicants (Committee on Food Protection, 1973; Hall, 1977; Liener, 1980; Ames, 1983). More recently, Ames and coworkers (Peto, 1984; Ames et al., 1987) devised a system of comparing the potency of carcinogens in rodent tests.

They use, as a measure, the TD_{50}, the daily dose rate in mg/kg body weight that halves the percent of tumor-free animals by the end of a standard lifetime. Using human exposure data from a variety of sources, they express each human exposure (daily lifetime dose in mg/kg body weight) as a percentage of the rodent TD_{50}. This percentage they call the HERP (Human Exposure Dose/Rodent Potency Dose).

The proposal of Ames and his coworkers is thoughtful and constructive. As they acknowledge, there remain in many specific instances large questions as to the relevancy of high-dose animal studies to human safety at exposures many orders of magnitude smaller. Moreover, the Ames system of rating potency is itself still a subject of debate. Its units of estimation, TD_{50} and HERPs, are unfamiliar and do not readily translate into the units and levels of risk that regulatory agencies use in performing their statutory function of controlling consumer exposure to carcinogens in foods and the environment. These risk expressions, such as "a lifetime risk of less than 1×10^{-6}" or "_____ excess deaths from cancer in an exposed population of _____," when used by regulatory agencies or in the popular press or scientific literature, often tend to communicate a misleading message. That misleading message is, first, an exaggerated estimate of the actual health threat and, second, a misleading impression of the precision of that estimate.

It will be a major point of this paper that these figures, so expressed, take on an apparent validity and precision that in fact they do not have. But until we can do better, or at least better understand them and their uncertainties, we are stuck with them. Moreover, we are persuaded that when QRA is used to compare risks, the ranking or comparison of relative risks is significantly less uncertain than the absolute values of the risk estimates themselves, a point also made by Ames and his coworkers. A better understanding and perspective on these matters are the objectives of this paper.

RISK ASSESSMENT

The design of carcinogenicity studies so that the results will be suitable for use in QRA has been discussed extensively elsewhere (Scientific Committee, 1980; Board of Scientific Counselors, 1984) and in this volume as well. Unfortunately, the data that have been used for QRA by no means always rise to the desired level of quality. In the comparisons that follow, the toxicological data used for the naturally occurring carcinogens were generally not of comparable quality to those used for added carcinogens for reasons that will be noted later. QRA is discussed more extensively by Dr. Flamm (see Chapter 15). An understanding of its basic elements, however, is necessary for the remainder of this chapter.

"Risk assessment" should be distinguished from "risk management." Risk assessment is "the characterization of the potential adverse health effects of human exposure to environmental hazards" (Committee on the Institutional Means for Assessment of Risks to Public Health, 1983). Risk management is "the process of evaluating alternative regulatory actions and selecting among them." Although the two activities can and should be distinguished, each process often affects the other. Risk assessment, as used by most regulatory agencies, has four steps:

1.   Hazard identification is the determination of whether or not an exposure to an agent can cause an increase in the incidence of an adverse health effect. The data to support such a determination are only rarely based on human exposures (epidemiological data). They usually come from studies in experimental animals, perhaps supported or initiated by the results of short-term in vitro tests or by inferences from structure/ activity comparisons. The quality of the data and the strength of the association should be described.

2.   Dose-response assessment is the process of estimating the possible relationship between the quantity to which humans may be exposed and any resulting adverse health effects. Because such data are seldom directly available, they must be inferred from animal studies. Animal studies typically use high doses to increase the probability of observing an adverse effect in a limited number of animals. It then becomes necessary to extrapolate, usually over several orders of magnitude, from the high doses used in the animal studies to the low doses to which humans are exposed. One must then generalize, across species, from the experimental animal to man. Such extrapolation should make use of any data on the dependence

of metabolism of the agent on the dose, and on data comparing metabolism of the agent in test animals and man. Unfortunately, such data are often not available. Because dose-response data are virtually never available at the typically low levels of human exposure, the results of dose-response assessment depend heavily on untestable assumptions about the shape of the dose-response curve much below the dose levels observed.

Different dose-response assumptions, often called "mathematical models," can fit the observed data equally well in the experimental dose range, but diverge dramatically at the far lower levels of human exposure. Regulatory agencies, out of concern for the public health consequences of their decisions, usually select a highly conservative model, i.e., one that leads to higher estimate of risk than other models would produce. The selection of the model for projecting low-dose response is only one of the many "inference options" in risk assessment, in which the choice of assumptions affects the outcome. It is however, one of the most weighty.

3. Exposure assessment attempts to measure or, failing that, to estimate the route, intensity frequency, and duration of actual or possible human exposure to the substance undergoing risk assessment. If it can be completely done, it will describe exposure differences among various population groups, with particular attention to those that may be most sensitive. The assumptions and uncertainties involved also should be described. Here as well, a desire to protect essentially all persons will usually dictate conservative inference options, i.e., those that increase risk estimates. Exposure assessment can be particularly useful in permitting comparisons of several possible regulatory control options for risk management.

4. Risk characterization, heretofore viewed as the final step if all are pursued, attempts to estimate the risk—the estimated incidence of a health effect under the conditions of human exposure. It thus combines the results of the dose-response and exposure assessments. The cumulative effects of the assumptions and uncertainties should be, but in fact seldom are, described. Usually, a series of inference options are chosen which, taken individually, are both reasonable and conservative. But far too often, when accumulated over the total risk assessment process, they can compound to produce an unrealistic and far more exaggerated estimate. Even more unfortunate, this unrealistic estimate is thereafter erroneously referred to as "the risk."

As discussed in Chapter 15 by Dr. Flamm, regulatory agencies use quantitative risk assessment because it is currently the best tool available to them for a job that must be done. However, all those associated with quatitative risk assessment—industry, regulatory agencies, academia, and the press—need to do a more effective job of risk communication. They have a responsibility to society to make sure that risk assessments are presented and discussed in a rational, socially responsible manner. Assumptions, points of scientific controversy, and significant gaps in knowledge must be explained. Quantitative risk assessment must be presented as a functional tool, an evolving scientific and policy process on which necessary public health decisions can be based. It is the principal point of this paper that the process of risk communication should include risk comparison. Such comparison is not only necessary for candid effective communication, it also will effect risk management.

Risk comparison should consist of comparing the estimates of the risk of a particular agent with estimates of the risks of alternative agents and with the risks of substances unavoidably and acceptably present as a result of natural occurrence. One must be cautioned, however, that the comparison of relative risks from several sources possess some degree of comparability. For example, it is not appropriate to compare the risk associated with consumption of naturally occurring or adventitious substances to that associated with a lightning strike. Further, the uncertainties in QRA, such as those that stem from low dose extrapolation or inadequate exposure data, often result in conservative inference options that produce risk estimates that are enormously exaggerated. However, these pressures toward conservatism in the face of uncertainty all tend in one direction—toward higher estimates of risk. Thus, comparison of such estimates, the *relative* ranking of risks, is very likely to be much less affected, much less in error, than the estimates of absolute value of risk. It thus gives a useful perspective on size of risk, and therefore on priority for seeking further data or for steps in risk management. This chapter examines, using actual animal data, human exposure estimates and parallel inference options, estimated risks of two pesticide residues. Folpet and ethylene dibromide (EDB), and three animal carcinogens that occur naturally in foods, either raw or as conventionally prepared: polynuclear aromatic hydrocarbons, found in broiled meats, smoked foods, coffee, and whiskies; allyl isothiocyanate, found in the *Brassica* species (broccoli, Brussels sprouts, cabbage, cauliflower, horseradish, and mustard); and safrol, found in various spices and herbs.

PESTICIDES

Folpet ((N-trichloromethyl) thiophthalimide)

Folpet is a fungicide used on lettuce, oranges and other citrus fruits, apples, and other small fruits. Pesticides are evaluated for safety and registered by the Office of Pesticide Programs, Environmental Protection Agency. Tolerances for pesticides in foods set by the EPA are enforced by the Food and Drug Administration. The FDA and EPA use slightly different methods of calculating risk and exposure.

Hazard identification.   In an oncogenicity study in Charles River CD-1 mice at doses of 0, 1000, 5000, and 12,000 ppm, duodenal adenocarcinomas were significantly elevated at the mid and high dose in both sexes (high dose: 45% in males, 39% in females vs. 0% in controls). Duodenal adenomas were significantly elevated at high dose, both sexes.

In an oncogenicity study in B6C3F1 mice, dose-related increases of duodenal carcinoma occurred in all treatment groups (0, 1000, 5000, and 10,000 ppm). There was a significant increase in papilloma of the non-glandular stomach in females. The maximum tolerated dose (MTD) appears to have been exceeded at high dose (25% decreased body weight); however, an oncogenic response was seen at all dose levels.

Mutagenicity studies were positive in vitro in bacteria, yeast, and mammalian systems. Folpet was both positive and negative for teratogenicity in the rabbit under different protocols, negative in the rat, and possibly teratogenic in the mouse.

EPA classified Folpet under Carcinogenicity Category B2 (probable human carcinogen), based on carcinoma and adenoma of the duodenum (relatively unusual site) in two strains of mice with additional supporting evidence provided from short-term tests. Folpet is a structural analog of captan, which also induced duodenal carcinoma in two mouse strains.

Dose-response assessment.   The EPA used the linearized multistage model for modeling the dose-response curve below the observable range of the mouse tumor data. For quantification of human risk, a Q_1^* of 3.5×10^{-3} $(\text{mg/kg/day})^{-1}$ was calculated. [The Q_1^* is a statement of risk. It is the slope of the dose response curve in the linear multistage model (Engler, 1986).]

Exposure assessment.   For calculating human risk, in the case of lettuce, orange juice, other citrus fruits, and apples, the EPA knew and used, in the exposure calculations, the percent of U.S. crop treated with Folpet. In the case of small fruits, the entire U.S. crop was assumed to have been treated with Folpet, which would have been unlikely. Treatment for all crops was assumed to have been at the maximum registered use level; this conservative assumption was thought to be warranted since actual Folpet residues in the crops cited were not known.

Risk characterization.   The following lifetime risk numbers were calculated using the Q_1^* value given above and with the exposure assumptions given above (Arne, 1988). The EPA's current position with regard to these risk figures, which could be construed to be fairly high for lettuce and small fruits, is that no additional registration of Folpet for new uses is to be allowed until additional crop residue and toxicology data become available to the EPA for analysis.

	Upper bound lifetime risk
Lettuce	2×10^{-6}
Orange juice	0.6×10^{-6}
Other citrus	0.1×10^{-6}
Apples	0.8×10^{-6}
Small fruits	2×10^{-6}
Total	5.5×10^{-6}

This total would be increased slightly if minor uses on other foods were included.

An alternative calculation of human risk is to use FDA actual Folpet measurements from the Total Diet Study and the EPA Q_1^* value. FDA's Total Diet Study uses approximately 234 foods for eight age-sex groups (infants, young children, male and female teenagers, male and female adults, and male and female older persons). These foods are analyzed for 11 essential minerals and more than 120 chemical contaminants (Pennington, 1983).

In the Total Diet Study, Market Baskets K64-K73 (April, 1988), the age-sex group consuming the highest Folpet residues across all 234 foods analyzed was the age 25–30 female group, where the Folpet total average daily intake was 0.26 µg or 0.00026 mg/person. Calculation of upper bound human risk then becomes:

$$0.00026 \text{ mg/60 kg person} \times 3.5 \times 10^{-3} = 1.5 \times 10^{-8}$$

This figure reflects food as the consumer actually receives it, with the effects of washing, peeling processing, cooking, etc. It is much lower than the highly conservative EPA risk figures calculated without actual residue data.

Ethylene Dibromide (EDB)

Ethylene dibromide (1,2-dibromoethane) is an effective nematocide and pesticide. Its major uses in the past were for

preplant soil fumigation for a wide variety of food and nonfood
    crops

postharvest fumigation for grains, fruits, and vegetables

fumigation of grain milling facilities and equipment

Human exposure occurred to applicators in agriculture and food processing and to the public at large from residues in treated foods.

Hazard identification. An NCI-sponsored intubation study reported
squamous cell carcinoma of the forestomach in both rats and mice, and in
both sexes. Later inhalation studies also found significant increases in
tumors of various sites in rats and mice. EDB showed mutagenic effects in
both prokaryotic (bacterial) and eukaryotic (higher organism) systems. In
its rebuttable presumption against registration, EPA therefore took the
position that EDB was a direct acting, genotoxic carcinogen.

Exposure assessment. Based at first on modeling of a "reasonable worst
case," and, later, on residue analyses, the EPA concluded that the dietary
burden for a 60 kg person consuming 1500g of total food per day was likely
to be 8.0×10^{-5} mg/kg body weight from bulk fumigation of grain, and
much smaller amounts from other uses.

Dose-response assessment and risk characterization. Using these figures and the "one-hit model with Weibull timing," the EPA concluded
that the total lifetime dietary risk approximated 3.9×10^{-3}, of which 3.3×10^{-3} was due to bulk fumigation of grain. It is primarily the choice of
model that causes this to be a conservative upper bound of risk.

NATURALLY OCCURRING COMPOUNDS

Polycyclic Aromatic Hydrocarbons (PAHs)

The designation PAH refers to hundreds of distinct molecular entities
ubiquitous in the modern environment. PAHs are formed during pyrolysis of organic substances, including the combustion of fossil fuels and
cooking of food, and are unavoidably present in air, water, and food.
Humans are exposed to PAHs on a daily basis by ingestion, inhalation,
and skin contact. PAHs do not occur individually, but as a complex mixture, whose composition varies widely from situation to situation.

Some individual PAHs have been shown to be carcinogenic in animal
testing; indeed some PAHs were among the earliest discovered animal

carcinogens and have been used as prototype compounds in carcinogenicity mechanism studies. However, many PAHs have not been tested for carcinogenicity at all, and others have given negative results in carcinogenesis testing. Adequate testing of all these compounds has not been performed.

One particular PAH—benzo(a)pyrene—has been chosen for illustrative purposes here because it is known to be carcinogenic based on a study of relatively good quality for quantitative risk assessment. It must be emphasized, however, that it is grossly inaccurate to assume that all PAHs have similar hazard, dose-reponse, or exposure profiles to benzo(a)pyrene.

Hazard identification.   In a study by Brune et al. (1981), benzo(a)pyrene was administred to Sprague-Dewey rats either as an admixture to the diet or by gavage in an aqueous 1.5% caffeine solution. Dissolved benzo(a)pyrene induced more tumors of the forestomach than undissolved benzo(a)pyrene (BaP); the 1.5% caffeine solution did not exert any carcinogenic activity under the conditions of this bioassay.

Dose-response assessment.   Data from only one dose group of rats were appropriate. This group of rats received BaP mixed in the diet 5 days/week at a level of 0.15 mg/kg body weight. This regimen was felt most likely to simulate chronic human exposure to BaP through food. Male rats and forestomach tumors were the basis of the calculation by a simple linear extrapolation commonly used by the FDA (Gaylor and Kodell, 1980). Potency of BaP was calculated by this method to be 9×10^{-1}.

Exposure assessment.   Human exposure to BaP was based on consumption of meat assumed to be charcoal broiled where BaP levels have been measured at 50 ppb. Actual consumption figures for charcoal broiled meat are not available. Per capita daily meat consumption in the United States is 197 g (U.S. Dept. of Commerce, 1987). We assume that 10 percent (20 g) is "charcoal" broiled. This is clearly a conservative assumption and overstates human exposure to BaP from charcoal broiled meat. Assuming this meat to contain 50 ppb BaP, estimated human consumption of BaP per day would be 1 μg or 0.001 mg (Lijinsky and Shubik, 1965).

Risk characterization.   Using the human exposure estimate above and a human body weight of 60 kg. the potency figure for BaP calculated above results in the following risk estimates:

$$\text{1 μg of BaP /60 kg person} \times 9 \times 10^{-1} = 1.5 \times 10^{-5}$$

The upper bond risk figure of 1.5×10^{-5} includes several conservative assumptions made where actual data were not available. These assumptions are: choosing BaP as representative for carcinogenic potency of all PAHs, using a linear extrapolation from one dose level point in the dose-response assessment, and overstating charcoal broiled meat consumption.

Allyl Isothiocyanate

Allyl isothiocyanate is the major component in volatile oil of mustard, a flavoring agent prepared from seeds of black mustard (*Brassica nigra*). Synthetically prepared allyl isothiocyanate and volatile oil of mustard are approved by the FDA for use as flavoring agents (Code of Federal Regulations, 1987a,b). Allyl isothiocyanate is also found in cabbage, broccoli, kale, cauliflower, and horseradish (Committee on Food Protection, 1973).

Hazard identification. A 2-year carcinogenesis bioassay of food-grade allyl isothiocyanate was conducted by the National Toxicology Program (National Toxicology Program, 1982). Twelve or 25 mg/kg body weight allyl isothiocyanate in corn oil was administered five times per week by gavage to groups of 50 F344/N rats and 50 B6C3F1 mice of each sex for 103 weeks. Groups of 50 rats and 50 mice of each sex received corn oil alone and served as vehicle controls. The NTP concluded that under the conditions of this bioassay, allyl isothiocyanate was carcinogenic for male F344/N rats, causing transitional-cell papillomas in the urinary bladder. The compound was not carcinogenic for B6C3F1 mice of either sex.

However, the relevance of this finding in mice to humans is not entirely clear. The progression of benign bladder papillomas in humans is not clearly established; such lesions do not always progress to malignancy. Also, bladder cancer in humans is rare; lifetime incidence of bladder cancer in U.S. males is approximately 1.5% (Flamm, 1988). Accordingly, for purposes of this paper, the dose-response assessment was adjusted arbitrarily to reflect concern for the human relevance of these bladder papillomas. While we consider this adjustment particularly appropriate in this case, it should be noted that this step has rarely been applied in other cases where data of questionable relevance have been used for risk assessment. The FDA has not performed a quantitative risk assessment using these data for regulatory purposes because the data have not been judged to be adequate for such purposes.

Dose-response assessment. The lowest-effect dose of 12 mg/kg body weight/day in male rats was selected. The number of benign papillomas (two) was arbitrarily divided by a factor of five to reflect their questionable relevance to humans. Potency was then calculated as follows:

$$0.4 \text{ benign papillomas ("corrected")}/49 \text{ male rats} \times 1/12 \text{ mg/kg body wt/day} \times 5 \text{ days/7 days per week} = 4.9 \times 10^{-4}$$

Exposure assessment. The mean human consumption of mustard oil (greater than 93% allyl isothiocyanate) was estimated to be 9.0 mg/person/day (Cramer, 1988).

Risk characterization. Using the potency figure calculated above and assuming a mean consumption of 9 mg/person/day allyl isothiocyanate and human body weight to be 60 kg, an extreme upper bound risk figure may be generated:

$$9/60 \times 4.9 \times 10^{-4} = 7.4 \times 10^{-5}$$

This human risk number has been generated for comparison purposes only and should not be construed to be a realistic estimate of human risk consumption of allyl isothiocyanate. In the opinion of the FDA, the carcinogenicity data were not of sufficient strength to support a quantitative risk assessment.

Safrol (4-Allyl-1,2-Methylenedioxybenzene)

Safrol is a natural plant constituent, found in oil of sassafras and certain other essential oils. A major source of human exposure to safrol is through consumption of spices, such as nutmeg, cinnamon, and black pepper, in which safrol is a constituent (Ioannides et al., 1981). Results of a chronic toxicity study completed in 1960 indicated that safrol should be classed as a weak hepatocarcinogen for the rat; safrol was then banned from all food use as an additive (Federal Register, 1960).

Hazard identification. The Food and Drug Administration has not performed a quantitative risk assessment for safrol because safrol was banned from use as a food additive before the development of this methodology. For purposes of this paper, a study by Long et al. (1963) was selected as being most appropriate for a demonstration of quantitative risk assessment.

In this study, five groups of Osborne-Mendel rats, 50 per group and evenly divided by sex, received 5000, 1000, 500, 100, or 0 ppm safrol in their diet for 2 years. The organ most severely affected was the liver, injury being moderate to severe at 5000 ppm, slight to moderate at 1000, slight at 500, and very slight at 100. At 5000 ppm hepatic tumorigenesis was significantly increased, and at 1000 ppm there were eight hepatic tumors, all benign. The authors of the study concluded that safrol was a low-grade hepatic carcinogen for the rat, perhaps acting on a basis of previous non-neoplastic damage.

Dose-response assessment. The lowest tumorigenic effect level was chosen (500 ppm or 25 mg/kg body weight/day). At this dose level one hepatic tumor appeared over control values. Using the Gaylor/Kodell linear extrapolation method, potency may be calculated:

$$1 \text{ tumor/50 animals} \times 1/25 \text{ mg/kg body weight/day} = 8 \times 10^{-4}$$

Exposure assessment. Mean total daily intake of safrol, based on reported analyses of nutmeg, basil, star anise, cinnamon, and black pepper, was estimated as 1.2 mg (National Academy of Sciences, 1979; McCormick & Co., 1982).

Risk characterization. Combining the potency estimate and the exposure estimate. upper bound risk was calculated:

$$1.2 \text{ mg mean daily intake/60 kg per person} \times 8 \times 10^{-4} = 1.6 \times 10^{-5}$$

This estimate of risk is probably inflated for two reasons. First, the exposure estimate is based partly on market product disappearance data, rather than actual analysis of human food as consumed. Second, the carcinogenicity of safrol is believed to be at least partly mediated through its metabolite. 1'-hydroxysafrol (Swanson et al., 1981; Ioannides, et al. 1981). This metabolite has been detected in the liver, urine, and bile of both rats and mice, but it is not presently known to what extent humans produce this metabolite or how important production of this metabolite is in the human carcinogenic process.

Estragole, which is structurally related to safrol and is also reported to be a rodent carcinogen, is hydroxylated to give 1'-hydroxyestragole, the proximate carcinogen (Miller et al., 1983). When comparative metabolic studies were done in mice and human volunteers, man excreted about 50 million times less of the proximate carcinogen than the mouse at the 500 mg/kg body weight doses, which was associated with hepatic tumors in the mouse (Caldwell, 1984).

Data such as these indicate that a more scientifically credible quantitative risk assessment should take into account metabolism and the dose of proximate carcinogen at the target organ rather than merely a delivered dose of a precursor.

DISCUSSION

QRA is an imperfect and evolving tool; its strengths, limitations, and uncertainties and, most of all, the limitations and uncertainties in the underlying data need constant emphasis—far more than they usually receive. Even with these problems, we believe that QRA is the best available tool for comparing the potential risks from different carcinogens. Such comparison is even more complex and difficult than we had at first expected, for reasons already mentioned and summarized below.

It is obvious that QRA does a better job of predicting risks when the data are of better quality. "Quality" in this sense refers to the criteria for toxicological data such as those embodied in the FDA "Redbook" (Food and Drug Administration, 1982). These include adequate numbers of animals, a minimum of three dose levels plus control, thorough pathology, adequate quality control, etc. The toxicological data on safrol are older and of poorer "quality" than the data on Folpet or allyl isothiocyanate, and the risk estimate for safrol may well be higher in proportion to this lower quality.

Criteria for quality also apply to data on exposure. Exposure data are tremendously important in understanding and predicting cancer risks from either naturally occurring or added chemicals in food. The exposure calculations with Folpet are a very significant case in point. Estimated risk dropped greatly when more realistic exposure estimates based on actual analyses of foods were substituted for EPA's assumptions that Folpet occurred at the tolerance level on every crop registered for Folpet use.

The example of estragole shows the potential value of data on dose dependency of metabolism and on comparative metabolism. Wherever possible, one should focus on the agent of actual interest—the ultimate carcinogen—and not on a more remote and inactive, but easy to measure, precursor.

The few estimates here presented are all conservative—perhaps exceedingly so. We cannot discard the possibility that the hundreds of naturally occurring carcinogens throughout the food supply may well be a significant cause of human cancer; *how* significant a cause is not easy to demonstrate.

Risk Comparison

It is interesting to note that the estimated upper bound risks from naturally occurring animal carcinogens (Table 8.2) are well within the range of the two pesticides and are slightly higher than the 1×10^{-6} level now often taken as the limit of acceptable risk. One can reasonably assume that a few other adventitious agents would be expected to give estimated upper-bound risks as high as that adduced for EDB. Considering the large number and widespread occurrence of naturally occurring carcinogens, one might reasonably expect the total risk from natural sources to substantially exceed that from human actions. That does not necessarily mean, however, that either the natural carcinogens or the adventitious ones are a significant cause of human cancer. Though possibly of quite different size, both risks may be insignificant contributors to human cancer incidence.

As mentioned earlier, we do not know how much of the overall risk from dietary sources is from initiators and how much from promoters, including the dietary promoter that has been most persuasively demonstrated—too many calories.

We do not know the relative contributions of carcinogens and anticarcinogens. Even less can we assess the overall contribution of those substances such as the antioxidants, which may be carcinogens at high doses and anticarcinogens at low doses. Beyond that are substances for which the risks are higher at both low doses and high doses than at intermediate exposures; the dose/response curve is not sigmoid, but U-shaped.

Potential Improvements

Risk assessment, for all its flaws, has appealing advantages. It provides a rationale for dealing with agents that may at least potentially cause effects at very low doses. Unlike the ADI, it attempts to give an estimate of risk.

TABLE 8.2 Upper-Bound Risk Estimates

Folpet	1.5×10^{-8}
EDB	3.9×10^{-3}
PAHs	1.5×10^{-5}
Allyl isothiocyanate	7.2×10^{-5}
Safrol	4.0×10^{-5}

And, also unlike the ADI, it provides an opportunity for—though not the assurance of—a science-based estimate of risk to be compared with a socially and politically based determination of an acceptable level of risk. The purpose of this exercise has been to illuminate the problems so that we may attempt to address them, not to provide an excuse for discarding the whole concept. The previous discussion foreshadows several areas of possible improvement we hope later to address.

It may even be possible, although certainly not easy, to sum risks from chemicals added to foods or the environment and sum risks from naturally occurring chemicals and to compare these sums.

Beyond these points, however, it is not sufficient merely to prepare a "conservative" estimate—an "upper bound"—of risk. Effective regulation and intellectual honesty compel one to estimate also, by the proper choice of inference options, the "most reasonable" or "most likely" risk, and the extreme lower bound of risk, at least for the potentially exposed population. The spread between these numbers, comparable to Doll and Peto's "range of acceptable estimates" would be an instructive lesson on the real precision—or lack of it—in the process. It would assist the essential process of risk comparison. It would begin to suggest what kinds of data could best serve to narrow the "range of acceptable estimates" of risk. In what we now conceive as one or more later papers in this vein, we expect to extend this comparison to other added and naturally occurring carcinogens and to explore in more detail these areas of potential improvement.

ACKNOWLEDGMENTS

The authors acknowledge with thanks the valuable help and suggestions of Dr. Gary Flamm and Dr. Greg Cramer of the Food and Drug Administration.

REFERENCES

Ames, B. N. 1983. Dietary carcinogens and anticarcinogens. *Science* 221: 1256.

Ames, B. N., Magaw, R., and Gold, L S. 1987. Ranking possible carcinogenic hazards. *Science* 236:271.

Arne, K. 1988. Telephone communication, June 10. U.S. EPA, Office of Pesticide Programs, Residue Chemistry Branch, Washington, DC.

Board of Scientific Counselors, National Toxicology Program. 1984.

Report of the NTP ad hoc Panel on Chemical Carcinogenesis Testing and Evaluation. U.S. Dept. of Health and Human Services, Public Health Services, Washington, DC.

Brune, H., Deutsch-Wenzel, R.P., Habs, M., Ivankovic, S., and Schmahl, D. 1981. Investigation of the tumorigenic response to benzo-a-pyrene in aqueous caffeine solution applied orally to Sprague-Dawley rats. *J. Cancer Res. Clin. Oncol.* 102: 153.

Caldwell, J. 1984. *Transcripts of the European Toxicology Forum,* September 18–21, 1984. pp. 124–131.

Code of Federal Regulations, Food and Drug Administration. 1987a. Essential oils, oleoresins, and natural extractives. 21 *CFR,* section 182.20. U.S. Govt. Printing Office, Washington, DC.

Code of Federal Regulations, Food and Drug Administration. 1987b. Synthetic flavoring substances and adjuvants. 21 *CFR.* section 172.515. U.S. Govt. Printing Office, Washington, DC.

Committee on Food Protection, Food and Nutrition Board, National Research Council. 1973. *Toxicants Occurring Naturally in Foods,* 2nd ed. National Academy of Sciences, Washington, DC.

Committee on the Institutional Means for Assessment of Risks to Public Health, National Research Council. 1983. *Risk Assessment in the Federal Government: Managing the Process.* National Academy Press, Washington, DC.

Cramer, G. M. 1988. Private communication, June 10. U.S. FDA, Washington, DC.

Doll, R. and Peto R. 1981. The causes of cancer: quantitative estimates of avoidable risks of cancer in the United States today. *JNCI* 66(6):1191, 1256.

Efron, E. 1984. *The Apocalyptics: Cancer and the Big Lie.* Simon and Schuster, New York.

Engler R. 1986. Memorandum, Summary of data on chemicals evaluated by Toxicology Branch Peer Review Committee, November 24. U.S. EPA, Office of Pesticides and Toxic Substances, Washington, DC.

Federal Register, 25 FR 12412, 1960.

Flamm, W. G. 1988. Private communication, June 10. U.S. FDA, Washington, DC.

Food and Drug Administration. 1982. *Toxicological Principles for the Safety Assessment of Direct Food Additives and Color Additives Used in Food.* U.S. FDA, Bureau of Foods, Washington, DC.

Gaylor, D. W. and Kodell, R. L. 1980. Linear interpolation algorithm for low dose assessment of toxic substances. *J. Environ. Pathol. Toxicol.* 4: 305.

Hall, R. L. 1977. Safe at the plate. *Nutrition Today* 12(6): 1.

Ioannides, C., Delaforge, M., and Parke, D. V. 1981. Safrole: Its metabolism, carcinogenicity and interactions with cytochrome P-450. *Food Cosmet. Toxicol.* 19: 657.

Land, H., Parada, L. F., and Weinberg, R. A. 1983. Cellular oncogenes and multistep carcinogenesis. *Science* 222: 771.

Liener, I.E. (Ed.) 1980. *Toxic Constituents of Plant Foodstuffs,* 2nd ed. Academic Press, London.

Lijinsky, W. and Shubik, P. 1965. Polynuclear hydrocarbon carcinogens in cooked meat and smoked food. *Ind. Med. Surg.* 34: 152.

Long, E. L., Nelson, A. A., Fitzhugh, O. G., and Hansen, W. H. 1963. Liver tumors produced in rats by feeding safrole. *Arch Path.* 75: 595.

McCormick & Company, Inc. 1982. In-house data.

Miller, E. C. Swanson, A. B. Phillips, D. H., Fletcher, T. L., Liem, A, and Miller J. A. 1983. Structure-activity studies of the carcinogenicities in the mouse and rat of some naturally occurring and synthetic alkenylbenzene derivatives related to safrole and estragole. *Cancer Research* 43: 1124.

National Academy of Sciences, 1979. The 1977 survey of industry on the use of food additives. National Academy of Sciences, Washington, DC.

National Toxicology Program. 1982. Technical Report Series No. 234. U.S. Dept. of Health and Human Services, Public Health Service, National Institute of Health, Washington, DC.

Pegg, A. E. 1977. Formation and metabolism of alkylated nucleosides: possible role in carcinogenesis by nitroso compounds and alkylating agents. *Adv. Cancer Res.* 25: 195.

Pennington, J. A. T. 1983. Revision of the total diet study food list and diets. *J. Am. Dietetic Assoc.* 82(2): 166.

Peto, R., Pike, M. C., Bernstein, L., Gold, L. S., and, Ames, B. N. 1984. The TD$_{50}$: A proposed general convention for the numerical description of the carcinogenic potency of chemicals in chronic-exposure animal experiments. *Environ. Health Perspect.* 58: 1.

Scientific Committee, Food Safety Council. 1980. *Proposed System for Food Safety Assessment.* Food Safety Council, Washington, DC.

Swanson, A. B., Miller, E. C., and Miller, J. A. 1981. The side-chain epoxidation and hydroxylation of the hepatocarcinogens safrole and estragole and some related compounds by rat and mouse liver microsomes. *Biochim. Biophys. Acta* 673: 504.

U.S. Department of Commerce. 1987. *Statistical Abstract of the United States.* pp. 648–649. U.S. Dept. of Commerce, Washintgon, DC.

9
Behavioral Disorders Associated with Food Components

Dian A. Gans

University of Wisconsin - Madison
Madison, Wisconsin

INTRODUCTION

Knowledge about the influence of diet on behavior is rapidly expanding at the present time, but concise definition of assumed relationships continues to be fraught with difficulty and uncertainty. This is due not only to scientists' unwillingness to investigate the simplistic theories put forth by overenthusiastic zealots, but also to scientists' incomplete understanding of the subtle and varied ways in which nutrients may affect behavior.

The belief that diet can alter behavior is an old one. Long before the disciplines of nutrition and psychology were formalized, people in various cultures thought certain foods had magical powers which could change behavior (Harper, 1988). Even today, popular claims about the behavioral effects of particular foods abound. For example, hyperactivity in children has been attributed to vitamin/mineral deficiencies, food additives, and sucrose. In addition, administrators in correctional facilities have changed residents' diets in the belief that significant improvements in antisocial behavior will be a natural outcome of the dietary manipulations. On occasion, seemingly contradictory types of behaviors have been ascribed to a single substance. Not only enhanced performance, but also negative consequences, such as nervousness, insomnia, and seizures have been attributed to the ingestion of caffeine. Some of these claims, such as the paradoxical, dose- and subject-dependent effects of caffeine, have been verified scientifically (Neims and von Borstel, 1983); others, especially the claims made about the adverse effects of sucrose, remain unsubstantiated (Behar et al., 1984; Gray, 1987).

INFLUENCE OF NUTRITIONAL STATUS ON BEHAVIOR

Despite the controversy, there is a large body of scientific evidence which demonstrates that mental performance and behavior can be influenced by nutritional status and, thus, indirectly by diet. Much of the evidence has been gained from research with animals other than humans. However, since human diet and behavior are the focus of this chapter, animal studies are cited only to illustrate specific points.

Protein-Energy Malnutrition

Effect of chronic protein-energy malnutrition on brain development and subsequent cognitive functioning has been studied extensively in animals (Levitsky, et al. 1979) and in humans (Hurley, 1980). Behavioral studies with animals have shown that malnourishment during critical periods of brain development can affect behavior; but malnutrition and isolation appear to exert synergistic effects that are evident at the biochemical, as well as the behavioral, level (Levine and Weiner, 1976; Levitsky and Barnes, 1972). Results from several retrospective studies of human populations that suffered from severe perinatal malnutrition (Anatov, 1947; Hertzig et al., 1972; Stein et al., 1975) support the animal observations. Since the behavioral deficits appear to be ameliorated through a combination of nutritional and psychosocial improvements in the environment, it remains difficult to assess the extent to which each affects behavior.

Acute protein-energy deprivation, such as from skipping a meal or fasting for a few days, may be more common in an affluent society than in a developing country (Kreusi and Rapoport, 1986), and these short-term deficits can also affect behavior. Breakfast appears to help school performance, as measured on behavioral tasks (Pollitt et al., 1982/83) and cognitive tasks (Pollitt et al., 1981). However, lunch may decrease perceptual sensitivity although evidence for a consistent effect is lacking (Craig, 1986). In general, when results of "fasting" studies are compared with those of "fed" studies in humans, performance appears to be better in the fed state (Kreusi and Rapoport, 1986).

Vitamins and Minerals

Deficiencies or excesses of specific micronutrients can have profound behavioral effects. In fact, behavioral abnormalities associated with deficiencies of several B vitamins (thiamin, niacin, pyridoxine, and vitamin B 12) helped define their essentiality in humans. For example, pellagra, the disease associated with niacin deficiency, leads to psychosis with delusions and hallucinations if left untreated. Unfortunately, this observation led to an unfounded and unsound treatment approach to the management of behavioral problems (APA, 1973). In the 1950s advocates of megavitamin therapy noted superficial similarities between the psychosis occurring in pellagra patients and the symptoms of schizophrenia. Thus, pharmacological doses of nicotinaminide, a physiologically active form of niacin, were given to schizophrenic patients with equivocal results. Subsequent controlled collaborative studies provided no support for the megavitamin concept (Ban and Lehmann, 1975). In fact, niacin itself has been implicated in behavioral changes when given in megadoses (Horwitt, 1980).

A number of trace minerals are essential for the development and function of brain. Maternal iodine deficiency during pregnancy can result in a deficit in cognitive function or even in severe mental retardation, depending upon timing and degree of deficiency (Sandstead, 1986). Iron deficiency has been associated with diminished neuropsychological function in children; these deficits have been interpreted as defects in attention and alertness (Pollitt et al., 1983). Inadequate zinc in rats' diets is associated with changes in brain neurotransmitter levels, which may relate to the abnormalities in neuropsychological functions observed in severe zinc deficiency in humans (Sandstead, 1986). Finally, copper deficiency results in nervous system injury in Menkes' disease, a lethal genetic condition of abnormal copper hemostasis in humans (Danks, 1983).

Lead and mercury are not considered essential to humans; on the contrary, they are toxic elements whose effects on neuropsychological function are of public health significance. The effects of mercury poisoning from contaminated food are particularly devastating; cerebral palsy in infants and gross motor and intellectual impairment in adults, as well as ataxia and visual effects. Lead intoxication, which probably affects more people than mercury poisoning, has been known since ancient times (Mahaffey et al., 1982) and can be due to either dietary or environmental contamination. Infants and children are particularly susceptible; sequelae range from deficits in attention and IQ to more serious consequences, such as convulsions and death (Weiss, 1981).

Precursor Control of Neurotransmitters

Neurotransmitters are the chemical messengers of the nervous system; some such as serotonin and catecholamines, are small molecules derived from dietary constituents: serotonin from the amino acid tryptophan and the catecholamines (dopamine and norepinephrine) from the amino acid tyrosine. Thus, it is reasonable to postulate that a neurone's ability to manufacture, store, and release neurotransmitters could be indirectly affected by the concentrations of appropriate dietary precursor amino acids.

Results from animal experiments about 15 years ago first suggested a causal relationship between dietary amino acid supply, brain neurotransmitter content, and subsequent behavioral change. It was then noted that changes in plasma tryptophan, produced either by intraperitoneal (i.p.) injections of tryptophan (Fernstom, and Wurtman 1971a) or injection of insulin or consumption of carbohydrate (Fernstrom and Wurtman, 1971b) could raise brain serotonin levels in rats. This observation seemed at odds with the then commonly held view that critical brain functions were isolated from peripheral influences. Furthermore, ingestion of a nonprotein substance, carbohydrate, actually produced a rise in the plasma concentration of tryptophan.

Fernstrom and Wurtman (1972) formulated and tested a hypothesis to attempt to resolve this paradox. They showed in rats that brain tryptophan and serotonin concentrations were not simply a reflection of plasma tryptophan levels, but also of the plasma concentrations of the other large neutral amino acids. Since carbohydrate ingestion elicited insulin secretion which increases amino acid uptake and protein synthesis in muscle, it effectively raised plasma tryptophan concentration by removing some of the amino acids, such as other large neutral amino acids, which compete with tryptophan. Insulin injection produced a similar response. Interestingly, protein consumption increased plasma tryptophan levels less than levels of several other amino acids because the ration of tryptophan to competing amino acids in dietary protein is almost always lower than this ratio in plasma (Fernstrom and Wurtman, 1972).

Subsequently, other investigators studied the effects of peripheral injections of serotonin or serotonin precursors on behavior in animals. Hodge and Butcher (1974) assessed isolation-induced measures of fighting (fight frequency, attack latency, and average fight duration) in mice after several drug regimes designed to enhance or impair serotonergic functioning. Mice injected i.p. with serotonin and a peripheral decarboxylase inhibitor engaged in fewer and shorter fights; injection of a putative tryptophan hydroxylase inhibitor was found to increase both fight frequency and locomotor activity for up to 8 hours. Further studies in rats utilizing lower i.p. doses of tryptophan (Taylor, 1976) showed a reduction of total active behavior such as rearing, walking, sniffing, and grooming immediately after treatment.

Dietary manipulation has also been used to study the effect of altering the availability of neurotransmitter precursors on animal behavior. Gibbons and coworkers (1979) found that if rats were maintained on a tryptophan-free diet for 4 to 6 days, mouse-killing behavior could be induced in nonkiller rats and killing facilitated in killer rats. Dietary repletion with tryptophan to levels found in rat chow modulated the killing response to control levels in terms of latency and topography. Behavior varied directly with brain serotonin concentrations; plasma tryptophan values were not reported. Then Chiel and Wurtman (1981), using diets in which the ratio of carbohydrate to protein was systematically varied, showed that spontaneous nocturnal activity patterns of rats changed significantly; as the ratio was increased, the rats were continuously more active. These and other animal studies suggest that the availability of tryptophan to brain may influence the amount of serotonin produced and that behavior may be modified by a change in the absolute amount of serotonin. However, it is not clear if the change in behavior is due solely to a change in serotonin content or to an effect of a dietary amino acid imbalance or to an inadequate amount of dietary protein.

Tyrosine delivered i.p. with a decarboxylase inhibitor (Wurtman et al., 1974) and tyrosine ingested as food (Gibson et al., 1982) have also been shown to influence brain catecholamine levels in rats. However, it is unclear if the rise in neurotransmitters was due to the precursor loading alone or if it was due to feeding itself. Brain catecholamine concentrations may increase due to activation of dopaminergic central nervous system neurones during eating, independent of changes in plasma and brain tyrosine (Sved, 1983).

Because dietary constituents, such as amino acids, as well as protein and carbohydrate, appear to influence brain content of neurotransmitters and their precursors and subsequent behavior in animals, it was natural to predict that they might modulate behavior in humans as well. Hartmann (1982/83) has shown that pharmacological doses of tryptophan will reduce sleep latency in individuals with insomnia; under some conditions, tryptophan can reduce sensitivity to pain (Seltzer et al., 1982/83). Recent work with healthy young males has produced evidence that large doses of tryptophan can reduce appetite or food consumption (Hrboticky et al., 1985). In another study with men (Lieberman et al., 1985), tryptophan increased drowsiness and fatigue but did not impair sensimotor performance on several tests. Tyrosine did not change subjects' self-reported mood states but did improve performance on a reaction time test. These results suggest that tryptophan may have significant sedative-like effects while tyrosine might be useful in treating depression. In fact, both amino acids have been undergoing extensive testing as either pharmacological agents or adjuvants in various treatment modalities for humans (Wurtman et al., 1981; Young, 1986; van Pragg and Lemus, 1986).

Researchers have also investigated the effect of dietary tyrosine and tryptophan on mood and performance in humans (Spring et al., 1982/83). A high carbohydrate food (sherbet) appeared to increase calmness in healthy males, but healthy females reported greater sleepiness. Older subjects responded differently to meals depending on the time of day, feeling less calm or more tense after a high protein meal (turkey) at breakfast as compared to a high carbohydrate meal. Unfortunately, these results are questionable because the study was not adequately blinded; both researchers and subjects were aware of the kind of food being eaten. Nevertheless, some of the effects of particular amino acids or particular macronutrients seem to occur consistently under defined conditions. As yet, the metabolic and neurochemical bases for these apparent effects of diet on behavior in humans have not been explained in biochemical terms.

NUTRITIVE SWEETENERS AND BEHAVIOR

Sweeteners have been available for human consumption since prehistoric times; perhaps the earliest used was date sugar (Tannahill, 1973) or honey (Newsome, 1986). Until the mid–nineteenth century, most dietary sugar consisted of sugars which occurred naturally as constituents in food, such as lactose in milk or glucose, fructose, and sucrose in fruits, cereals, and vegetables. Then, as food processing techniques made refined sugars less expensive and more available, per capital consumption of sweeteners, as

TABLE 9.1 U.S. Per Capita Consumption of Caloric Sweeteners

Calendar year	Refined sugar	Total corn sweeteners[b]	Honey/ edible syrups	Total caloric sweeteners
1975	89.2	27.5	1.4	118.1
1977	94.2	31.2	1.4	126.8
1979	89.3	36.4	1.4	127.1
1981	79.4	44.5	1.2	125.1
1983	71.1	52.2	1.3	124.6
1985[a]	61.8	64.2	1.4	127.4

[a]Estimated.
[b]Includes high fructose corn syrup.
Source: USDA/ERS (1985).

measured by disappearance data, rose to about 100 lb/year during the first 30 years of this century and remained at that level until the mid-1970s (Table 9.1). Since that time, total sugar (total caloric sweetener) intake has risen moderately to an average of about 125 lb/year for each person in the United States. Concomitantly, sucrose use has decreased while that of corn sweeteners has increased. This increased use of corn sweeteners and other sugar substitutes, such as aspartame (N-aspartyl-phenylalanine-methylester), is reflected in the relatively low position held by the United States in per capita sucrose consumption among a group of economically developed countries with high per capita income (Table 9.2).

Unlike sucrose, with its long and intimate association with human diets, aspartame was introduced into the U.S. food supply in 1981 after 16 years of lengthy legal and scientific scrutiny (Hattan et al., 1983). Although aspartame is a dipeptide, it is categorized as a nutritive sweetener by the U.S. Food and Drug Administration (FDA) because it contributes the same number of calories per gram as sugar and is, of course, sweet. However, since it is approximately 200 times as sweet as sucrose, it contributes insignificant amounts of energy to the foods to which it is added (Newsome, 1986).

The FDA set the acceptable daily intake (ADI) for aspartame at 50 mg/kg body weight when the product was initially approved for human consumption (FDA, 1981), a value which included the then proposed usage in soft drinks. ADI is based on human and animal studies and represents a daily consumption level that is considered safe by a 100-fold factor. The actual level of consumption of aspartame in the U.S. population has been

TABLE 9.2 Per Capita Sucrose Consumption in Selected Developed Countries

Country	Refined sugar
Israel	129
Iceland	118
New Zealand	118
Australia	113
Ireland	106
Sweden	102
Denmark	99
Canada	95
Switzerland	95
Finland	94
Netherlands	91
United Kingdom	89
United States	64

Source: Ahlfeld (1986/87).

estimated by several groups to be less than 34 mg/kg in 99% of the population (Table 9.3). Comprehensive evaluations of the safety and health effects of both sucrose (Glinsman et al., 1986) and aspartame (Stegink, 1984; Dews, 1987) have appeared recently; therefore, they will not be discussed herein. The remainder of this section will focus on results from scientific studies which were undertaken to explore some of the subtle associations that have been postulated to occur between each of these two nutritive sweeteners and subsequent behavior.

TABLE 9.3 Summary of Projected Aspartame Intake

Source	Aspartame projected maximum intake (mg/kg body weight)
FDA (1974)	22–28
MRCGF (1976) and MRCA (1976)	25–34
Stegink et al. (1977)	23–25

Source: Stegink et al. (1987).

Aspartame and Behavior

Aspartame is already being used to sweeten many types of food products (Table 9.4), and use petitions are currently pending on a number of others (Andres, 1987). Because of its expanding availability in food products and because it contains an amino acid (phenylalanine) that is an indirect precursor to central nervous system catecholamines, some researchers have suggested that there should be concern about potential behavioral changes that could result from aspartame ingestion.

In order for aspartame to affect behavior, a hypothetical sequence of complex biochemical events has been postulated to occur. Initially, the phenylalanine moiety of aspartame could change blood levels of phenylalanine, once the substituted dipeptide has been ingested, the peptide bond cleaved, and phenylalanine absorbed. Changes in plasma phenylalanine concentration could, in turn, influence the concentration of plasma tyrosine, its metabolite, and subsequently the concentration of brain tyrosine. Since tyrosine is a precursor of dopamine and norepinephrine, concentrations of these neurotransmitters could also be altered; mood states or behavior modified by these central nervous system compounds could thus be susceptible to change. This sequence, while physiologically and biochemically feasible, has not been demonstrated in humans, and results from animal experiments do not support an aspartame-behavior link. Results from rat studies published shortly after FDA approval of aspartame showed that gavage administration of aspartame to adult rats can effect rises in both brain phenylalanine and tyrosine (Fernstrom et al., 1983; Yokogoshi et al., 1984), but rates of formation of

TABLE 9.4 Food Product Categories Sweetened by Aspartame: FDA Approved

Breath mints	Instant breakfast mix
Carbonated soft drinks	Instant coffee and tea mixes
Cereal	Milk flavor additive
Chewable multivitamins	Over-the-counter pharmaceuticals
Chewing gum	Powdered soft drinks
Cocoa mix	Puddings and pie fillings
Cookie/cracker fillings	Shake mix
Fresh/frozen fruit drinks	Tabletop sweetener
Frozen novelties on a stick	Tea beverages
Gelatin dessert	Topping mix

Sources: IFIC (1986), Holmer et al. (1987).

monoamine neurotransmitters were minimally affected (Fernstrom et al., 1983). In both studies, the highest dose employed (200 mg/kg) was comparable to that representing the 99th percentile of intake when aspartame replaces sucrose in the diet of humans. In addition, results from experiments with rats fed single-meal abuse doses of aspartame (530 mg/kg) in conjunction with a carbohydrate meal suggest that the normal cabohydrate-induced rise in brain tryptophan can be blunted (Fernstrom et al., 1986). Thus, studies with whole rat brain preparations, including those noted above, have demonstrated that aspartame can change the biochemical milieu of the brain. Furthermore, evidence from a recent mouse study (Coulombe and Sharma, 1986) suggests that aspartame may alter concentrations of neurotransmitters and metabolites in specific brain regions. Despite this suggestive evidence from animal studies that, under very specific circumstances, aspartame can alter the neurotransmitter concentrations in either whole brain or certain groups of neurones, little evidence exists to suggest that subsequent behavior is altered in rodents (Butcher and Voorhes, 1984) or in subhuman primates (FDA, 1983; Suomi, 1984).

Similarly, studies of aspartame ingestion in humans offer little or no evidence for an aspartame–behavior link, although some studies have shown that aspartame can induce significant rises in plasma phenylalanine concentrations. Abuse doses of aspartame (100 mg/kg) have been shown to cause statistically significant elevations of plasma phenylalanine in both normal and phenylketonuric (PKU) heterozygote subjects (Stegnik et al., 1980). In addition, smaller, single-consumption doses of aspartame (10 mg/kg) in PKU heterozygote subjects have been reported safe, despite statistically significant elevations in plasma phenylalanine concentrations (Caballero et al., 1986).

Data from studies of either acute (Stengik et al., 1988) or chronic ingestion (Stegnik, 1984) of aspartame-sweetened beverages in normal individuals indicate that the phenylalanine portion of aspartame is readily metabolized when administered at levels likely to be ingested. Furthermore, in a study of adults heterozygous for PKU, acute doses of aspartame (10 mg/kg) in beverages did not cause plasma phenylalanine concentrations to rise significantly from baseline values (Stegnik et al., 1987).

Childhood Hyperactivity.   Studies of the effects of aspartame on behavior in humans are limited, and, in most studies, no behavioral effect of aspartame has been documented. In one group of studies relating to childhood hyperactivity, aspartame has been used as a placebo for sucrose; in mose of these studies, doses of aspartame were low (10 mg/kg). Wolraich and coworkers (1985) reported no significant difference in behavior in hyperactive boys between the ages of 7 and 12 after sucrose or aspartame double-blind challenges across a number of valid laboratory measures. Other research groups have reported similar results. Ferguson et al. (1986) found no significant behavioral differences after ingestion of aspartame and sucrose either in a group of boys and girls diagnosed "sugar-responsive" by parents or in a group of normal preschool boys and girls. Kreusi et al. (1987), working with younger male subjects, concluded that it was unlikely that either sugar or aspartame was a clinically significant cause of aggressive behavior.

A few studies have shown that aspartame ingestion appears to modify behavior. Results from studies in which subjects consumed high doses of aspartame (Kreusi and Rapoport, 1986) or aspartame as a component of Nutrasweet™ (Goldman et al., 1986) suggest that certain subgroups of preschool children may be less active or exhibit improved attention following aspartame as compared to following sugar ingestion. Opposite effects of low doses of aspartame have also been reported; Conners (1984) reported that activity in children may increase after aspartame ingestion as compared to sucrose. Interpretation of these seemingly paradoxical behavioral effects is problematic because aspartame has been used as a "control" for sucrose, when in actuality both sucrose and aspartame constitute treatments. Thus, the observed effects may be due to a caloric effect or to some effect of sucrose itself; alternatively, aspartame may mediate different behavioral effects in different groups of subjects in a manner similar to caffeine.

Control of Food Intake. Concern about behavioral effects of aspartame has also focused on changes in eating behavior, i.e., changes in kilocalorie intake in weight loss diets. Since aspartame is a food component with a few kilocalories per unit of sweetness, it becomes important to know if aspartame ingestion can have an influence on eating behavior in addition to, and separate from, its role in reducing dietary energy intake (Dews, 1987).

Well-controlled studies on caloric dilution of diets with aspartame have shown that both normal weight and obese individuals can lose weight when the diets are aspartame-diluted (Porikos and Pi-Sunyer, 1984; Knopp et al., 1986). However, an epidemiological survey of women 50 to 69 years old showed that their use of sugar substitutes, including aspartame, was positively correlated with weight gain and increased body weight (Stellman and Garfinkel, 1986). Cautious interpretation of these results is in order, because such findings may mean that persons with excess body weight use artificial sweeteners to avoid weight gain, rather than that use of artificial sweeteners necessarily predates weight gain.

Results from a recent pilot study suggest that aspartame may have both appetite-stimulating (motivation to eat) and appetite-suppressing (decrease in pleasantness of eating) effects on mood (Blundell and Hill, 1986). Neither subject weights nor food intake data were reported. Despite these paradoxical effects, the authors tentatively concluded that the subjects were left with a "residual hunger " after ingestion of aspartame as compared to glucose. They further speculated that these ambiguous signals may lead to confusion, a loss of control over appetite, and disordered eating patterns.

Experiments designed to investigate possible neurobehavioral effects of aspartame offer no evidence that either aspartame or phenylalanine affects food selection and subjective feelings (Ryan-Harshman et al., 1987). Phenylalanine or aspartame in doses up to 10 g did not affect lunchtime energy intake and macronutrient selection in normal weight males 29 to 35 years old. Furthermore, subjective feelings of hunger, mood, and arousal were not affected. Both plasma phenylalanine and tyrosine were increased, and amino acid ratios suggest that brain uptake of both amino acids could be increased, but no changes in subjective feelings directly associated with eating could be documented which correlated with the changes in plasma amino acid concentrations.

Current scientific evidence suggests that aspartame may have subtle and paradoxical, effects on mood states associated with eating, but there is no consensus as to the underlying biochemical mechanisms that may be involved. Furthermore, there is no consensus as to whether any changes in mood, if indeed they do exist, influence food intake, nor is there agreement that use of sugar substitutes, such as aspartame, does or does not alter normal levels of food intake. Obviously, more research is needed to understand fully the hedonic properties of aspartame, as well as its utility in weight reduction diets.

Sugar and Behavior

Proponents of a nutrition–behavior connection have suggested a number of diet-related explanations for the link: reactive hypoglycemia, food allergies or sensitivities, eating sugar, drinking milk and vitamin/mineral excesses or deficiencies (Gray, 1987). Claims that sugar is the specific nutrient responsible for unusual behavior have received widespread attention (Brody, 1984; Schoenthaler, 1985; Harper and Gans, 1986); but such claims are based mainly on anecdotal reports (Schauss, 1981), misinterpretation of scientific literature (Hippchen, 1981), or flawed interpretation of questionable data (Schoenthaler, 1985).

To date, no credible research exists relating antisocial behavior to sucrose consumption. Unfortunately, this has not deterred staff at some detention and correctional facilities from changing institutional diets by eliminating or reducing sugar in the belief that such modification can prevent or correct undesirable behavior (Gray, 1987). In addition, despite the lack of supporting evidence, some pediatricians and family practitioners continue to recommend a sugar-restricted diet for their hyperactive pediatric patients (Bennett and Sherman, 1983), and parents continue to focus the blame for their children's behavioral problems on refined sugar (Varley, 1984).

There is in the scientific literature, however, information from two seemingly unrelated areas of research that suggests that there may be a sucrose–behavior connection. Studies of both childhood hyperactivity and adult criminality may offer clues to a clearer definition of the possible links between sucrose ingestion and antisocial or disruptive behavior.

Childhood hyperactivity.   Interest in a dietary approach to treatment of abnormal behavior stems partially from the hypothesis that naturally occurring salicylates and artificial food colors and dyes in foods might be associated with hyperactivity and learning disabilities in children (Feingold, 1974). Despite anecdotal, case-study evidence that 50 to 70% of hyperactive children showed dramatic improvement on restricted diets, subsequent double-blind studies have not confirmed the utility of additive- and salicylate-free diets (Harley et al., 1978a, b; Gross, 1984; David, 1987). Furthermore, a recent meta-analysis (a statistical technique which allows rigorous integration of information from a cohesive body of literature) of 23 diet-hyperactivity studies offers negligible support for the efficacy of such diets (Kavale and Forness, 1983).

Critics of this additive-salicylate research have noted that the children's normal diets were not only high in additives and dyes, but also in refined sugars. Thus, they suggested that any improvement in behavior may have been due to the inadvertant elimination of sugar (Prinz et al., 1980). It is conceivable that sucrose or other simple sugars could have either a direct or an indirect effect on hyperactivity. If certain children whose carbohydrate metabolism may be faulty react adversely to sucrose, a direct physiological or behavioral reaction to it should be termed a food intolerance or idiosyncrasy, rather than an allergy, which is solely an immunologically mediated response to a food constituent, usually a protein (Atkins, 1986). Such a reaction appears to be uncommon; only one such report has appeared in the scientific literature (Gross, 1984). Under double-blind challenge conditions, a hyperkinetic boy and his mother were found to be intolerant of sucrose, but not glucose, lactose, or saccharin. Shortly after drinking sucrose-flavored lemonade, the mother became irritable and developed a headache; the son became easily frustrated, hyperactive, and difficult to control. Unfortunately, this interesting dyad was lost to further investigation, so no biochemical data are available to help define the etiology of their condition. Thus, popular books to the contrary (Yudkin, 1972; Dufty, 1975), there is little scientific evidence to support claims that humans are intolerant of sugar (Glinsman et al., 1986).

Results from several correlational studies (Prinz et al., 1980; Prinz and Riddle, 1986; Wolraich, 1986) do, however, offer weak suggestive evidence for a relationship between sugar intake and hyperactivity. Cautious interpretation of such data is in order, though, because correlational results do not justify statements about cause and effect. In these studies, the magnitude of the effects were small and were not comparable across studies; many behavioral measures showed no relation to sucrose intake. Significant decrements in behavior were restricted to measures collected in a single laboratory setting in a hospital; thus, no statement about the practical significance (e.g., in a home or school environment) of the adverse effects of sugar can be made (Milich et al., 1987).

Whether or not sucrose intake has adverse effects on hyperactive children can be addressed objectively only with experimental studies in which sugar intake is systematically manipulated. To date, although several adequately controlled challenge studies have been completed, no one single study has been able to deal with all of the issues of design, such as characteristics of the sample, appropriate nutritional and behavioral measures, optimum time course, number of responders, correct sucrose dose, prior food intake (including sugar), and placebo effects (Milich et al., 1987). Thus, results of these studies are conflicting and at times irreconcilable. However, two general conclusions seem appropriate. First, in most studies with hyperactive children (Gross, 1984; Wolraich et al., 1985) or in those with mixed groups of hyperactive and normal children (Behar et al., 1984; Rapoport, 1986; Kreusi et al., 1987), there is no convincing evidence that sucrose ingestion adversely affects hyperkinetic behavior, directly or indirectly. If any effects did occur, they appear to be in the direction of improved performance (Behar, et al. 1984). Second, individual children may respond adversely to sucrose (Gross, 1984; Ferguson et al., 1986), and this reaction may be evident only in young or preschool children (Goldman et al., 1986). In any event, the biochemical and metabolic causes for such reactions remain undefined, although several research groups have advanced the theory that reactive hypoglycemia and/or changes in brain metabolites may be the connection between sucrose ingestion and exacerbation of hyperactivity in children.

Adult criminality. Although no concise theoretical explanation has emerged from the hyperactivity studies with children, research with adult criminals habitually violent under the influence of alcohol is beginning to offer provocative evidence that abnormalities in carbohydrate metabolism may in some way be related to antisocial behavior (Virkkunen, 1987). However, it is important to note that these studies, too, are correlational and cannot be used to support allegations that sucrose ingestion causes violent behavior. Virkkunen and colleagues (Virkkunen, 1982; Virkkunen and Huttunen, 1982) first noted that during an oral glucose tolerance test, when compared to control subjects, the blood glucose concentrations of particular subgroups of violent male criminals fell to significantly lower values and the velocity of return to the original baseline value was different depending on the psychopathological state of the subjects. In further studies, Virkkunen has also been able to differentiate criminals into behavioral subtypes by their metabolic responses to a load of glucose. Enhanced insulin secretion was found to be associated with one type of antisocial personality disorder (Virkkunen, 1983); low blood glucose has been correlated with a subgroup of arsonists who display a particular set of behaviors in connection with their fire-setting activity (Virkkunen, 1984). In recent work, Virkkunen and Narvanen (1987) have begun to explore the possibility that unusual responses to glucose may alter plasma amino acid profiles and subsequently brain neurotransmitter levels. Unfortunately, the measure chosen (plasma serotonin) for the level of brain serotonin may produce erroneous results, because serotonin is also produced by peripheral tissues (blood platelets, small intestine, and mast cells). In addition, too much importance may have been placed on the level of one amino acid (tryptophan), whereas the whole plasma amino acid profile must be considered in predicting possible brain neurotransmitter changes. Finally, almost all of Virkkunen's experimental subjects were alcoholics; it is conceivable that the abnormalities in both their behavior and their carbohydrate metabolism could be related directly to their history of alcohol abuse.

Virkkunen incorrectly refers to his subjects as exhibiting reactive hypoglycemia (e.g., Virkkunen, 1982, 1987). Relative hypoglycemia is an uncommon medical condition, but some have claimed that it is quite prevalent in criminal populations, with estimates as high as 90% of all incarcerated individuals being affected (Gray and Gray, 1983). In order to diagnose clinical reactive hypoglycemia, blood glucose levels must drop below a specified value (40 to 50 mg/dL), adrenergic symptoms must occur at the glucose nadir, and these symptoms must appear after meals and be alleviated by food within about 10 to 15 minutes (Sherwin and Felig, 1981).

In his earlier papers, Virkkunen makes no mention of meeting the diagnostic criteria for reactive hypoglycemia (e.g., Virkkunen, 1982, 1983); in his most recent work, he mentions adrenergic symptoms, but does not document their occurrence or frequency and, of course, did not measure their disappearance after ingestion of food (Virkkunen and Narvanen, 1987). It would be more correct scientifically to say that his subjects were exhibiting "low blood glucose," rather than "reactive hypoglycemic tendencies."

Unfortunately, popular wisdom has already assumed a cause and effect relationship between the ingestion of sucrose, reactive hypoglycemia, and criminal behavior. Some of the popularization of this misinformation in the United States can be traced to 1977 when Barbara Reed—then a probation officer in Ohio—appeared before the United States Senate Select Committee on Nutrition and Human Needs (Reed, 1977) and testified concerning her high success rate with eliminating recidivism to crime with dietary manipulation. Most of Reed's evidence consisted of anecdotal reports, not substantiated with empirical research. She "diagnosed" reactive hypoglycemia only with a questionnaire of doubtful validity borrowed from schizophrenia research. Her follow-up on the parolees included undefined measures of blood constituents and unreliable analytical methodology: handwriting and hair analyses (Hambidge, 1982).

To date, the only papers published dealing with the interaction of sugar and juvenile deliquent behavior have been written by one person and have appeared in a quasi-scientific, non–peer-reviewed journal, the International Journal of Biosocial Research (Schoenthaler, 1985). Schoenthaler has concluded that poor institutional diets, particularly those high in sucrose, are a primary cause of hypoglycemia and that these diets can lead to antisocial behavior. Some of the modifications that he made in the institutional diets resulted in less sugar being served; others represented a substitution of one sugar-containing food for another (Harper and Gans, 1986). The studies were neither controlled nor double-blinded, and, most importantly, neither the amount of sugar served nor individual or group dietary intakes were reported in Schoenthaler's early studies. Attempt to correct the methodological flaws have not been successful, mainly due to misunderstanding of the concepts of placebo, double-blind challenge, and rigorously correct experimental design (Schoenthaler, 1987).

Conclusions

Almost any food ingredient can produce potentially harmful effects, depending upon dose and previously existing conditions, be they psychological or physiological. However, clearly there is little, if any scientific support for claims that ingestion of either sucrose or aspartame at current intake levels is responsible for hyperactivity or behavioral problems related to criminality. Any recommendations to eliminate sugar or aspartame from institutional diets in hope of preventing or treating these problems are unfounded. However, future questions about other diet–behavior relationships will continue to engage researchers; much of the current difficulty and uncertainty in interpretation of results can be avoided in future studies by first recognizing and defining the salient theoretical and methodological issues and devising a concise, but flexible, framework within which to approach all research questions relating to the effect of diet upon behavior.

TOWARDS A MORE OBJECTIVE METHODOLOGY

Historically, the main sources of information about diet–behavior interactions have been anecdotes and speculations not supported by empirical evidence. Scientific investigation into the behavioral effects of nutrients remains difficult because the effects may be subtle (Lieberman et al., 1982/83) and the research methodology, of necessity, must draw on a variety of disciplines, such as nutrition, metabolism, neurochemistry, and behavior (Dews, 1982/83). Critical evaluation of diet–behavior studies is problematic for the same reasons (Schwab and Conners, 1986). Thus, a framework for comparing and critiquing these interdisciplinary studies is still evolving as investigators continue to refine their own specialized techniques and learn to function effectively as a member of a team of specialists.

Nutritional Assessment

The scope of a comprehensive assessment of nutritional status continues to change as new methodologies become available; the objective remains the same: to identify individuals and population groups at risk for malnutrition. In a monograph written for health workers, Jelliffe (1966) identified four forms of malnutrition: (1) undernutrition due to a lack of enough food; (2) overnutrition caused by an excess of food; (3) deficiency states due to a lack of specific nutrients; and (4) dietary imbalance resulting from disproportionate amounts of nutrients. The relevant information is derived from medical, social, and dietary history-taking and from measurements of a wide range of nutritional and metabolic variables and should address all the various forms of malnutrition.

The medical-social history of a subject can provide information on socioeconomic circumstances, accessibility and selection of food, dietary patterns or habits, and general state of health. It is a well-accepted fact that lifestyle factors, such as disease and current or past drug and alcohol use, can influence nutrient availability and utilization.

Physical measurements (height, weight, body circumferences, fat folds) allow indirect, and more importantly, noninvasive estimates of body composition. Such measurements may be associated with specific nutritional deficiencies or may be simple indices of a generally malnourished state. For children, physical growth is one of the best indicators of nutritional status (Robbins and Trowbridge, 1984) when measures, both direct and derived, are compared with those from age- and culture-specific healthy populations.

Although dietary assessment is difficult and one's first inclination might be to abandon the entire undertaking (Mann et al., 1962), it is the only way to discover what people eat over the short term and usually eat over the long term. Then, once a reliable and valid measure of dietary intake is determined, the nutrients consumed are generally compared with some accepted standard, such as the Recommended Dietary Allowances (NAS/NRC, 1980).

Finally, laboratory assessments of tissue samples or body excreta are a valuable, and arguably indispensible, part of any nutritional evaluation. Measurements include levels of nutrients or metabolites in specific tissues, nutrient or metabolite excretion rate, and changes of enzyme levels related to intakes of specific nutrients or in response to a nutrient load (Pi-Sunyer and Woo, 1984).

It would be ideal to have one simple, quick test to identify individuals at risk for malnutrition. Unfortunately, such an analysis does not exist; currently, a comprehensive evaluation using a number of nutritional measures appears to be the most reliable approach.

Behavioral Assessment

The conflicts between popular wisdom and expert opinion over the nature and magnitude of the effects of diet on behavior cannot be resolved without methodologically rigorous behavioral research. Sprague (1981) has suggested that the area is so immense that the scope of the research should be limited to those areas already controversial and of interest to those who formulate public policy. In addition, it should be restricted to theories amenable to testing with currently available behavioral techniques and focused on populations presumed to be "at risk."

The above limitations suggest that standard behavioral measures be used, ones already demonstrated to be valid and reliable and for which normative value ranges exist. It must be recognized, however, that standard measures may not yet exist for particular dimensions of behavior, and new measurement techniques may need to be developed. Even when a behavioral concept is clearly defined operationally, one must also appreciate that many other methodological problems can plague the research. In studies of diet–behavior interactions in groups of children, especially delinquent adolescents, these issues can appear at first glance to be overwhelming.

Guidelines for Nutrient–Behavior Research

Early diet–behavior research with children dealt with the effects of particular diet regimes, such as the purported salicylate- and additive-free Feingold diet (Conners et al., 1976; Harley et al., 1978a, b). Other studies, some more recent, have focused on the short-term effects of individual nutrients, such as megavitamins (Rimland et al., 1978), specific food additives (Swanson and Kinsbourne, 1980), and sucrose (Otto et al., 1982; Behar et al., 1984) on cognition and behavior. In a recent review article, Schwab and Conners (1986) have discussed concisely the issues of methodology and evaluation for future studies of pediatric nutrient-behavior relationships and have offered criteria for evaluation of past and future research. These guidelines, as summarized in Table 9.5, might well serve as a preliminary basis for diet and behavior research in other age groups.

First, the hypothesis, and evidence used for its basis, should be stated clearly. Subject recruitment and selection procedures should include a description of demographic characteristics and medical history, as well as exclusion/inclusion criteria for both experimental and control groups. Several aspects of presentation of both challenge substance and placebo merit consideration; dosage and form of substance, order, timing and duration of substance administration issues, as well as past dietary intake, can all influence behavioral variables. In addition, dependent behavioral measures themselves should be not only valid, reliable, and replicable, but also should be ones sensitive to the hypothesized effects of the food challenge. Several types of behavioral measures are appropriate: observation, rating scales, activity monitoring, mood states, and laboratory tests of performance, attention, and cognitive functioning. Blood analyses and

TABLE 9.5   Criteria for Evaluation of Pediatric Diet–Behavior Research

Hypothesis
  States study hypothesis and rationale clearly.
  Identifies unique biochemical basis(es) for interaction.
Subject description
  Defines recruitment methods and exclusion/inclusion criteria.
  Includes all relevant and necessary demographic characteristics.
  Identifies current and past medications.
  Defines matching procedure used in selecting control group.
Food challenge presentation
  Defines dosage level (rationale and dose/weight).
  Describes challenge carrier (free of physiological and behavioral effects, ease of
    consumption by subjects).
  Describes placebo (free of physiological and behavioral effects, matched to
    challenge).
  Defines nutrient consumption prior to challenge.
  Describes method of counterbalancing challenge administration (within sub-
    ject design).
  Randomizes assignment of subjects to groups (between subjects design).
  Allows for wash-out between administrations of challenge.
Dependent measures
  Describes measures (related to and sensitive to hypothesis, multiple, valid, reli-
    able, replicable, age-appropriate).
  Plans administration of measures to coincide with anticipated effects of
    challenge.
  Calculates interrater reliabilities.
  States that raters are blind to challenge.
  Presents baseline scores for measures.
Conclusions
  Describes conclusions based on hypothesis and derived from data.
  Discusses correlations between unrelated measures.
  Compares results with other studies.
  Discusses clinical (practical) significance of effects.

Source: Schwab and Conners (1986).

other measures of metabolism, such as urinary metabolites, can provide
important biochemical correlates to the behavioral observations.

   Finally, conclusions must be based on the hypothesis and be derived
from the results. Results from several unrelated measures should correlate
with one another and should be compared with results from other studies.
The author's last caveat is perhaps the most important: statistical significance need not always imply or mean practical or clinical significance

(Conners and Blouin, 1982/83). It may be scientists' hesitancy or inability to communicate this subtle, but substantial, difference in types of significance to a less-than receptive public that is at the heart of the discrepancy between scientific evidence and popular belief about the nature of diet–behavior relationships.

ACKNOWLEDGMENTS

The author gratefully acknowledges the critical and skeptical comments of Dr. Alfred E. Harper on an earlier version of this chapter. Supported in part by gift funds from the Food Research Institute, University of Wisconsin, Madison.

REFERENCES

Ahlfeld H. (Ed.). 1986/87. *World Sugar Statistics,* p. 74-75. F. O. Licht, Ratzeburg, W. Germany.

Anatov, A. N. 1947. Children born during the seige of Leningrad in 1942. *J. Pediatrics* 30: 250–259.

Andres, C. 1987. Twin prong aspartame expansion. *Food Processing* 48(2): 40–43.

APA. 1973. *Task Force Reports: Megavitamins and Orthomolecular Therapy in Psychiatry.* American Psychiatric Association, Washington, DC.

Atkins, F. M. 1986. Food allergy and behavior: Definitions, mechanisms, and a review of the evidence. *Nutr. Rev.* (suppl.) 44: 104–11.

Ban, T. A. and Lehmann, H. E. 1975. Nicotinic acid in the treatment of schizophrenia. *Canadian Psychiatric Assoc. J.* 20: 103–112.

Behar, D., Rapoport, J. L., Adams, A. J., Berg, C. J., and Cornblath, M. 1984. Sugar challenge testing with children considered behaviorally sugar reactive. *Nutrition & Behavior* 1: 277–288.

Bennett, F. C. and Sherman, R. A. 1983. Management of childhood "hyperactivity" by primary care physicians. *J. Developmental & Behavioral Pediatrics* 4: 88–93.

Blundell, J. E. and Hill, A. J. 1986. Paradoxical effects of an intense sweetener (aspartame) on appetite. *Lancet* 1: 1092–1093.

Brody, J. E. 1984. Diet therapy for behavior is criticized as premature. *New York Times,* Dec. 4, p. 21, 24.

Butcher, R. E. and Vorhees, C. A. 1984. Behavioral testing in rodents given food additives. In *Aspartame: Physiology and Biochemistry.* (Ed.) SteginK, L. D. and Filer, L. J., p. 379–404. Marcel Dekker, New York.

Caballero, B., Mahon, B. E., Rohr, F. J., Levy, H. C., and Wurtman, R. J. 1986. Plasma amino acid levels after single-dose aspartame consumption in phenylketonuria, mild hyperphenylalanemia and heterozygous state for PKU. *J. Pediatrics* 109: 668–671.

Chiel, H. J. and Wurtman, R. J. 1981. Short-term variations in diet composition change the pattern of spontaneous motor activity in rats. *Science* 213: 676–678.

Conners, C. K., Goyette, C. H., Southwick, D. A., Lees, J. M., and Adrulonis, P. A. 1976. Food additives and hyperkinesis: A controlled double-blind experiment. *Pediatrics* 58: 154–166.

Conners, C. K. and Blouin, A. G. 1982/83. Nutritional effects on behavior of children. *Psychiatric Res.* 17: 193–202.

Conners, C. K. 1984. Experimental studies of nutrient effects on brain, cognition and behavior in children. Paper presented at Diet and behavior: A multidisciplinary evaluation, Arlington, V. A. November 27–29.

Coulombe, R. A. and Sharma, R. P. 1986. Neurochemical alterations induced by the artificial sweetener aspartame (Nutrasweet). *Toxicology & Applied Pharmacology* 83: 79–85.

Craig, A. 1986. Acute effects of meals on perceptual and cognitive efficiency. *Nut. Rev.* (Suppl.) 44: 163–171.

Danks, D. M. 1983. Hereditary disorders of copper metabolism in Wilson's disease and Menkes' disease. In *The Metabolic Basis of Inherited Disease,* 5th ed., (Ed.) Stanbury, J. B., Wynngaarden, J. B., Frederickson, D. S., Goldstein, J. L., and Brown, M. J. p. 1251–1268. McGraw-Hill, New York.

David, T. T. 1987. Reactions to dietary tartrazine. *Archives of Disease in Childhood* 62: 119–122.

Dews, P. B. 1982/83. Comments on some major methodologic issues affecting analysis of the behavioral effects of foods and nutrients. *J. Psychiatric Res.* 17: 223–225.

Dews, P. B. 1987. Summary report of an international aspartame workshop. *Food & Chemical Toxicology* 25(7): 549–552.

Dufty, W. 1975. *Sugar Blues.* Warner Books, New York.

FDA. 1974. Title 21-Food and drugs. Chapter 1—Food and Drug Administration, Department of Health, Education, and Welfare. Subchapter B—Food and food products. Part 121—Food additives. Subpart D—Food additives permitted in food for human consumption. Aspartame. *Federal Register* 39: 27317–37320.

FDA. 1981. Aspartame: Commissioner's final decision. *Federal Register* 46(142): 38284–38308. July 24, p. 38289.

FDA. 1983. Food additives permitted for direct addition to food for human consumption. Aspartame: final rule. *Federal Register* 48(132): 31376–31382. July 8, p. 31380.

Feingold, B. F. 1974. *Why Your Child is Hyperactive.* Random House, New York.

Ferguson, H. B., Stoddard, C., and Simeon, J. G. 1986. Double-blind challenge studies of behavioral and cognitive effects of sucrose-aspartame ingestion in normal children. *Nutr. Rev.* (Suppl.) 44: 141–150.

Ferstrom, J. D. and Wurtman, R. J. 1971a. Brain serotonin content: Physiological dependence on plasma tryptophan levels. *Science* 173: 149–152.

Fernstrom, J. D. and Wurtman, R. J. 1971b. Brain serotonin content: Increase following ingestion of carbohydrate diet. *Science* 174: 1023–1025.

Fernstrom, J. D. and Wurtman, R. J. 1972. Brain serotonin content: Physiological regulation by plasma neutral amino acids. *Science* 178: 414–416.

Fernstrom, J. D., Fernstrom, M. H., and Gillis, M. A. 1983. Acute effects of aspartame on large neutral amino acids and monoamines in rat brains. *Life Sciences* 32: 1651–1658.

Fernstrom, J. D., Fernstrom, M. H., and Grubb, P. E. 1986. Effects of aspartame ingestion on the carbohydrate-induced rise in tryptophan hydroxylation rate in rat brain. *Amer. J. Clin. Nutr.* 44: 195–205.

Gibbons, J. L., Barr, G. A., Bridge, W. H., and Leibowitz, S. F. 1979. Manipulations of dietary tryptophan: Effects on mouse killing and brain serotonin in the rat. *Brain Res.* 169: 139–153.

Gibson, D. J., Deibel, S. M., Young, S. M., and Binik, Y. M. 1982. Behavioral and biochemical effects of tryptophan, tyrosine and phenylalanine in mice. *Psychopharmacology* 76: 118–121.

Glinsman, W. H., Iransquin, H., and Park, Y. K. 1986. *Evaluation of Health Aspects of Sugars Contained in Carbohydrate Sweeteners: Report of Sugars Task Force 1986.* Executive summary, p. 148–152. Food and Drug Administration. U.S. Government Printing Office, Washington, DC.

Goldman, J. A., Lerman, R. H., Contois, J. H., and Udall, J. N. 1986. Behavioral effects of sucrose on preschool children. *J. Abnormal Child Psychiatry* 14: 565–577.

Gray, G. E. 1987. Crime and diet: Is there a relationship? *World Rev. Nutr. & Dietetics* 49: 66–86.

Gray, G. E. and Gray L. K. 1983. Diet and juvenile delinquency. *Nutrition Today* 18(3): 14–17, 20–22.

Gross, M. D. 1984. The effect of sucrose on hyperkinetic children. *Pediatrics* 74: 876–878.

Hambidge, K. M. 1982. Hair analyses: Worthless for vitamins, limited for minerals. *Amer. J. Clin. Nutr.* 36: 943–949.

Harley, J. P., Matthews, C. G., and Eichman P. 1978a. Synthetic food colors and hyperactivity in children: A double-blind challenge experiment. *Pediatrics* 62: 975–983.

Harley, J. P., Ray. R. S., Tomasi, L., Eichman, P. L., Matthews, C. G., Chen, P., Cleeland, C. S., and Traisman, E. 1978b. Hyperkinesis and food additives: Testing the Feingold hypothesis. *Pediatrics* 61: 818–828.

Harper, A. E. 1988. Killer french fries: The misguided drive to improve the American diet. *The Sciences,* January/February.

Harper, A. E. and Gans, D. A. 1986. Claims of antisocial behavior from consumption of sugar: An assessment. *Food Technol.* 40: 141–149.

Hartmann, E. 1982/83. Effects of L-tryptophan on sleepiness. *J. Psychiatric Res.* 17: 107–113.

Hattan, D. G., Henry, S. H., Montgomery, S. B., Bleiberg, M. J., Rulis, A. M., and Bolger, P. M. 1983. Role of the Food and Drug Administration in regulation of neuroeffective food additives. In *Nutrition and the Brain,* Vol. 6, (Ed.) Wurtman, R. J. and Wurtman, J. J., p. 31–99. Raven Press, New York.

Hertzig, M. E., Birch, H. G., Richardson, S. A., and Tizard, J. 1972. Intellectual levels of school children severly malnourished during the first two years of life. *Pediatrics* 49: 814–824.

Hippchen, L. J. 1981. Some possible biochemical aspects of criminal behavior. *Intl. J. Biosocial Res.* 2: 37–42.

Hodge, G. K. and Butcher, L. L. 1974. 5-Hydroxytryptamine correlates of isolation induced aggression in mice. *European J. Pharmacology* 28: 326–337.

Holmer, B. H., Kedo, A., and Shazer, W. R. 1987. FDA approves four new aspartame uses. *Food Technol.* 41(7): 41–49.

Horwitt, M. K. 1980. Niacin. In *Modern Nutrition in Health and Disease,* 6th ed. (Ed.) Goodhart, R. S. and Shils, M. E., p. 208. Lea and Febiger, Philadelphia.

Hrboticky, N., Leiter, L. A., and Anderson, G.H., 1985. Effects of L-tryptophan on short term food intake in lean men. *Nutr. Res.* 5: 595–607.

Hurley, L. S. 1980. *Developmental Nutrition,* p. 76–109. Prentice-Hall, Inc., Englewood Cliffs, NJ.

IFIC. 1986. *Aspartame Safety Issues: A Scientific Update.* International Food Information Council, Washington, DC.

Jelliffe, D. B. 1966. *The Assessment of the Nutritional Status of the Community.* World Health Organization, Geneva.

Kavale, K. A. and Forness, S. R. 1983. Hyperactivity and diet treatment: A meta-analysis of the Feingold hypothesis. *J. Learning Disabilities* 16: 324–330.

Knopp, R. H., Brandt, K., and Arky, R. A. 1976. Effects of aspartame in young persons during weight reduction. *J. Toxicology & Environmental Health* 2: 417–428.

Kreusi, M. J. P. and Rapoport, J. L. 1986. Diet and human behavior: How much do they affect each other? In *Ann. Rev. Nutr.* Vol. 6, (Ed.) R. E. Olson, E. Beutler, and H. P. Broquist, p. 113–130 Annual Reviews Inc., Palo Alto, CA.

Kreusi, M. J. P., Rapoport, J. L., Cummings, E. M., Berg, C. J., Ismond, D. R., Flament, M., Yarrow, M., and Zahn-Waxler, C. 1987. Effects of sugar and aspartame on aggression and activity in children. *Amer. J. Psychiatry* 144: 1487–1490.

Levine, L. and Wiener, S. 1976. A critical analysis of data on malnutrition and behavioral deficits. *Adv. Pediatrics* 22: 113–136.

Levitsky, D. A. and Barnes, R. H. 1972. Nutritional and environmental interactions in the behavioral development of the rat: Long-term effects. *Science* 176: 68–71.

Levitsky, D. A., Goldberger, L., and Massaro, T. F. 1979. Malnutrition, learning and animal models of cognition. In *Nutrition: Pre- and Postnatal Development.* (Ed.) Winick, M., p. 273. Plenum Press, New York.

Lieberman, H. R., Corkin, S., Spring, B. J., Growdon, J. M., and Wurtman, R. J. 1982/83. Mood, performance and pain sensitivity: *J. Psychiatric Res.* 17: 135–146.

Lieberman, H. R., Corkin, S., Spring, B. J., Wurtman, R. J., and Growdon, J. H. 1985. The effects of dietary neurotransmitter precursors on human behavior. *Amer. J. Clin. Nutr.* 42: 366–370.

Mann, G. V., Pearson, G., Gordon, T., and Dawber, T. R. 1962. Diet and cardiovascular disease in the Framingham study. I. Measurement of dietary intake. *Amer. J. Clin. Nutr.* 11: 200–255.

Mahaffey, K. R., Annest, J. L., Roberts, J., and Murphy, R. S. 1982. National estimates of blood lead levels: United States 1976–1980. *New England J. Med.* 307: 573–579.

Milich, R., Wolraich, M., and Lindgren, S. 1987. Sugar and attention deficit disorder. In *Nutrients and Brain Function,* (Ed.) Essman, W. B., p. 138–150. Karger, New York.

MRCA (Market Research Corporation of America). 1976. Consumption of sweeteners in the United States and projected consumption of aspartame. A report to General Foods by the Market Research Corporation of America. Food and Drug Administration. Hearing Clerk File, Administrative Record, Aspartame 75F-0355, file vol. 103.

MRDGF (Market Research Department of General Foods). 1976. Potential aspartame consumption estimation. Research summary. Prepared by the Market Research Department of General Foods, Food and Drug Administration, Hearing Clerk File, Administrative Record, Aspartame 75F-0355, file vol. 103. March.

NAS/NRC. 1980. *Recommended Dietary Allowances,* 9th ed., National Academy of Sciences/National Research Council. National Academy of Sciences, Washington, DC.

Neims, A. H. and von Borstel, R. W. 1983. Caffeine: Metabolism and biochemical mechanisms of action. In *Nutrition and the Brain,* Vol. 6. (Ed.) Wurtman, R. J. and Wurtman, J. J., p. 1–30. Raven Press, New York.

Newsome, R. L. 1986. Sweeteners: Nutritive and non-nutritive. *Food Technol.* 40(8): 195–206.

Otto, P. L., Sulzbacher, S. I., and Worthington-Roberts, B. S. 1982. Sucrose-induced behavior changes of persons with Prader-Willi syndrome. *Amer. J. Mental Deficiency* 86: 335–341.

Pi-Sunyer, F. X. and Woo, R. 1984. Laboratory assessment of nutritional status. In *Nutrition Assessment: A Comprehensive Guide for Planning Intervention,* (Ed.) M. D. Simko, C. Cowell, and J. A. Gilbride, p. 139–174. Aspen Systems Corporation, Rockville, MD.

Pollitt, E., Leibel, R. L., and Greenfield, D. 1981. Brief fasting, stress and cognition in children. *Amer. J. Clin. Nutr.* 34: 1526–1533.

Pollitt, E., Leibel, R.L., and Greenfield, D. 1983. Iron deficiency and cognitive test performance in preschool children. In *Nutrition and the*

Brain, Vol. (Ed.) Wurtman, R. J. and Wurtman, J. J., p. 137–146. Raven Press, New York.

Pollitt, E., Lewis, N. S., Garza, C., and Shulman, R. 1982/83. Fasting and cognitive function. *J. Psychiatric Res.* 17: 169–174.

Porikos, K. P. and Pi-Sunyer, F. X. 1984. Regulation of food intake in human obesity: Studies with caloric dilution and exercise. *Clinics in Endocrinology & Metabolism* 13(3): 547–561.

Prinz, R. J., Roberts, W. S., and Hantman, E. 1980. Dietary correlates of hyperactive behavior in children. *J. Consulting Clin. Psychology* 48: 760–769.

Prinz, R. J. and Riddle, D. B. 1986. Associations between nutrition and behavior in 5-yr old children. *Nutr. Rev.* (Suppl.) 44: 151–157.

Rapoport, J. L. 1986. Diet and hyperactivity. *Nutr. Rev.* (Suppl.) 44: 158–162.

Reed, B. 1977. Testimony presented before U.S. Senate Select Committee on Nutrition and Human Needs, 95th Congress: *Diet Related to Killer Diseases. V: Nutrition and Mental Health.* U.S. Government Printing Office, Washington, DC.

Rimland, B., Callaway, E., and Dreyfus, P. 1978. The effect of high doses of vitamin B-6 on autistic children: A double-blind crossover study. *Amer. J. Psychiatry* 135: 472–475.

Robbins, G. E. and Trowbridge, F. L. 1984. Anthropometric techniques and their application. In *Nutrition Assessment: A Comprehensive Guide for Planning Intervention,* (Ed.) Simko, M. D., Cowell, C., and Gilbride. J. A., p. 69. Aspen Systems Corporation, Rockville, MD.

Ryan-Harshman, M., Leiter, L. A., and Anderson, G. H. 1987. Phenylalanine and aspartame fail to alter feeding behavior, mood and arousal in men. *Physiology & Behavior* 39: 247–253.

Sandstead, H. H. 1986. Nutrition and brain function: Trace elements. *Nutr. Rev.* (Suppl.) 44: 37–41.

Schauss, A. G. 1981. *Diet, Crime and Deliquency.* Parker House, Berkeley, CA.

Schoenthaler, S. J. 1985. Institutional nutritional policies and criminal behavior. *Nutr. Today* 20: 16–24.

Schoenthaler, S. J. 1987. Malnutrition and maladaptive behavior: Two correlational analyses and a double-blind placebo-controlled challenge in five states. In *Nutrients and Brain Function,* (Ed.) Essman, W. B., p. 198–218. Karger, New York.

Schwab, E. K. and Conners, C. K. 1986. Nutrient-behavior research with children: Methods, considerations, and evaluations. *J. Amer. Dietetics Assoc.* 86: 319–324.

Seltzer, S., Dewart, D., Pollack, R. L., and Jackson, E. 1982/83. The effects of dietary tryptophan on chronic maxillofacial pain and experimental pain tolerance. *J. Psychiatric Res.* 17: 181–186.

Sherwin, R. S. and Felig, P. 1981. Hypoglycemia. In *Endocrinology and Metabolism.* (Ed.) Felig, P., Baxter, J. D., Broadaus, A. E., and Frohman, L. A., p. 869. McGraw-Hill, New York.

Sprague, R. L. 1981. Measurement and methodology of behavioral studies: the other half of the nutrition and behavior equation. In *Nutrition and Behavior.* (Ed.) Miller, S. A., p. 269–275.

Spring, B., Maller, O., Wurtman, J., Digman, L., and Cozolino, L. 1982/83. Effects of protein meals on mood and performance: Interactions with sex and age. *J. Psychiatric Res.* 17: 155–167.

Stegink, L. D., Filer, L. J., and Baker, G. L. 1977. Effect of aspartame and aspartate loading upon plasma and erythrocyte free amino acid levels in normal adult volunteers. *J. Nutrition* 107: 1837–1845.

Stegink, L. D., Filer, L. J., Baker, G. L., and McDonnell, J. E. 1980. Effect of an abuse dose of aspartame upon pplasma and erythrocyte levels of amino acids in phenylketonuric heterozygous and normal adults. *J. Nutrition* 110: 2216–2224.

Stegink, L. D. 1984. The aspartame story: A model for the clinical testing of a food additive. *Amer. J. Clin. Nutr.* 46: 204–215.

Stegink, L. D., Wolf-Novak, L. C., Filer, L. J., Bell, E. F., Zeigler, E. E., Krause, W. A., and Brummel, M. C. 1987. Aspartame-sweetened beverage: Effect on plasma amino acid concentration in normal and adults heterozygous for phenylketonuria. *J. Nutr.* 117: 1989–1995.

Stegink, L. D., Filer, L. J., and Baker, G. L. 1988. Repeated ingestion of aspartame-sweetened beverage: Effect on plasma amino acid concentrations in normal adults. *Metabolism* 37(3) 246–251.

Stein, Z., Susser, J., Saenger, G., and Marolla, F. 1975. *Famine and Human Development: The Dutch Hunger Winter of 1944/45.* Oxford University Press, New York.

Stellman, S. D. and Garfinkel, L. 1986. Artificial sweetener use and one-year weight change among women. *Preventive Medicine* 15(2): 195–202.

Suomi, S. J. 1984. Effects of aspartame on the learning test performance of young stumptail macaques. In *Aspartame: Physiology and Biochemistry,* (Ed.) Stegink L. D. and Filer, L. J., p. 425–445. Marcel Dekker, New York.

Sved, A. F. 1983. Precursor control of the function of monoaminergic neurons. In *Nutrition and the Brain,* Vol. 6. (Ed.) Wurtman, R. J. and Wurtman, J. J., p. 259. Raven Press, New York.

Swanson, J. M. and Kinsbourne, M. 1980. Food dyes impair performance of hyperactive children on a laboratory learning test. *Science* 207: 1485–1487.

Tannahill, R. 1973. *Food in History.* Stein and Day, New York.

Taylor, M. 1976. Effects of L-tryptophan and L-methionine on activity in the rat. *Br. J. Pharmacology* 58: 117–119.

USDA/ERS. 1985. *Sugars and Sweeteners: Outlook and Situation Report.* USDA, Economic Research Service, Washington, DC., September.

van Pragg, H. M. and Lemus, C. 1986. Monoamine precursors in the treatment of psychiatric disorders. In *Nutrition and the Brain,* Vol. 7. (Ed.) Wurtman, R. J. and Wurtman, J. J. Raven Press, New York.

Varley, C. K. 1984. Diet and behavior of children with attention deficit disorder. *J. Amer. Academy of Child Psychiatry* 23: 182–185.

Virkkunen, M. 1982. Reactive hypoglycemia tendency among habitually violent offenders. *Neuropsychobiology* 8: 35–40.

Virkkunen, M. 1983. Insulin secretion during the glucose tolerance test in antisocial personality. *Br. J. Psychiatry* 142: 598–604.

Virkkunen, M. 1984. Reactive hypoglycemia tendency among arsonists. *Acta Psychiatrica Scandinavica* 69: 445–462.

Virkkunen, M. 1987. Metabolic dysfunctions among habitually violent offenders: Reactive hypoglycemia and cholesterol levels. In *The Causes of Crime: New Biological Approaches.* (Ed.) Mednick, S. A., Moffitt T. E., and Stack, S. A., p. 293–311. Cambridge University Press. Cambridge.

Virkkunen, M. and Huttunen, M. O. 1982. Evidence for abnormal glucose tolerance test among violent offenders. *Neuropsychobiology* 8: 30–34.

Virkkunen, M. and Narvanen, S. 1987. Plasma insulin, tryptophan and serotonin levels during the glucose tolerance test among habitually violent and impulsive offenders. *Neuropsychobiology* 17: 19–23.

Weiss, B. 1981. Behavior as a common focus of toxicology and nutrition. In *Nutrition and Behavior,* (Ed.) Miller, S. A., p. 95–107. The Franklin Institute Press, Philadelphia.

Wolraich, M. L. 1986. Behavioral effects of sugars. Paper presented at Searle-UCLA Symposium, *Amino Acids in Health and Disease: New Perspectives,* Keystone, CO, 30 May–4 June.

Wolraich, M. L., Milich, R., Stumbo, P., and Schultz, F. 1985. Effects of sucrose ingestion on the behavior of hyperactive boys. *J. Pediatrics* 106: 675–682.

Wurtman, R. J., Hefti, F., and Melamed, E. 1981. Precursor control of neurotransmitter synthesis. *Pharmacological Rev.* 32: 315–335.

Wurtman, R. J., Larin, F., Mostafopour, S., and Fernstrom, J. D. 1974. Brain catechol synthesis; Control by brain tyrosine concentration. *Science* 185: 183–184.

Yokogoshi, H., Roberts, C. H., Caballero, B., and Wurtman, R. J. 1984. Effects of aspartame and glucose administration on brain and plasma levels of large neutral amino acids and brain 5-hydroxyindoles. *Amer. J. Clin. Nutr.* 40: 1–7.

Young, S. N. 1986. The clinical psychopharmacology of tryptophan. In *Nutrition and the Brain,* Vol. 7. (Ed.) Wurtman, R. J. and Wurtman, J. J., p. 49–88. Raven Press, New York.

Yudkin, J. 1972. *Sweet and Dangerous.* Peter W. Hyden, New York.

10
Food Allergies and Sensitivities

Steven L. Taylor, Julie A. Nordlee, and John H. Rupnow

University of Nebraska-Lincoln
Lincoln, Nebraska

INTRODUCTION

Food allergies and sensitivities have been the subject of confusion and controversy. Numerous physiological and emotional ailments have been attributed to unconfirmed food sensitivities. (King, 1984; Rippere, 1984; Rix et al., 1984; Pearson et al., 1983; Selner and Staudenmayer, 1986). Although the incidence of food allergy has been estimated between 0.3 and 7.5% of the population (Taylor, 1985; Bahna and Gandhi, 1983; Golbert, 1972; Wood, 1986), it is viewed by the public as being a major health concern. Sloan and Powers (1986) conducted a survey of 200 metropolitan women regarding their concerns about food safety. Thirty percent indicated that they or someone in their immediate family had a food sensitivity. As expected, when asked to identify the illness most feared from artificial food ingredients, most (55%) reported a fear of possible cancer. However, 26% percent reported a fear of allergic reactions. Although the actual incidence of clinically significant food sensitivity is probably less than 1% of the population (Taylor, 1985), unwarranted concern and misinformation may lead to the unnecessary removal of nutritionally important foods.

There are several different types of individualistic adverse reactions to foods generically termed "food allergies" by both physicians and the

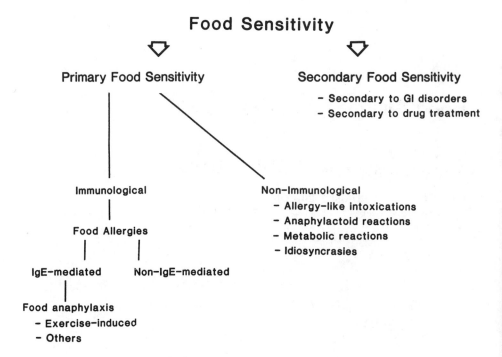

FIG. 10.1 A classification scheme for primary food allergies and sensitivities.

public. The mechanisms that result in food sensitivity are varied and should carry descriptive terms. Although there has been an effort to develop common language concerning adverse reactions to foods and food additives (Anderson, 1986) a set of definitions has not been universally accepted. Food sensitivities can be defined as any abnormal physiological response occurring among a minority of consumers that is attributed to the ingestion of a food or food additive. Food sensitivities may be organized into two broad groups (Fig. 10.1):

Immunological Food Sensitivities (Food Allergies)

The term "food allergy" should only be used to identify true immunologically based adverse reactions. Although the occurrence of food allergies was documented by Hippocrates, it was not until the 1970s that involvement of the immune system in food allergy was demonstrated. Prausnitz and Kustner (1921) subcutaneously injected a normal individual with a fish extract and noted no adverse reaction. However, when the normal individual was first inoculated with serum from another person with fish allergy and then injected with the fish extract, there was an inflammatory skin reactioin. This indicated that the blood of the allergic sufferer contained some substance that sensitized them to the allergen in fish. In 1966, the unknown substance was identified as immunoglobulin E or IgE (Ishizaka et al., 1966). In normal individuals, the usual immunological response to a food protein is IgG, IgM, or IgA formation rather than IgE formation (Taylor, 1986a). Although other types of immunological mechanisms may occur in food allergies, the IgE-mediated mechanism is, by far, the most well documented and completely understood.

Celiac disease will be discussed later as a possible non–IgE-mediated, yet true, food allergy involving other elements of the immune system.

Nonimmunological Food Sensitivities

In contrast to true food allergies, many of the individualistic adverse reactions to food do not involve the immune system.

Anaphylactoid reactions are the result of substances in food that cause mast cells and basophils to spontaneously release histamine and other mediators of allergic reactions. However, unlike true food allergies, there appears to be no involvement of the IgE or other immunoglobulins, and prior exposure is not a prerequisite (Taylor, 1985).

Metabolic food disorders are adverse reactions to a food or food additive that occur through some effect of the substance on the metabolism of the individual (Anderson, 1986). Two of the most common examples of metabolic food disorders are lactose intolerance and favism which are quite common in many parts of the world.

Idiosyncratic reactions is the term used to describe a variety of individual food sensitivities thought to have nonimmunological, but unknown, mechanisms (Taylor, 1985). Many of the reported adverse reactions to food additives are placed in this category owing to the lack of understanding of their modes of action. The involvement of sulfites (Stevenson and Simon, 1981) in asthma is well documented. However, the extent to which chocolate causes migraine headaches (Monro et al., 1980; Egger et al., 1983; Perkin and Hartje, 1983), food coloring agents and sugar cause hyperkinesis, (Stare et al., 1980; Harper and Gans, 1986), BHA and BHT cause hives (Juhlin et al., 1972), and monosodium glutamate causes the headache, facial flush, and chest pain termed "Chinese Restaurant Syndrome" (Kenney, 1979) in sensitive individuals is less certain. Although the prevalence of these mechanistically mysterious reactions is thought to be more common than true food allergy, the actual number of sensitive individuals is unknown.

TRUE FOOD ALLERGIES

True food allergy or food hypersensitivity, the immunologically mediated adverse reactions resulting from the ingestion of a food or food additive, is manifested in only a minor proportion of the population. Evidence indicates that heredity and other physiological factors are significant in predisposing individuals to food allergies. Almost 65% of patients with clinically documented allergy have first degree relatives with atopic disease (Chandra, 1987). Conditions that increase the permeability of the intestine to macromolecules such as viral gastroenteritis, premature birth and cystic fibrosis, tend to increase the risk of development of food allergy (Taylor, 1986a).

The vast majority of true food allergies are caused by naturally occurring substances in foods, mostly proteins. The nature and identity of some of the known food allergens will be discussed later. Only a few contaminants or additives are implicated in true food allergies, and the overall impact of allergic reactions to these categories of foodborne chemicals is infinitesimal by comparison to naturally occurring substances. Where naturally occurring proteins exist as components of food additives or inadvertent, unlabelled contaminants of other foods, a risk exists to those consumers with food allergies. Perhaps the only food additive associated with true food allergies is papain (Mansfield and Bowers, 1983). This proteolytic enzyme, a component of meat tenderizers, is a known allergen, although not a very common one. Penicillin is one of the few food contaminants associated with true, IgE-mediated food allergies (Minikin and Lynch, 1969; Dewdney and Edwards, 1984), although the trace residues of penicillin in dairy and meat products currently are not known to present any hazard to penicillin-allergic consumers (Dewdney and Edwards, 1984).

Mechanisms

Hypersensitivity reactions are based on four different immunological mechanisms (Types I, II, III, and IV) as first described by Coombs and Gell (1975). These mechanisms apply to all types of hypersensitivity such as reactions to pollens, mold spores, animal danders, insect venoms, and drugs as well as foods. The type I mechanism, also called immediate hypersensitivity, is the one that involves the formation of IgE as mentioned earlier. Type II reactions have not yet been demonstrated to be associated with food hypersensitivities. Type III, or immune complex responses, and Type IV, or delay hypersensitivity, may also have some role in food hypersensitivity (Paganelli et al, 1984; Bjorksten, 1984; Kay and Ferguson, 1984), but further studies are required to determine a cause-and-effect role of food and these immune responses in atopic individuals.

IgE-mediated allergies. In Type I reactions (Fig. 10.2), the offending food substance triggers production by the B lymphocytes of specific IgE antibodies. It is this step which distinguishes allergic and nonallergic individuals. Nonallergic individuals will not respond to an exposure of foreign food protein with the production of an allergen-specific IgE. The harm that IgE causes allergic sufferers is mediated by the mast cells and basophils. Once formed, the IgE antibodies bind to the surface of these cells. On subsequent exposure, the offending substance cross-links two IgE molecules on the surface of the mast cell or basophil which causes the sensitized cell to degranulate. The granules in mast cells and basophils contain most of the important mediators of the allergic reaction. While over 40 substances have been identified as mast cell and basophil mediators, histamine is responsible for most of the immediate effects

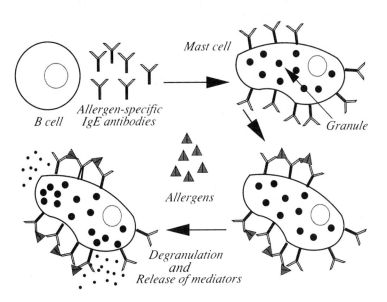

FIG. 10.2 The type I, IgE-mediated allergic reaction.

causing inflammation, pruritis, and contraction of the smooth muscles in the blood vessels, gastrointestinal tract, and respiratory tract. Other important mediators include a variety of prostaglandins and leukotrienes, which cause the slower-developing responses observed in some cases of food allergy (e.g., late-phase asthmatic reactions).

Histamine and other mediators may cause a myriad of symptoms ranging from somewhat mild and annoying to life-threatening. These symptoms are listed in Table 10.1. Not all of these symptoms are experienced by any one atopic individual, the type of symptoms will vary from one individual to another, and the severity of the symptoms may vary from one occasion to another due to the amount of the offending food ingested and the length of time since the last previous exposure. Systemic anaphylaxis is sometimes a fatal allergic reaction to food which involves many organ systems. Symptoms may include tongue swelling and itching, palatal itching, throat itching and tightness, nausea, abdominal pain, vomiting, diarrhea, dyspnea, wheezing, cyanosis, chest pain, urticaria, angioedema, hypotension and shock (Taylor, 1985). Anaphylactic shock is the most common cause of death in the occasional fatalities associated with true food allergies (Yunginger et al., 1988).

IgG$_4$-mediated allergies. It has been suggested, but not proven, that a subclass of IgG antibodies termed IgG$_4$ may be involved in certain types of food allergy. This role was speculated when it was demonstrated that patients with atopic eczema to egg and/or milk proteins had elevated levels of IgG$_4$, that these immunoglobulins could bind to basophils, and that antibody directed against IgG$_4$ would cause the basophil to degranulate and release histamine (Merrett et al., 1984; Shakib et al., 1984). However, the allergen itself was not able to mediate the release of histamine from IgG$_4$-bound basophils (Van Toorenenbergen and Aalberse, 1982). Also, food-specific IgG$_4$ antibodies were often detectable in the sera of healthy individuals in the population (Shakib et al., 1984; Layton and

TABLE 10.1 Symptoms of IgE-Mediated Food Allergies

Cutaneous: urticaria (hives), eczema, dermatitis, pruritis, rash

Gastrointestinal: nausea, vomiting, diarrhea, abdominal cramps

Respiratory: asthma, wheezing, rhinitis, bronchospasm

Other: anaphylactic shock, hypotension, palatal itching, swelling including tongue, larynx

Stanworth, 1984; Shakib et al., 1975) and the clinical significance of this subclass of IgG in food allergy has not been determined.

Exercise-induced food allergy.   A syndrome characterized by exertion-related development of allergy-like symptoms was first described in 1936 (Grant et al., 1936). Recently, there has been recognition that in certain individuals, the exercise must be preceded or followed by the ingestion of specific foods. Shellfish (Maulitz et al., 1979), peach (Buchbinder et al., 1983), wheat (Kushimoto and Aoki, 1985), celery (Kidd et al., 1983) and solid food (Kidd et al., 1983) have been incriminated in food-dependent, exercise-induced anaphylaxis. Although the mechanism is unknown, enhanced mast cell responsiveness to physical stimuli may be involved (Sheffer et al., 1983). Symptoms are individualistic and similar to those involved in other food allergies. With awareness of the existence of this syndrome, and the recent emphasis on physical activity, it is expected that reports of this condition will increase.

Diagnosis of Food Allergies

Food hypersensitivity may be diagnosed in a number of ways. However, self-diagnosis and parental diagnosis are frequently erroneous and unreliable. Confirmation of a true food allergy must involve careful medical evaluation. This evaluation consists of initially determining if, in fact, an adverse reaction occurs following the ingestion of a suspected food. Suspect foods may be determined from the patient's history or by a food and activity diary, logging when, what and how much of various foods and their ingredients are consumed, and recording any untoward reaction over a period of time. This information gives physicians a starting place in their "Holmesian" pursuit of the offending culprit.

The physician must then determine if the suspected food actually causes an adverse reaction after ingestion. The best and most reliable way to determine this cause-and-effect relationship is by the double-blind food challenge (DBFC). In this test, the individual patient and the physician do not know whether the suspect food or a placebo food is being administered. This test is free from the biases associated with single-blind challenges and open challenges. The following caveat must be heeded for any kind of oral challenge if the affected individual experiences life-threatening symptoms: No minimum or "safe dose" has been scientifically determined for allergic individuals with life-threatening symptoms. Oral challenges should not be performed with exquisitely sensitive individuals who present with life-threatening symptoms.

Once a cause-and-effect relationship has been established, the physician must determine if the reaction is IgE-mediated. This may be ascertained by employing the skin prick test or the radio-allergosorbent test (RAST). Sometimes the skin prick test is used as a screening procedure to determine what foods should be suspected when no suspect food can be determined from a history or food diary. The skin prick test is simple and is based on the existence of mast cells in the skin adjacent to blood vessels. An extract containing the allergen of the suspect food is placed on the skin, usually on the inside of the forearm or on the back, and the site is pricked or scratched to allow the entry of the allergen. A wheal-and-flare response is the result of IgE cross linking by the specific allergen, thereby releasing histamine and other mediators that cause an increase in vascular permeability, local edema and itching. The result is usually seen within 20 minutes. The RAST is based on the presence of serum IgE specific for an allergen. Serum from the sensitive individual is reacted with the allergen, usually in the form of a crude extract, which has been bound to a solid matrix. Any IgE that recognizes the allergen and binds to it is detected by radioactively labelled antibody against human IgE.

There are any number of controversial diagnostic tests including sublingual challenges and cytotoxic testing. These tests cannot be recommended since no scientific proof exists that they are of any diagnostic value.

Due to the lack of a standardized definition of food hypersensitivity until recently, the prevalence of true food allergies is unknown. Most estimates of the prevalence of food allergies are based on anecdotal reports (self or parental diagnosis) or clinical impression without the benefit of a complete medical diagnosis (Taylor, 1985; Bahna and Gandhi, 1983; Golbert, 1972; Wood, 1986). Sampson (1988), citing various studies including a major clinical investigation by Bock (1987), suggests adverse reactions to foods occur in probably 4% to 6% of infants and 1% to 2% in young children. In adults, reproducible adverse reaction to foods probably occur in less than 1% of the population (Taylor, 1985, 1987). Popular perceptions of the incidence of food allergies as cited earlier are erroneously high.

True food allergies are thought to occur with higher frequency in infants because of the increased permeability of the newborn intestinal tract and the lack of maturity of the immune system (Kleinman and Walker, 1984). Allergen exposure may occur *in utero* (Michel et al., 1986) or through the presence of traces of potentially allergenic proteins in breast milk (Gerrard, 1984). Most infants outgrow their IgE-mediated food allergies within a few weeks or months (Bock, 1982). The mechanism involved in this loss of sensitivity is not precisely known. However, evidence of allergen-specific IgE may persist even after loss of sensitivity to an oral challenge (Taylor, 1986a). Thus, the mechanism may involve the development of blocking antibodies, especially secretory IgA antibodies or the maturity of the intestinal tract coupled with a decrease in its permeability (Taylor, 1986a; Kleinman and Walker, 1984; Taylor et al., 1987b). Some food allergies tend to be more persistent than others. For example, peanut allergy is much more likely to persist than cows' milk allergy (Bock, 1982).

Nature and Chemistry of Food Allergens

In true food allergies, the known allergens are usually naturally occurring proteins found in the food (Taylor et al., 1987b). In theory, any food with a protein moiety has the potential of sensitization, and upon subsequent exposure, causing a reaction in the atopic individual. Surprisingly, only a few categories of foods are most commonly associated with food hypersensitivity (Table 10.2). These foods are cows' milk, eggs, legumes (peanuts and soybeans), crustacea (shrimp, crab, lobster), molluscs (clams, oysters, scallops), fish, wheat, and tree nuts. Frequently implicated foods such as chocolate, strawberries and citrus fruits do not give positive results in double-blind food challenges in children with atopic dermatitis (Sampson, 1988). In infants and young children, cows' milk allergy is the most common and is usually short lived (Taylor, 1986a; Sampson, 1988, Bock, 1982). Other allergies common in this age group are allergies to peanuts, eggs and soybeans (Sampson, 1988; Bock 1982). Since these foods are commonly consumed in early childhood, this may increase the prevalence of hypersensitivity to these foods. In American adults, peanuts and

TABLE 10.2 Common Allergenic Foods

Infants:
  Cows' milk
  Eggs
  Legumes—peanuts and soybeans
  Wheat
Adults:
  Legumes—peanuts and soybeans
  Crustacea—shrimp, crab, lobster
  Molluscs—clams, oysters, scallops
  Fish
  Tree nuts
  Eggs
  Wheat

crustacea are likely to be the most common allergenic foods (Taylor, 1987). Frequent exposure may have something to do with why these foods are most commonly associated with true food allergy. However, the inherent immunogenicity of the protein must also play an important role because some commonly eaten, proteinaceous foods such as beef, pork, and chicken are rarely implicated in true food allergies (Taylor, 1987). Because of differences in the diet in other countries, the incidence of true food allergies to other foods is higher. For example, soybeans are a common allergenic food in Japan, and codfish are a common allergenic food in Scandanavian countries.

Few food allergens have been purified and characterized (Table 10.3). Some commonly allergenic foods are complex mixtures of allergens, such as cows' milk. Cows' milk contains a total protein level of 30-35 grams/liter (Swaisgood, 1985). The six major protein classes are α_{s1}-caseins, α_{s2}-caseins, β-caseins, γ-caseins, β-lactoglobulins, and α-lactalbumins (Swaisgood, 1985). Numerous studies have evaluated the allergenicity of these proteins in allergic individuals by skin testing and oral challenges (Goldman et al., 1963a,b; Lebenthal, 1975; Davidson et al., 1965; Gjesing et al., 1986; Bleumink and Young, 1968; Kuitunen et al., 1975; Baldo, 1984). From these studies, it can be stated that multiple allergens exist in cows' milk and the major proteins are the major allergens with β-lactoglobulin, α-lactalbumin, and casein being the most prevalent allergens (Taylor, 1986a; Taylor et al., 1987b). Some cows' milk allergens (serum albumin and immunoglobulins) are heat-labile (Hanson and Mansson, 1961). Caseins, however can retain their antigenicity for 15 minutes at 120°C, and α-lactalbumin and β-lactoglobulin are stable at 100°C (Hanson and Mansson, 1961).

Some investigators report cross-reactivity between species of fish, and this may be explained by the character of an allergen purified from codfish termed allergen M (Taylor et al., 1987b). This allergen is well characterized and is a sacroplasmic protein belonging to a group of proteins known as parvalbumins. Parvalbumins bear a close structural resemblance between different fish species (Aas, 1966). This may explain some of the cross-reactivity observed between fish species (Tuft and Blumstein, 1946).

Allergen M contains 113 amino acid residues and one glucose moiety, has a molecular weight of 12,328 and an isoelectric point of 4.75 (Elsayed and Bennich, 1975). The three-dimensional structure is known and apparently contains several IgE-binding sites (Elsayed and Apold, 1983; Elsayed et al., 1980). Synthetic polypeptides of the sequence of the domains of the allergen M molecule have the ability to bind IgE from the sera of cod-allergic individuals (Elsayed and Apold, 1983; Elsayed et al., 1980).

TABLE 10.3   Known Allergenic Food Proteins

Food	Allergenic Proteins
Cows' milk	Casein β-Lactoglobulin α-Lactalbumin Others
Egg whites	Ovomucoid Ovalbumin Ovotransferrin (conalbumin)
Egg yolks	Lipoprotein Livetin
Peanuts	Peanut I Lectin-reactive glycoprotein Arachin Conarachin
Soybeans	β-Conglycinin (7S fraction) Glycinin (11S fraction) 2S Fraction Kunitz trypsin inhibitor Unidentified 20kD protein
Codfish	Allergen M (parvalbumin)
Shrimp	Antigen II
Green peas	Albumin fraction
Rice	Glutelin fraction Globulin fraction
Cottonseed	Glycoprotein fraction
Tomato	Several glycoproteins

Allergen M is extremely resistant to physical destruction (Elsayed and Aas, 1971) and would therefore be expected to retain its allergenic activity through most processing and cooking treatments.

Little information is known about allergens causing reactions to crustacea. Many species of shrimp, crab, and lobster are edible, and it is highly probable that some shared and some unique allergens exist in crustacea.

Of the few purifications attempted, an Antigen II was purified from an unspecified species of cooked shrimp (Hoffman et al., 1981). Antigen II has a molecular weight of 38,300 with 341 amino acid residues and 4% carbohydrate. Its isoelectric point is 5.4–5.8. IgE from the serum of all 11 individuals in the study (Hoffman et al., 1981) bound Antigen II in the RAST. Other allergens have been identified, but no attempts have been made to purify them (Nagpal et al., 1985; Lehrer et al., 1985). Shared major allergens between shrimp, crab and lobster have been demonstrated by crossed radio-immunoelectrophoresis (CRIE) (Lehrer et al., 1985).

The protein composition of egg whites and yolks is well known (Powrie and Nakai, 1985). Several studies utilizing CRIE (Langeland, 1982; Hoffman, 1983; Langeland 1985) and skin testing (Bleumink and Young, 1969, 1971) indicate that ovalbumin, ovomucoid and conalbumin (ovotransferrin) may be the significant egg white allergens. Allergenicity of the egg yolk is associated with the lipoprotein fraction, livetin fraction, and several proteins in the low density lipoprotein fraction (Anet et al., 1985). Cross reactions were observed between egg white and egg yolk using RAST-inhibition (Anet et al., 1985). Cooking does not destroy the allegenicity of eggs, but does decrease the allergenicity for some allergic individuals (Anet et al., 1985). The effects of other processing and cooking on the allergens in eggs have not been investigated.

Peanuts contain 25%-28% protein which has been classified into three groups: arachin, conarachin and albumins. Arachin and conarachin are not well defined with regard to their protein and polypeptide composition and molecular weight. Part of the confusion is due to the ability of arachin and conarachin to undergo reversible and non-reversible association dependent upon pH, ionic strength, protein concentration and storage temperature of the isolated protein fractions. Multiple allergens have been identifed in peanuts by CRIE and Western blotting; seven to 16 allergens seem to be present (Barnett et al., 1983; Meier-Davis et al., 1987). Sachs et al. (1981) purified peanut I, an acidic glycoprotein that may be a subfraction of either arachin or conarachin, and claimed that it was a major peanut allergen. The allergenicity was determined by RAST inhibition. CRIE and RAST results indicate α-arachin (major subfraction of arachin), conarachin I and a conanavalin A-reactive glycoprotein bind IgE of allergic individuals (Heinen and Neucere, 1975; Kemp et al., 1985; Barnett and Howden, 1986). A lectin-reactive glycoprotein may be one of the major allergens since it is reactive with over 50% of the serum of a group of peanut-allergic individuals (Kemp et al., 1985; Barnett and Howden, 1986). In all likelihood, peanuts probably contain multiple allergens and perhaps several major allergens. The major allergenic activity of peanuts is heat-stable (Barnett and Howden, 1986) and usual processing does not destroy allergenicity (Nordlee et al., 1981).

Soybeans contain 32%–42% protein in two major fractions, the globulin and the whey. The major globulins are glycinin or the 11S fraction and β-conglycinin or the 7S fraction. A minor fraction, the 2S fraction, contains several tryspin inhibitors. Allergenic activity has been found in the 2S, 7S, and 11S fractions by RAST, RAST-inhibition, and Western blotting (Shibasaki et al., 1980; Broadbent et al., 1988; Burks et al., 1988; Herian et al., 1989). As with peanuts, soybeans seem to contain multiple allergens. Herian et al (1989) showed that adults with soybean allergy fall into at least two categories based on their IgE-binding patterns with electrophoretically separated soybean proteins. Sera from Category I patients with allergies to peanuts and soybeans display IgE binding to several proteins with electrophoretic migration similar to β-conglycinin. The sera from Category II patients with allergy only to soybeans display IgE binding to an unidentified protein with a molecular weight of about 20,000.

The allergens in green peas are localized in the albumin fraction (Malley et al., 1975, 1976). The allergenicity of the albumin fraction is heat-stable and gave positive skin tests in allergic individuals. Much more time and effort will be necessary to isolate, purify, and characterize the allergens of green peas.

Several allergenic glycoproteins have been isolated from ripe tomatoes (Bleumink et al., 1966) that cause skin reactivity in allergic individuals. Though cottonseed is only of minor importance to the food industry, it possesses allergenic activity. The allergenic fraction was characterized as a complex mixture of glycoproteins ranging in molecular weight from 5,000 to 18,000 (Spies, 1977).

The allergens in rice have been partially characterized (Shibasaki et al., 1979). Both of the major protein fractions of rice, glutelin, and globulin, were capable of binding IgE from the serum of rice-allergic individuals. Three subfractions of the globulin fraction also bound IgE in the RAST. The ability to bind IgE was decreased when the fractions were heated.

The most active allergens of sesame seeds were identified by density gradient ultracentrifugation and had molecular weights ranging from 8000 to 62,000 daltons (Malish et al., 1981). These allergens were not further characterized.

Treatment of True Food Allergies

The major mode of treatment for all food allergies and sensitivities is the specific avoidance diet. If allergic to peanuts for example, one simply avoids peanuts. While such diets can be quite successful, adherence can be troublesome. The construction of avoidance diets and the difficulties faced by consumers with such diets have been extensively reviewed elsewhere (Taylor et al., 1986a, 1987a).

Patients with true food allergies often pose three basic questions as they begin to construct a specific avoidance diet.

1. Will trace levels of the food elicit reactions or increase sensitization?
2. Do all foods and food ingredients made from the offending food contain the allergens?
3. Are cross-reactions likely to occur between closely related species?

In answer to the first question, trace levels of the offending food can elicit adverse reactions (Table 10.4). Many examples of mostly anecdotal experiences are reported in Table 10.4. However, several incidents have been well investigated and confirmed (Yunginger et al., 1988; Yunginger et al., 1983; Fries, 1982) lending credibility to the anecdotal reports. For all practical purposes, no safe level of the offending food can be tolerated by individuals with true food allergies. Essentially, complete avoidance must be maintained. Foods may become contaminated with trace amounts of other foods through a wide variety of means. Such contamination is especially important to individuals who are exquisitely sensitive to the of-

TABLE 10.4 Events Reported to Cause Reactions or Increase Sensitivity of Some Food-Allergic Individuals Who Demonstrate Exquisite Sensitivity

Traces of the offending food contaminating other foods, due to
  inadequate cleaning of processing equipment
  attempts to remove the offending food from a mixture by the allergic individual or others
  direct and indirect contact between two foods, e.g., using the same serving utensil or cooking vessel for several different foods

Touching utensils, bottles, etc. contaminated with the offending food

Kissing lips of person who has just eaten the offending food

Opening packages containing the offending food

Inhalation of vapors from cooking the offending food

Transfer of food allergens from mother to infant via breast milk

Transfer of food allergens from husband to wife via sperm during intercourse

Transfer of food allergens from mother to fetus during pregnancy

fending food and who experience life-threatening symptoms. No avoidance diet would provide absolute safety for these individuals, but strict adherence to a well-constructed avoidance diet will minimize the chances of a reaction.

Traces of food allergens may also increase the level of sensitization to the offending food. Presumably, such an exposure would trigger formation of additional allergen-specific IgE and the sensitization of larger numbers of mast cells and basophils. Thus, the tolerance level to the offending food could decrease. Upon subsequent exposure, the likelihood and severity of a reaction increases.

If one is allergic to a food, must he or she avoid all products derived from that food or foods that are closely related? No generalized statement can be made on this topic since few studies have been conducted. Cross-reactivity to closely related foods in the few investigations seems to be a very individualistic phenomenon (Herian et al., 1989; Waring et al., 1980; Daul et al., 1988). Individuals with a mollusc allergy are often told to avoid all seafood including crustacea and fish. Considering the distant taxonomic relationships between edible seafoods, it is unlikely that molluscs would cross-react with fish or crustacea (Taylor et al., 1987a). However, some peanut-allergic individuals are allergic to other legumes, such as soybeans (Herian et al., 1989). Cross-reactions are known to occur between different species of avian eggs(Langeland, 1983) and between cows' milk and goats' milk (Juntunen and Ali-Yrkko, 1983). Cross-reactions are also reported to occur between certain types of pollens and certain foods (Halmepuro et al., 1984).

When considering foods derived from a food causing an allergic reaction, the presence of the allergen is important. In a study by Nordlee et al. (1981) the allergenicity of peanut products was determined by RAST-inhibition. The extracts of most processed peanut products retained their ability to bind specific IgE from peanut-allergic sera indicating the peanut allergens are highly heat-stable. Double-blind challenge testing to determine the allergenicity of peanut, soybean, and sunflower oils indicate that the oils did not cause allergic reactions in sensitive individuals (Taylor et al., 1981; Bush et al., 1985; Halsey et al., 1986). As more allergens are purified and characterized, more information will be available to determine cross reactivity with related foods and the presence of the allergens in foods derived from a food known to cause an allergic reaction.

Celiac Disease—An Example of Delayed Hypersensitivity?

Celiac disease, also known as celiac sprue or gluten-sensitive enteropathy, is a malabsorption syndrome that occurs in certain individuals following the ingestion of wheat, rye, barley, and sometimes oats (Kasarda, 1978; Hartsook, 1984). The ingestion of these grains somehow triggers damage to the absorptive epithelial cells in the small intestine. Thus, the absorption of nutrients by these cells is impaired. The symptoms of celiac disease are typical of a malabsorption syndrome: diarrhea, bloating, weight loss, anemia, bone pain, chronic fatigue, weakness, muscle cramps, and, in children, failure to grow (Strober, 1986).

Celiac disease is an inherited trait, but its inheritance is complex and poorly understood. Celiac disease occurs in about 1 of every 3000 individuals in the U.S. (Kasarda, 1978; Hartsook, 1984). The disease occurs with differing frequencies in other parts of the world. However, celiac disease is certainly one of the most common food allergies and/or sensitivities in the world.

Despite its prevalence and a rather substantial research effort, the pathogenesis of celiac disease remains a mystery. Celiac disease is not necessarily a form of true food allergy. It is definitely not an IgE-mediated food allergy (Strober, 1986). However, abnormal immunological responses are observed with celiac disease (Strober, 1986). It is unknown whether these immunological responses are a primary factor in the pathogenesis of celiac disease or merely a secondary phenomenon associated with the altered intestinal function. Strober (1986) has suggested that celiac disease may result from an immunocytotoxic reaction mediated by intestinal lymphocytes. However, while the explanation is consistent with clinical observations, it has not yet been clearly established as the pathogenic mechanism.

Celiac disease is associated with the naturally occurring protein fractions of wheat, rye, barley, and oats. Specifically, the gliadin fraction of wheat protein and the equivalent prolamin fractions of barley, rye, and oats are responsible for the damage (Kasarda, 1978). These grains are closely related genetically (Kasarda, 1978) and it is likely that the cross-reactivity is due to the conservation of reactive peptide sequences in these complex protein fractions.

The treatment of celiac disease typically involves the total avoidance of wheat, rye, barley, and oats and all products produced from these grains (Hartsook, 1984). Like other true food allergies, the symptoms of celiac disease can be triggered by ingestion of rather small quantities of these grains. A safe tolerance level cannot yet be estimated, so complete avoidance is the prudent choice. However, adherence to these strict avoidance diets can be quite difficult. Questions also remain about the necessity of excluding ingredients prepared from wheat, rye, barley, and oats if the ingredients contain no intact proteins (Taylor, 1987). Examples might include wheat starch, rye whiskey, malt extract, and hydrolyzed vegetable protein. In the absence of data demonstrating the safety of these ingredients for celiac patients, most will likely continue to avoid these products.

FOOD SENSITIVITIES

Food sensitivities occur through many different mechanisms. Like true food allergies, they affect only a limited number of individuals in the population. While true food allergies involve abnormal immunological responses to certain food constituents, especially proteins, food sensitivities can occur through any of a host of nonimmunological mechanisms (Taylor, 1985, 1987). As noted earlier, the three major classes of nonimmunological food sensitivities are (1) anaphylactoid reactions, (2) metabolic food disorders, and (3) idiosyncratic reactions. Several examples of the nonimmunological food sensitivities are provided in Table 10.5.

Most of the nonimmunological food sensitivities are caused by foodborne substances other than proteins. While the vast majority of true food allergies can be attributed to naturally occurring proteins in foods, the nonimmunological food sensitivities are associated with both naturally occurring and additive substances (Table 10.5). Anaphylactoid reactions are thought to involve naturally occurring substances, although none of these chemicals has yet been identified. Occasionally, histamine poisoning (also known as scombroid fish poisoning) is included as an example of an anaphylactoid reaction (AAAI and NIAID, 1984) or as a separate category of nonimmunological food sensitivity (Taylor, 1987). However, histamine poisoning is actually a foodborne intoxication associated with the ingestion of foods containing unusually high levels of histamine. The histamine is formed during bacterial spoilage (Taylor et al., 1978). Everyone is susceptible to histamine poisoning, so it does not truly fit into this review of food allergies and sensitivities. It is frequently included because the symptoms resemble those encountered with food allergies, and it is often misdiagnosed as true food allergy. Histamine poisoning has been described in several recent reviews (Taylor, 1986b; 1988; Taylor et al., 1984) and will not be discussed further here. The known metabolic food disorders involve naturally occurring substances exclusively. Idiosyncratic reactions can involve either food additives or naturally occurring substances. However, the situation is complicated by the fact that the evidence supporting the existence of some of these illnesses is far from complete. Food additives appear to be a focus of concern for unexplained maladies, but the possible role of naturally occurring substances in these

TABLE 10.5 Some Causative Substances (Naturally Occurring and Additive) Associated with Nonimmunological Food Sensitivities

Type of reaction	Specific illness	Known, suspected or speculated causative substance(s)
Naturally occurring substance:		
Anaphylactoid reaction	—	Unknown substances in strawberries, shellfish
Metabolic food disorder	Lactose intolerance	Lactose
	Favism	Vicine and convicine
Idiosyncratic reaction	Migraine headache	Chocolate, cheese
	Celiac disease	Wheat, rye, barley, oats
Additive substance:		
Anaphylactoid reaction	—	None known
Metabolic food disorder	—	None known
Idiosyncratic reaction	Asthma	Sulfites, tartrazine, monosodium glutamate
	Urticaria	BHA, BHT, benzoates, tartrazine, parabens, aspartame
	Migraine headache	Aspartame
	Behavioral disorders	Food colorants, sugar
	Chinese restaurant syndrome	Monosodium glutamate

conditions has received considerably less attention. Still, food additives play a definite role in several well-documented and serious idiosyncratic reactions; sulfite-induced asthma is a prime example.

Anaphylactoid Reactions

In true food allergies, the release of mediators from the mast cells and basophils is mediated by IgE as discussed earlier. In anaphylactoid reactions, the release of mediators from these cells occurs through an as yet undefined, but nonimmunological, mechanism. While histamine poisoning is sometimes classified as an anaphylactoid reaction, it is clearly a distinct illness because histamine poisoning involves the ingestion of exogenous histamine rather than the release of histamine from mast cells and basophils in vivo.

In anaphylactoid reactions, it is presumed that some substance in the implicated food destabilizes the mast cell membranes causing a spontaneous release of the histamine contained therein. Actually, none of these histamine-releasing substances has ever been isolated or identified in foods. Therefore, the evidence for the existence of anaphylactoid reactions is largely circumstantial and anecdotal. The most persuasive evidence for the existence of anaphylactoid reactions is the lack of evidence for immunological involvement in a few types of food allergy.

The best example is probably strawberry "allergy." Strawberries are well known to cause adverse reactions (frequently urticaria) in some individuals. Yet, strawberries contain little protein, no strawberry allergen has ever been identified, and no evidence has been obtained for the existence of strawberry-specific IgE. The symptoms of strawberry "allergy" are reminiscent of a true food allergy, so in vivo release of histamine and other mediators seems likely to occur. Strawberries also contain only traces of histamine, so histamine poisoning is not a likely explanation. Thus, by a process of elimination, nonimmunological release of the mast cell and basophil mediators seems a plausible explanation. However, it must be emphasized that this mechanism has not been proven in strawberry "allergy" or any other food sensitivity.

Metabolic Food Disorders

Metabolic food disorders involve genetically determined deficiencies that either affect the host's ability to metabolize a food component or enhance the sensitivity of the host to some foodborne chemical via an altered metabolic pattern. An example of the former is lactose intolerance, caused by a deficiency of intestinal β-galactosidase and characterized by an inability to digest lactose. An example of the latter is favism, where a genetic deficiency in erythrocyte glucose-6-phosphate dehydrogenase causes an increased sensitivity to several hemolytic factors in fava beans. These two are by far the most common metabolic food disorders. Celiac disease, already discussed as a possible form of food allergy, could conceivably be a metabolic food disorder. However, no genetic defect has ever been demonstrated in celiac disease.

Lactose intolerance. In normal digestive processes, lactose, a disaccharide and the principal naturally occurring sugar in milk, is hydrolyzed into its constituent monosaccharides, galactose and glucose, in the intestinal mucosa. The monosaccharides can then be absorbed and used metabolically as energy sources. In cases of lactose intolerance, the key enzyme, known as β-galactosidase or lactase, involved in this hydrolytic process is absent or present at diminished levels (Kocian, 1988; Sandine and Daly, 1979).

Since lactose cannot be absorbed in the small intestine unless it is hydrolyzed to galactose and glucose, it passes into the colon in individuals with lactose tolerance. The large numbers of bacteria present in the colon metabolize the lactose to CO_2, H_2, and H_2O (Taylor, 1987). The hallmark symptoms of lactose intolerance—abdominal cramping, flatulence, and frothy diarrhea (Bayless et al., 1975) are the result of this bacterial action. The symptoms vary in intensity with the individual's level of intestinal lactase activity and the amount of lactose ingested.

Lactose intolerance affects a substantial number of people worldwide. Only about 6–12% of Caucasians are affected (Sandine and Daly, 1979). However, lactose intolerance is much more prevalent in other ethnic groups and races affecting as many as 60–90% of Greeks, Arabs, Jews, black Americans, Hispanics, Japanese, and other Asians (Kocian, 1988; Sandine and Daly, 1979; Houts, 1988). Lactose intolerance can have its onset at any age, occurring as early as the age of 3 (Simoons, 1980). Lactose intolerance tends to worsen with age so it is more common and more severe among the elderly, although symptomatic lactose intolerance usually has its onset at an earlier age (Taylor, 1987; Kocian, 1988; Houts, 1988). The level of intestinal lactase activity is usually sufficient at birth to allow the digestion of lactose in mother's milk. But, those individuals born with an inherited deficiency of intestinal lactase suffer a decline in lactase activity as they age. At some point, symptoms may begin to develop following the consumption of dairy products.

Lactose intolerance can also occur secondary to another intestinal illness or infection (Metcalfe, 1984). For example, secondary lactose intolerance occasionally occurs after a bout with viral gastroenteritis. Secondary lactose intolerance is often a short-term illness. Once the gastrointestinal damage has been repaired, intestinal function returns to normal and secondary lactose intolerance disappears (National Dairy Council, 1978).

A clinical diagnosis of lactose intolerance is usually established by the lactose tolerance test (LTT). Classically, the LTT has involved the oral administration of 50 g of lactose to a fasting individual (Taylor, 1987; Kocian, 1988). Blood glucose or breath hydrogen levels are measured to determine whether lactose is being absorbed. Gastrointestinal symptoms are also monitored.

The LTT has been frequently criticized in recent years (Taylor, 1987; National Dairy Council, 1978). The 50g dose of lactose is the focus of the criticism. To obtain 50g of lactose from fluid milk, one would need to consume one liter or more of milk, an unlikely circumstance. Many individuals, diagnosed as lactose intolerant on the basis of the 50g challenge, can tolerate the smaller quantities of lactose contained in more reasonable amounts of milk (National Dairy Council, 1978; Bayless, 1981; Newcomer, 1981; Stephenson and Latham, 1974). Newcomer (1981) concluded that only 19% of lactase-deficient individuals were intolerant to 8 oz of milk containing 12g of lactose. As a result of such concerns, lower doses of lactose have become more common in the diagnosis of lactose intolerance. Solomons et al. (1980) use 360 mL of milk with 18g of lactose and the measurement of breath hydrogen as a more reasonable test for lactose intolerance. Another diagnostic approach would be the use of sequential, increasing doses of lactose in the challenge to obtain a better perspective on the individual patient's tolerance for lactose in the diet (Taylor, 1987). Use of this type of diagnostic procedure might help to clarify the extent to which lactose intolerance worsens with age in affected individuals.

Lactose may not be responsible for all cases of mild intolerance. True cows' milk allergy has already been discussed. In addition, several investigators have identified individuals with normal capacities for lactose digestion who experience the same symptoms as lactose-intolerant individuals when challenged with 8-12 oz of milk (Haverberg et al., 1980; Kwon et al., 1980; Rosado et al., 1987). These investigators have speculated that substances other than lactose in milk may be responsible for some cases of milk intolerance. One possibility would be a milk protein intolerance distinct from IgE-mediated cows' milk allergy and possibly similar mechanistically to celiac disease (Ford et al., 1983; Anon., 1981).

The usual treatment for lactose intolerance is the avoidance of dairy products containing lactose. However, lactose-intolerant individuals may be able to tolerate some dairy products and some lactose, although the degree of tolerance varies widely. Individuals identified as intolerant to 50g oral challenges with lactose may, in some cases, be able to tolerate reasonable amounts of most dairy products. Several alternatives exist for individuals with greater degrees of lactose intolerance. Some will be able to tolerate small, divided doses of milk. Lactose-hydrolyzed milk is also available in the marketplace (Paige et al., 1975). This product is effective, but its sweet taste limits acceptance. The addition of β-galactosidase to milk at the time of ingestion also seems to be effective (Rosado et al., 1984;

Barillas and Solomons, 1987; Kim and Gilliland, 1983). Presumably, the enzyme retains its activity in vivo and hydrolyzes the ingested lactose in the gut. Martin and Savaiano (1988) have demonstrated that the tolerated amount of lactose increases when the lactose is consumed with a meal. Lactose-intolerant individuals appear to tolerate yogurt and acidophilus milk better than other dairy products (Gallagher et al., 1977; Kolars et al., 1984). Apparently, these fermented dairy products contain active β-galactosidase, which is able to autodigest the lactose (Kolars et al., 1984; Martini et al., 1987). The level of lactase activity varies from one brand of yogurt to another, so some brands are more easily tolerated than others (Wytock and DiPalma, 1988). The incorporation of tolerated levels of dairy products into the diets of lactose-intolerant individuals is important, because dairy products are excellent from a nutritional perspective, especially with respect to calcium (Taylor, 1987). Birge et al. (1967) suggested that osteoporosis may result from the inadequate calcium intakes associated with dairy product–avoidance diets.

Favism. Some individuals will suffer from acute hemolytic anemia following the ingestion of fava or broad beans (*Vicia faba*) or inhalation of the pollen from the plant (Mager et al., 1980). This condition is known as favism. The symptoms of favism are consistent with those of a hemolytic disease: pallor, fatigue, dyspnea, nausea, abdominal and/or back pain, fever, and chills. In severe cases, hemoglobinuria, jaundice, and renal failure can occur. The onset time is quite rapid, ranging between 5 and 24 hr. The disease is usually self-limited with a prompt and spontaneous recovery following avoidance of further exposure. Favism is most prevalent when the *V. faba* plant is blooming, causing elevated levels of airborne pollen. An increase in favism is noted later in the season when the fava beans are available in the market.

Favism affects individuals with an inherited deficiency of the enzyme glucose-6-phosphate dehydrogenase (G6PDH) in their red blood cells. G6PDH is a critical enzyme in erythrocytes. It is essential to maintain adequate levels of the reduced form of glutathione (GSH) and nicotinamide adenine dinucleotide phosphate (NADPH). GSH and NADPH help to prevent oxidative damage to erythrocytes. The red blood cells of individuals with a deficiency of erythrocyte G6PDH are thus susceptible to oxidative damage.

Fava beans contain several naturally occurring oxidants, including vicine and convicine (Fig. 10.3), which are able to damage the red blood cells of individuals with G6PDH deficiency (Mager et al., 1980). These oxidants damage the erythrocyte membrane, causing the characteristic hemolytic anemia. The mechanism of this metabolic food disorder is

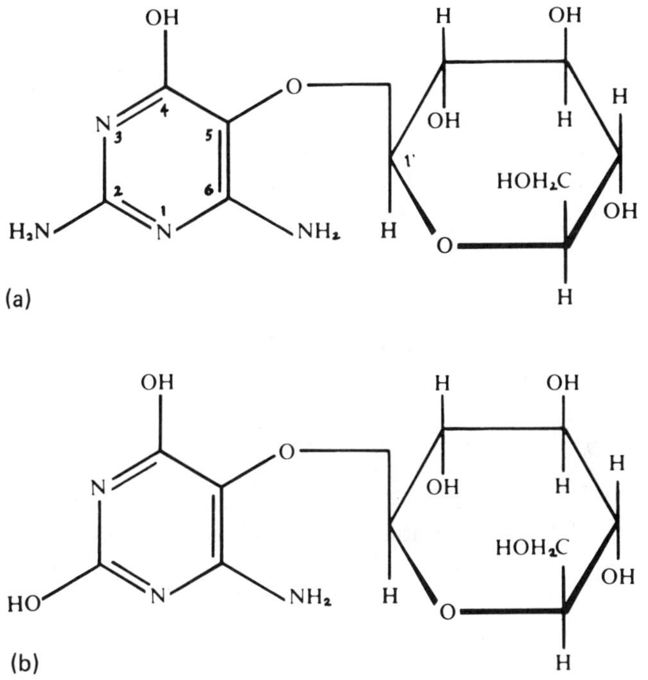

FIG. 10.3 Structures of the naturally occurring oxidants (a) vicine and (b) convicine of fava beans.

quite distinct from that of lactose intolerance. With favism, the genetic deficiency causes an increased susceptibility to the oxidative toxins in fava beans.

G6PDH deficiency is the most common enzymatic defect in humans worldwide, affecting about 100 million people (Mager et al., 1980). The greatest prevalence of G6PDH deficiency occurs among Oriental Jews in Israel, Sardinians, Cypriot Greeks, American blacks, and certain African populations. The trait is virtually absent among Caucasians, North American Indians, and Eskimos. Despite the high incidence of G6PDH deficiency, favism is not especially common. Favism occurs primarily in the Mediterranean area, the Middle East, China, and Bulgaria where the genetic trait is fairly common and where the broad beans grow and are frequently consumed

G6PDH deficiency is not necessarily a very serious condition. However, individuals with G6PDH deficiency must avoid fava beans.

Idiosyncratic Reactions

Many adverse reactions to foods that affect certain individuals in the population occur through unknown mechanisms (Taylor, 1987). Conceivably, a large number of different mechanisms could be involved in these idiosyncratic reactions. Similarly, the symptoms associated with this wide variety of illnesses range from the trivial to severe, life-threatening reactions.

Food idiosyncrasies fall into three categories: (a) illnesses whose association with specific foods or food ingredients is well documented, (b) illnesses whose association with specific foods or food ingredients have not been firmly established or, in some cases remain controversial, and (c) illnesses widely believed by consumers to be associated with specific foods or food ingredients despite considerable evidence to the contrary. Table 10.6 contains a partial list of food idiosyncrasies in each category.

Celiac disease (Kasarda, 1978) and sulfite-induced asthma (Bush et al., 1986a) would be good examples of well-documented idiosyncratic reactions to foods. In both cases, substantial evidence from challenge studies has confirmed the association with foods. Despite the well documented association with foods, the mechanisms of the reactions remain unknown. Celiac disease was previously discussed as a possible non–IgE-mediated form of true food allergy, but this mechanism has not been firmly established. Actually, only a few of the many possible food idiosyncrasies

TABLE 10.6 Partial List of Food-Associated Idiosyncratic Reactions

Category	Reaction	Implicated food or ingredient
Proven	Asthma	Sulfites
	Celiac disease	Wheat, rye, barley, oats
	Urticaria	Aspartame
Unproven	Chronic urticaria	BHA, BHT, benzoates
	Asthma, urticaria	Tartrazine
	Migraine headache	Many foods, aspartame
	Aggressive behavior	Sugar
	Chinese restaurant syndrome	Monosodium glutamate
	Asthma	Monosodium glutamate
Disproven	Hyperkinesis	Food-coloring agents

have been definitely linked to the ingestion of specific foods or food ingredients.

In the vast majority of food idiosyncrasies, the role of specific foods or food ingredients remains to be firmly established. With many of these reactions, carefully controlled challenge studies have not been conducted to examine the role of foods or food ingredients. For example, the role of sugar in aggressive behavior has not been carefully tested (Harper and Gans, 1986). The existence of many of these illnesses is based solely on unconfirmed, anecdotal reports. Some of these may truly exist, but others may be psychosomatic or attributable to causes other than foods. The role of psychological disorders in perceived reactions to foods has been the subject of several notable studies (King, 1984; Rippere, 1984; Rix et al., 1984; Pearson et al., 1983; Selner and Staudenmayer, 1986). In some cases, the symptoms are so subjective that confirmation of the responses is difficult. Examples would include food-induced migraines and "Chinese restaurant syndrome." In other cases, the results of several challenge studies are not in agreement. Examples would include the alleged roles of tartrazine (FD&C Yellow #5) in asthma and butylated hydroxytoluene (BHT) and butylated hydroxyanisole (BHA) in chronic urticaria.

Occasionally, the alleged role of foods or food ingredients in an idiosyncratic reaction is received with considerable fanfare. When the reaction is subsequently shown not be associated with the specific food or food ingredient, the consuming public may not accept the new findings. The classical example in this category is the role of artificial food colorants in hyperkinesis in children. Food colorants were first implicated as causative factors in hyperkinesis by Dr. Benjamin Feingold on the basis of poorly controlled trials and anecdotal experiences (Feingold, 1975). However, the Feingold hypothesis received considerable publicity, and many consumers became convinced of the relationship. Subsequently, several well-controlled trials revealed that few, if any, hyperkinetic children were adversely affected by these food colorants (Stare et al., 1980; Harley et al., 1978a,b). However, some consumers persist in their beliefs regarding a role for food colorants in this condition. Other reactions may soon fall into this category including the role of monosodium glutamate in Chinese restaurant syndrome and the role of tartrazine in asthma.

The role of specific foods or food ingredients in many of these idiosyncratic reactions remains to be established. Double-blind food challenges (DBFC) are advocated as a preferred method for assessing the role of foods or ingredients in these reactions. A positive DBFC confirms the causative role of the specific food or ingredient in the reaction, although it cannot reveal the mechanism of the adverse reaction. A negative DBFC may indicate that foods are not involved in the reaction or at least that the specific food or ingredient was wrongly incriminated. DBFCs should not be used in cases of life-threatening reactions unless special precautions are taken.

Obviously, a complete discussion of all of the food-associated idiosyncratic reactions is beyond the scope of this chapter. Instead, several idiosyncratic reactions will be highlighted as examples.

Sulfite-induced asthma.   Sulfites are widely used in foods for a variety of purposes: to prevent enzymatic and nonenzymatic browning, as broad spectrum antimicrobial agents, as dough conditioning agents, to provide antioxidant protection, and as bleaching agents in the processing of maraschino cherries and hominy (Taylor et al., 1986b). As a result, sulfite residues are present in a variety of foods at levels ranging from a few ppm to >1000 ppm in dried fruits. The foods and beverages with the highest sulfite levels as consumed would include dried fruits other than dark raisins or prunes (500–2500 ppm), nonfrozen lemon and lime juices (150–800 ppm), wine (20–350 ppm), molasses (125 ppm), dehydrated potatoes (30–90 ppm), shrimp (<10–100 ppm), white and pink grape juices (50–250 ppm), and sauerkraut juice (100 ppm). Sulfites can also occur naturally in foods, especially fermented foods, but the residues of naturally occurring sulfites are usually low (Taylor et al., 1986b).

Sulfites are very reactive chemicals (Taylor et al., 1986b). They tend to react with other food components such as reducing sugars, proteins, amino acids, aldehydes, and ketones. As a consequence, very little free, unreacted sulfite remains in most foods. Instead, residual sulfites tend to be bound to other organic constituents either reversibly or irreversibly. Sulfites can also be oxidized to sulfate in food matrices. Sulfites can also be lost as volatile SO_2 especially from acidic foods and beverages.

Sulfites have been used for centuries with little evidence of harm to consumers. However, in recent years, sulfites have been implicated as triggers for asthmatic reactions in some sensitive individuals (Stevenson and Simon, 1981; Bush et al., 1986a; Baker et al., 1981). The reactions typically occur within a few minutes after ingestion of a provoking dose of sulfite. The reactions can be quite severe on occasion. The U.S. Food and Drug Administration has received reports of over 20 deaths alleged to be due to sulfited foods since 1982.

Asthma is the most prominent and severe symptom attributed to the ingestion of sulfited foods. Other symptoms have been reported, but these reports are largely anecdotal and unverified (Bush et al., 1986a). The role of sulfites in asthma has been verified by numerous investigators through the use of double-blind challenge procedures (Bush et al., 1986a). Double-blind challenges have been conducted with sulfite in capsules and in acidic beverages. In acidic beverages, volatilization of SO_2 occurs; sulfite-sensitive asthmatics are more likely to respond to sulfited, acidic beverages than to capsules (Delohery et al., 1984). This increased sensitivity seems to be due to the inhalation of SO_2 vapors while swallowing (Delohery et al., 1984).

The prevalence of sulfite-induced asthma is quite low. Bush et al. (1986b) concluded from challenges of over 200 asthmatics that sulfite sensitivity occurs in only 1–2% of all asthmatics. Severe asthmatics, defined as those requiring steroid-based drugs, are most likely to be sulfite-sensitive; the prevalence in this subpopulation is 4–7% (Bush et al., 1986b). None of the mild asthmatics included in this large clinical trial were confirmed to be sulfite sensitive (Bush et al., 1986b). While other investigators have estimated a higher prevalence of sulfite sensitivity among asthmatics, these estimates may have been based mostly on challenges of steroid-dependent asthmatics rather than a representative cross-section of the asthmatic population (Buckley et al., 1985; Simon et al., 1982).

The pathogenesis of sulfite-induced asthma is not understood. Multiple mechanisms may be involved including IgE-mediated reactions, hyperreactivity to inhaled SO_2, and sulfite oxidase deficiency (Taylor et al., 1986b; Simon, 1986). The hyperreactivity to SO_2 inhaled while swallowing seems to be the most common mechanism (Delohery et al., 1984). However, this mechanism does not explain all adverse reactions to sulfites.

Sulfite-sensitive asthmatics must avoid highly sulfited foods and beverages. The individual tolerance for sulfites among sulfite-sensitive asthmatics is variable. In controlled challenges with capsules and/or acidic beverages, the threshold level of sulfite ranges from 3 to 130 mg of SO_2 equivalents (Taylor et al., 1986b). Sulfite-sensitive asthmatics seem to be even more tolerant of sulfites in foods (Taylor et al., 1988). Perhaps the increased tolerance is due to the bound forms of sulfite which predominate in most foods. Sulfite-sensitive asthmatics are especially sensitive to sulfited lettuce (Taylor et al., 1988; Howland and Simon, 1985). Lettuce contains a preponderance of free sulfite (Martin et al., 1986) and may represent an especially hazardous food for sulfite-sensitive asthmatics.

The FDA has recently promulgated several regulations for the protection of sulfite-sensitive asthmatics. One regulation requires the declaration of sulfites on the label of any food containing in excess of 10 ppm total SO_2. The FDA also banned the use of sulfites on fresh fruits and vegetables other than potatoes. This ban prevents the use of sulfite in salad bars in restaurants. FDA has also proposed a ban on the use of sulfites in fresh potatoes. Sulfite use in shrimp has been limited to a level that will result in sulfite residues not exceeding 100 ppm total SO_2.

Tartrazine-induced asthma and urticaria.   In 1958, Speer stated that tartrazine (FD&C Yellow #5) caused asthma in some children. No data were presented to support this conclusion. In 1959, Lockey presented anecdotal evidence on three patients who reported urticaria (hives) after the ingestion of yellow-colored drugs. Nonblinded challenges with tartrazine provoked various types of reactions including urticaria (Lockey, 1959). Mounting evidence, mostly from anecdotal reports or nonblinded or open challenges with tartrazine, led the Food and Drug Administration to require the specific labelling of FD&C Yellow #5 on food products in 1979 (FDA, 1979). The evidence at that time suggested that between 50,000 and 100,000 individuals in the United States might be at risk from ingestion of tartrazine (FDA, 1979). In particular, a small percentage of aspirin-intolerant asthmatics seemed to constitute the risk group for tartrazine-induced asthma (Samter and Beers, 1968). Today, the failure to properly declare FD&C Yellow #5 on food labels is perhaps the most frequent cause of food recalls.

Since the FDA action in 1979, numerous additional clinical trials have been conducted on tartazine-induced asthma and urticaria (Robinson, 1988). Many of these trials were conducted in double-blind fashion, and they represent a strong test of the hypothesis that tartrazine is involved in the causation of asthma and urticaria. The results of these and the earlier trials on the effects of tartrazine have been extensively reviewed by Stevenson et al. (1986) and Simon (1986). The results of the double-blind oral challenges with tartrazine have indicated that tartrazine plays virtually *no* role in either asthma or urticaria. However, the criteria used by these investigators has been criticized as possibly too restrictive (Robinson, 1988).

With respect to asthma, most of the double-blind trials with tartrazine have failed to identify any tartrazine-sensitive subjects even when the patient population was comprised of aspirin-intolerant asthmatics (Simon, 1986; Stevenson et al., 1986). The few studies identifying tartrazine-sensitive asthmatics were complicated by withholding bronchodilators from patients with unstable airway disease (Spector et al., 1979). Stevenson et al. (1986) conclude that tartrazine-induced asthma does not exist and that the early reports were simply exacerbations of asthma in patients with unstable airways who had been deprived of their bronchodilators.

With regard to urticaria, a very small number of tartrazine-sensitive individuals has been identified in double-blind, placebo-controlled trials (Simon, 1986; Stevenson et al., 1986; Settipane et al., 1976). Most of the studies with tartrazine on urticarial patients are complicated by the failure to blind the challenge, a lack of placebo controls, and the withholding of antihistamines which are essential for the control of symptoms in patients with chronic urticaria (Stevenson et al., 1986). Tartrazine is, at worst, a cause of urticaria in only a few of the many individuals with this symptom.

Other food additives in chronic urticaria. Chronic urticaria is a disease with few known causes. Most patients with this illness are forced to exist on chronic medication with antihistamines.

In the search for causative agents in chronic urticaria, considerable attention has been focused on food additives: tartrazine, sunset yellow (FD&C Yellow #6), sodium benzoate, benzoic acid, parabens, butylated hydroxyanisole (BHA), and butylated hydroxytoluene (BHT). Numerous clinicians have concluded that these additives play a causative role in chronic urticaria (Juhlin et al., 1972, 1981; Doeglas, 1975; Thune et al., 1975; Ros et al., 1976; Rudzki et al., 1980; Gibson and Clancy, 1980; Ortolani et al., 1984).

However, the studies cited above are all significantly flawed in one respect or another (Simon, 1986). The most frequent flaws were lack of placebo controls in challenge studies, omission of positive placebo challenge data, and the withholding of antihistamines for up to 5 days prior to challenge (Simon, 1986). The withholding of antihistamines may be especially critical. If hives are observed in such challenge studies, are they the result of the additive challenge or the withdrawal of the medication? With additive-avoidance diets, the claims of significant improvement in chronic urticaria are complicated by a lack of placebo controls, questions about the formulation of such diets, adherence to the diets, and simultaneous changes in medical treatments for the condition.

The conclusion is that the evidence implicating various food additives in chronic urticaria is suspect. Changes in the use and regulation of any of these food additives on the basis of this type of evidence is unwarranted.

REFERENCES

Aas, K. 1966. Studies on hypersensitivity to fish. Allergologicial and serological differentiation between various species of fish. *Int. Arch. Allergy* 30: 257–267.

American Academy of Allergy and Immunology and National Institute of Allergy and Infectious Diseases. 1984. *Adverse Reactions to Foods,* U.S. Dept., of Health and Human Services, NIH Publ. No. 84-2442, Washington, D.C. 110 pp.

Anderson, J. A. 1986. The establishment of common language concerning adverse reactions to foods and food additives. *J. Allergy Clin. Immunol.* 78: 140–144.

Anet, J., Back, J. F., Baker, R. S., Barnett, D., Burley, R. W., and Howden, M. E. H. 1985. Allergens in white and yolks of hen's egg. A study of IgE binding by egg proteins. *Int. Arch. Allergy Appl. Immunol.* 77: 364–371.

Anonymous. 1981. Exploring cow's milk and soy protein sensitivity in human infants. *Nutr. Rev.* 39: 305–307.

Bahna, S. L. and Gandhi, M. D. 1983. Milk hypersensitivity. I. Pathogenesis and symptomology. *Ann. Allergy* 50: 218–224.

Baker, G. J., Collett, P., and Allen, D. H. 1981. Bronchospasm induced by metabisulphite-containing foods and drugs. *Med. J. Aust.* 2: 614–616.

Baldo, B. A. 1984. Milk allergies. *Aust. J. Dairy Technol.* 39: 120–128.

Barillas, C. and Solomons, N. W. 1987. Effective reduction of lactose maldigestion in preschool children by direct addition of β-galacto-sidases to milk at mealtime. *Pediatrics* 79: 766–772.

Barnett, D., Baldo, B. A., and Howden, M. E. H. 1983. Multiplicity of allergens in peanuts. *J. Allergy Clin. Immunol.* 72: 61–68.

Barnett, D. and Howden, M. E. H. 1986. Partial characterization of an allergenic glycoprotein from peanut (*Arachis hypogaea* L.). *Biochim. Biophys. Acta* 882: 97–105.

Bayless, T. M. 1987. Lactose malabsorption, milk intolerance, and symptom awareness in adults. In *Lactose Digestion: Clinical and Nutritional Implications,* D.M. Paige and T. M. Bayless (Ed.) The Johns Hopkins University Press, Baltimore, MD., 117–123.

Bayless, T. M., Rothfeld, B., Massa, C., Wise, L., Paige, D., and Bedine, M. S. 1975. Lactose and milk intolerance: clinical implications. *N. Engl. J. Med.* 292: 1156–1159.

Birge, S. T., Kentman, H. T., Cuatrecasas, P., and Whedon, G. D. 1967. Osteoporosis, intestinal lactose deficiency and low dietary calcium intake. *N. Engl. J. Med,* 276: 445–448.

Bjorksten, B. 1984. Atopic allergy in relation to cell-mediated immunity. *Clin. Rev. Allergy* 2: 95–106.

Bleumink, E., Berrens, L., and Young, E. 1966. Studies on the atopic allergen in ripe tomato fruits. I. Isolation and identification of the allergen. *Int. Arch. Allergy Appl. Immunol.* 30: 132–145.

Bleumink, E. and Young, E. 1969. Studies on the atopic allergen in hen's egg. I. Identification of the skin reactive fraction in egg white. *Int. Arch. Allergy Appl. Immunol* 35: 1–19.

Bleumink, E. and Young, E. 1971. Studies on the atopic allergen in hen's egg. II. Further characterization of the skin-reactive fraction in egg-white; immuno-electrophoretic studies. *Int. Arch. Allergy Appl. Immunol.* 40: 72–88.

Bleumink, E. and Young, E. 1968. Identification of the atopic allergen in cow's milk. *Int. Arch. Allergy Appl. Immunol.* 34: 521–543.

Bock, S. A. 1987. Prospective appraisal of complaints of adverse reactions of foods in children during the first 3 years of life. *Pediatrics.* 79: 683–688.

Bock, S. A. 1982. The natural history of food sensitivity. *J. Allergy Clin. Immunol.* 69: 173–177.

Broadbent, J. B., Taylor, S., Adam, E. H., and Sampson, H. A. 1988. Western blot and dot blot analyses of immunologic cross-reactivity in legume allergic patients. *J. Allergy Clin. Immunol.* 81: 189.

Buchbinder, E. M., Bloch, K. J., Moss, J., and Guiney, T. E. 1983. Food-dependent, exercise-induced anaphylaxis. *J. Am. Med. Assoc.* 250: 2973–2974.

Buckley, C. E., Saltzman, H. A., and Sieker, H. O. 1985. The prevalence and degree of sensitivity to ingested sulfites. *J. Allergy Clin. Immunol.* 75: 144.

Burks, A. W., Jr., Brooks, J. R., and Sampson, H. A. 1988. Allergenicity of major component proteins of soybean determined by enzyme linked immunosorbent assay (ELISA) and immunoblotting in children with atopic dermatitis and positive soy challenges. *J. Allergy Clin. Immunol.* *81*: 1135–1142.

Bush, R. K., Taylor, S. L., and Busse, W. W. 1986a. A critical evaluation of clinical trials in reactions to sulfites. *J. Allergy Clin. Immunol.* 78: 191–202.

Bush, R. K., Taylor, S. L., Holden, K., Nordlee, J. A., and Busse, W. W. 1986b. The prevalence of sensitivity to sulfiting agents in asthmatics. *Am. J. Med.* 81: 816–820.

Bush, R. K., Taylor, S. L., Nordlee, J. A., and Busse, W. W. 1985. Soybean oil is not allergenic to soybean-sensitive individuals. *J.Allergy Clin. Immuno.* 76: 242–245.

Chandra, R. K. 1987. Food allergy: setting the theme. In *Food Allergy,* R. K. Chandra (Ed.). Nutrition Research Education Foundation, St. John's, Newfoundland, pp. 3–5.

Coombs, R. R. A. and Gell, P. H. G. 1975. Classification of allergic reactions responsible for clinical hypersensitivity and disease. In *Chemical Aspects of Immunology,* P. G. H. Gell, R. R. A. Coombs, and P. J. Lachmann (Ed.), Blackwell Scientific, Oxford, 761–782.

Daul, C. B., Morgan, J. E., O'Neil, C. E., and Lehrer, S. B. 1988. Species-specific shrimp allergens. *J. Allergy Clin. Immunol.* 81: 189.

Davidson, M., Burnstine, R. C., Kugler, M. M., and Bauer, C. H. Malabsorption defect induced by ingestion of beta lactoglobulin. *J. Pediatr.* 66: 545–554.

Delohery, J., Simmul, R., Castle, W. D., and Allen, D. 1984. The relationship of inhaled sulfur dioxide reactivity to ingested metabisulfite sensitivity in patients with asthma. *Am. Rev. Resp. Dis.* 130: 1027–1032.

Dewdney, J. M. and Edwards, R. G. 1984. Penicillin hypersensitivity - is milk a significant hazard?: a review. *J. Royal Soc. Med.* 77: 866–877.

Doeglas, H. M. 1975. Reactions to aspirin and food additives in patients with chronic urticaria, including the physical urticarias. *Br. J. Dematol.* 93: 135–144.

Egger, J., Carter, C. M., Wilson, J., Turner, M. W., and Soothill, J. F. 1983. Is migraine food allergy? A double-blind controlled trial of oligoantigenic diet treatment. *Lancet* ii: 865–868.

Elsayed, S. and Aas, K. 1971. Characterization of a major allergen (cod) Observations on effect of denaturation on the allergenic activity. *J. Allergy* 47: 283–291.

Elsayed, S. and Apold, J. 1983. Immunochemical analysis of cod fish allergen M: locations of the immunoglobulin binding sites as demonstrated by the native and synthetic peptides. *Allergy* 38: 449–459.

Elsayed, S. and Bennich, H. 1975. The primary structure of allergen M from cod. *Scand. J. Immunol.* 4: 203–208.

Elsayed, S., Titlestad, K., Apold, J., and Aas, K. 1980. A synthetic hexadecapeptide derived from allergen M imposing allergenic and antigenic reactivity. *Scand. J. Immunol.* 12: 171–175.

Feingold, T. 1975. *Why Your Child is Hyperactive.* Random House, New York.

Food and Drug Administratioin. 1979. FD&C Yellow No. 5; labeling in food and drugs for human use. *Fed. Reg.* 44: 37212–37221.

Ford, R. P. K., Hill, D. J., and Hosking, C. S. 1983. Cow's milk hypersensitivity: immediate and delayed onset clinical patterns. *Arch. Dis. Child.* 58: 856–862.

Fries, J. H. 1982. Peanuts: allergic and other untoward reactions. *Ann. Allergy* 48: 220–226.

Gallagher, C. R., Molleson, A. L., and Caldwell, J. H. 1977. Lactose intolerance and fermented dairy products. *Cult. Dairy Prod. J.* 10(1): 22–24.

Gerrard, J. W. 1984. Allergies in breastfed babies to foods ingested by the mother. *Clin. Rev. Allergy* 2: 143–149.

Gibson, A. and Clancy, R. 1980. Management of chronic idiopathic urticaria by the identification and exclusion of dietary factors. *Clin. Allergy* 10: 699–704.

Gjesing, B. Osterballe, O., Schwartz, B., Wahn, U., and Lowenstein, H. 1986. Allergen-specific IgE antibodies against antigenic components in cow milk and milk substitutes. *Allergy* 41: 51–56.

Golbert, T. M. 1972. Food allergy and immunologic diseases of the gastrointestinal tract. In *Allergic Diseases: Diagnosis and Management,* R. Patterson (Ed.). Lippincott, Philadelphia, PA, pp. 355–379.

Goldman, A. S., Sellars, W. A., Halpern, S. R., Anderson, D. W., Furlow, T. E., and Johnson, C. H. 1963a. Milk allergy. II. Skin testing of allergic and normal children with purified milk proteins. *Pediatrics* 32: 572–579.

Goldman, A. S., Anderson, D. W., Sellars, W. A., Saperstein, S., Kniker, W. T., and Halpern, S. R. 1963b. Milk allergy. I. Oral challenge with milk and isolated milk proteins in allergic children. *Pediatrics* 32: 425–433.

Grant, R. T., Pearson, R. S. B., and Corneau, W. J. 1936. Observations on urticaria provoked by emotion, by exercise, and warming of the body. *Clin. Sci.* 2: 253–272.

Halmepuro, L., Vuontela, K., Kalimo, K., and Bjorksten, F. 1984. Cross-reactivity of IgE antibodies with allergens in birch pollen, fruits, and vegetables. *Int. Arch. Allergy Appl. Immunol.* 74: 235–240.

Halsey, A. B., Martin, M. E., Ruff, M. E., Jacobs, F. O., and Jacobs, R. L. 1986. Sunflower oil is not allergenic to sunflower seed-sensitive patients. *J. Allergy Clin. Immunol.* 78: 408–410.

Hanson, L. A. and Mansson, I. 1961. Immune electrophoretic studies of bovine milk and milk products. *Acta Pediatr. Scand.* 50: 484–490.

Harley J. P., Ray, R. S., Tomasi, L., Eichman, P. L., Matthews, C. G., Chun, R., Cleeland, C. S., and Traisman, E. 1978a. Hyperkinesis and food additives: testing the Feingold hypothesis. *Pediatrics* 61: 818–828.

Harley, J. P., Matthews, C. G., and Eichman, P. 1978b. Synthetic food colors and hyperactivity in children: a double-blind challenge experiment. *Pediatrics* 62: 975–983.

Harper, A. E. and Gans, D. A. 1986. Diet and behavior - an assessment of reports of agressive, antisocial behavior from consumption of sugar. *Food Technol.* 40: 142–149.

Hartsook, E. I. 1984. Celiac sprue: sensitivity to gliadin. *Cereal Foods World* 29: 157–158.

Haverberg, L., Kwon, P. H., and Scrimshaw, N. S. 1980. Comparative tolerance of adolescents of differing ethnic backgrounds to lactose-containing and lactose-free dairy drinks. I. Initial experience with a double-blind procedure. *Am. J. Clin. Nutr.* 33: 17–21.

Heiner, D. C. and Neucere. N. J. 1975. RAST analyses of peanut allergens. *J. Allergy Clin. Immunol.* 55: 82–83.

Herian, A. M., Taylor, S. L., and Bush, R. K. 1989. Food Research Institute, University of Wisconsin, Madison.

Hoffman, D. R., Day, E. D., and Miller, J. S. 1981. The major heat stable allergen from shrimp. *Ann. Allergy* 47: 17–22.

Hoffman, D. R. 1983. Immunochemical identification of the allergens in egg white. *J. Allergy Clin. Immunol.* 71: 481–486.

Houts, S. S. 1988. Lactose intolerance. *Food Technol.* 42(3): 110–113.

Howland, W. C. and Simon, R. A. 1985. Restaurant-provoked asthma: ? sulfite sensitivity. *J. Allergy Clin Immunol.* 75: 145.

Ishizaka, K., Ishizaka, T., and Hornbrook, M. 1966. Physicochemical properties of a human reaginic antibody. IV. Presence of a unique immunoglobulin as a carrier of reaginic activity. *J. Immunol.* 97: 75–85.

Juhlin, L. 1981. Recurrent urticaria: clinical investigation of 330 patients. *Br. J. Dermatol.* 104: 369–381.

Juhlin, L., Michaelson, G., and Zetterstrom, O. 1972. Urticaria and asthma induced by food-and-drug additives in patients with aspirin hypersensitivity, *J. Allergy Clin. Immunol.* 50: 92–98.

Juntunen, K. and Ali-Yrkko, S. 1983. Goat's milk for children allergic to cow's milk. *Kiel Milchwirt. Forschungsberg.* 35: 439–440.

Kasarda, D. D. 1978. The relationship of wheat protein to celiac disease. *Cereal Foods World* 23: 240–244.

Kay, R. A. and Ferguson, A. 1984. Intestinal T cells, mucosal cell-mediated immunity and their relevance to food allergic disease. *Clin. Rev. Allergy* 2: 55–68.

Kemp, A. S., Mellis, C. M., Barnett, D., Sharota, E., and Simpson, J. 1985. Skin test, RAST and clinical reactions to peanut allergens in children. *Clin. Allergy* 15: 73–78.

Kenney, R. A. 1979. Placebo-controlled studies of human reaction to oral monosodium L-glutamate. In *Glutamic Acid: Advances in Biochemistry and Physiology,* L. J. Filer, Jr., S. Garattini, M. R. Kare, W. A. Reynolds, and R. J. Wurtman (Ed.). Raven Press, New York, pp. 363–373.

Kidd, J. M., Cohen, S. H., Sosman, M. D., and Fink, J. N. 1983. Food dependent exercise-induced anaphylaxis. *J. Allergy Clin. Immunol.* 71: 407–411.

Kim, H. S. and Gilliland, S. E. 1983. *Lactobacillus acidophilus* as a dietary adjunct for milk to aid lactose digestion in humans. *J. Dairy Sci.* 66: 959–966.

King, D. S. 1984. Psychological and behavioral effects of food and chemical exposure in sensitive individuals. *Nutr. Health* 3: 137–151.

Kleinman, R. E. and Walker, W. A. 1984. Antigen processing and uptake from the intestinal tract. *Clin. Rev. Allergy* 2: 25–37.

Kocian, J. 1988. Lactose intolerance. *Int. J. Biochem.* 20: 1–5.

Kolars, J. C., Levitt, M. D., Aouji, M., and Savaiano, D. A. 1984. Yogurt—an autodigesting source of lactose. *N. Engl. J. Med.* 310: 1–3.

Kuitunen, P., Visakorpi, J. K., Savilahti, E., and Pelkonen, P. 1975. Malabsorption syndrome with cow's milk intolerance. Clinical findings and course in 54 cases. *Arch. Dis. Child.* 50: 351–356.

Kushimoto, H. and Aoki, T. 1985. Masked type I wheat allergy. *Arch. Dermatol.* 121: 355–360.

Kwon, P. H., Rorick, M. H., and Scrimshaw, N. S. 1980. Comparative tolerance of adolescents of differing ethnic backgrounds to lactose-containing and lactose-free dairy products. II. Improvement of a double-blind test. *Am. J. Clin. Nutr.* 33: 22–26.

Langeland, T. 1982. A clinical and immunological study of allergy to hen's egg white. III. Allergens in hen's egg white studies by crossed radio-immunoelectrophoresis (CRIE). *Allergy* 37: 521–530.

Langeland, T. 1983. A clinical and immunological study of allergy to hen's egg white. VI. Occurrence of proteins cross-reacting with allergens in hen's egg white as studied in egg white from turkey, duck, goose, seagull, and in hen egg yolk, and hen and chicken sera and flesh. *Allergy* 39: 399–412.

Langeland, T. 1985. Allergy to hen's egg white in atopic dermatitis. *Acta Derm. Venereol.* Suppl. 114: 109–112.

Layton, G. T. and Stanworth, D. R. 1984. The quantitation of IgG$_4$ antibodies to three common food allergens by ELISA with monoclonal antiIgG$_4$. *J. Immunol. Meth.* 73: 347–356.

Lebenthal, E. 1975. Cow's milk protein allergy. *Pediatr. Clin. North Am.* 22: 827–833.

Lehrer, S. B., McCants, M. L., and Salvaggio, J. E. 1985. Identification of crustacea allergens by crossed radioimmunoelectrophoresis. *Int. Arch.*

Allergy Appl. Immunol. 77: 192–194.

Lockey, S. D. 1959. Allergic reactions due to FD&C Yellow No. 5 tartrazine, and aniline dye used as coloring and identifying agent in various steroids. *Ann. Allergy* 17: 719–721.

Mager, J., Chevion, M., and Glaser, G. 1980. Favism. In *Toxic Constituents of Plant Foodstuffs,* 2nd ed., I. E. Liener (Ed.). Academic Press, New York., 265–294.

Malish, D., Glovsky, M. M., Hoffman, D. R., Ghekiere, L., and Hawkins, J. M. 1981. Anaphylaxis after sesame seed ingestion. *J. Allergy Clin. Immunol.* 67: 35–38.

Malley, A., Baecher, L., Mackler, B., and Perlman, F. 1976. The isolation of allergens from the green pea. *J. Allergy Clin. Immunol.* 56: 282–290.

Malley, A., Baecher, L., Mackler, B., and Perlman, F. 1975. Further characterization of a low-molecular weight allergen fragment isolated from the green pea. *Clin. Exp. Immunol.* 25: 159–164.

Mansfield, L. E. and Bowers, C. H. 1983. Systemic reaction to papain in a nonoccupational setting. *J. Allergy Clin. Immunol.* 71: 371–374.

Martin, L. B., Nordlee, J. A., and Taylor, S. L. 1986. Sulfite residues in restaurant salads. *J. Food Prot.* 49: 126–129.

Martini, M. C. and Savaiano, D. A. 1988. Reduced intolerance symptoms from lactose consumed during a meal. *Am. J. Clin. Nutr.* 47: 57–60.

Martini, M. C., Bollweg, G. L., Savaiano, D. A., and Levitt, M. D. 1987. Lactose digestion by yogurt β-galactosidase: influence of pH and microbial integrity. *Am. J. Clin. Nutr.* 45: 432–436.

Maulitz, R. M., Pratt, D. S., and Shocket, A. L. 1979. Exercise-induced anaphylactic reaction to shellfish. *J. Allergy Clin. Immunol.* 63: 433–435.

Meier-Davis, S., Taylor, S. L., Nordlee, J., and Bush, R. 1987. Identification of peanut allergens by immunoblotting. *J. Allergy Clin. Immunol.* 79: 218.

Merrett, J., Barnetson, R. St. C., Burr, M. L., and Merrett, T. G. 1984. Total and specific IgG$_4$ antibody levels in atopic eczema. *Clin. Exp. Immunol.* 56: 645–652.

Metcalfe, D. D. 1984. Food hypersensitivity. *J. Allergy Clin. Immunol.* 63: 749–762.

Michel, F. B., Bousquet, J., Dannaeus, A., Hamburger, R. N., Bellanti, J. A., Businco, L. M., and Soothill, J. 1986. Preventive measures in early childhood allergy. *J. Allergy Clin. Immunol.* 78: 1022–1027.

Minikin, W. P. and Lynch, P. J. 1969. Allergic reactions to penicillin in milk. *J. Am. Med. Assoc.* 209: 1089-1090.

Monro, J., Rostoff, J., Carini, C., and Zilkha, K. 1980. Food allergy in migraine. Study of dietary exclusion and RAST. *Lancet* ii: 1-4.

Nagpal, S., Metcalfe, D. D., and Subba Rao, P. V. 1985. Isolation of allergenic constituents from shrimp (*Penaeus indicus.*). *Ann. Allergy* 55: 306A.

National Dairy Council. 1978. Perspective on milk intolerance. *Dairy Council Digest* 49: 31-36.

Newcomer, A. D. 1981. Immediate symptomatic and long-term nutritional consequences of hypolactasia. In *Lactose Digestion: Clinical and Nutritional Implications,* D. M. Paige and T. M. Bayless (Ed.). The John Hopkins University Press, Baltimore, MD., 124-133.

Nordlee, J. A., Taylor, S. L., Jones, R. T., and Yunginger, J. W. 1981. Allergenicity of various peanut products as determined by RAST inhibition. *J. Allergy Clin. Immunol.* 68: 376-382.

Ortolani, C., Pastorello, E., Luraghi, M. T., Della-Torre, F., Bellani, M., and Zanussi, C. 1984. Diagnosis of intolerance to food additives. *Ann. Allergy* 53: 587-591.

Paganelli, R., Matricardi, P. M., and Aiuti, F. 1984. Interactions of food antigens, antibodies, and antigen-antibody complexes in health and disease. *Clin. Rev. Allergy* 2: 69-78.

Paige, D. M., Bayless, T. M., Huang, S. -S., and Wexler, R. 1975. Lactose hydrolyzed milk. *Am. J. Clin. Nutr.* 28: 818-822.

Pearson, D. J., Rix, K. J. B., and Bentley, S. J. 1983. Food allergy: how much in the mind? *Lancet* i: 1259-1961.

Perkin, J. E. and Hartje, J. 1983. Diet and migraine: a review of the literature. *J. Am. Diet. Assoc.* 83: 459-463.

Powrie, W. D. and Nakai, S. 1985. Characteristics of edible fluids of animal origin: eggs. In *Food Chemistry,* 2nd ed., O. R. Fennema (Ed.). Marcel Dekker, New York, pp. 829-855.

Prausnitz, C. and Kustner, H. 1921. Studies on hypersensitivity. *Zbl. Bakt.* 1: 160-169.

Rippere, V. 1984. Some varieties of food tolerance in psychiatric patients. An overview. *Nutr. Health* 3: 125-136.

Rix, K. J. B., Pearson, D. J., and Bentley, S. J. 1984. A psychiatric study of patients with supposed food allergy. *Br. J. Psychiatry* 145: 121-126.

Robinson, G. 1988. Tartrazine - the story so far. *Food Chem. Toxicol.* 26: 73-78.

Ros, A. M., Juhlin, L., and Michaelson, G. 1976. A following study of patients with recurrent urticaria and hypersensitivity to aspirin. benzoates and azo dyes. *Br. J. Dermatol.* 95: 19–24.

Rosado, J. L., Solomons, N. W., Lisker, R., Bourges, H., Anrubio, G., Garcia, A., Perez-Briceno, R., and Aizupuru, E. 1984. Enzyme replacement therapy for primary adult lactase deficiency: effective reduction of lactose malabsorption and milk intolerance by direct addition of β-galactosidase to milk at mealtime. *Gastroenterology* 87: 1072–1082.

Rosado, J. L., Allen, L. H., and Solomons, N. W. 1987. Milk consumption, symptom response, and lactose digestion in milk intolerance. *Am. J. Clin. Nutr.* 45: 1457–1460.

Rudzki, E., Czubalski, K., and Grzywa, Z. 1980. Detection of urticaria with food additivies intolerance by means of diet. *Dermatologica* 161: 57–62.

Sachs, M. I., Jones, R. T., and Yunginger, J. W. 1981. Isolation and partial characterization of a major peanut allergen. *J. Allergy Clin. Immunol.* 67: 27–34.

Sampson, H. A. 1988. IgE-mediated food intolerance. *J. Allergy Clin. Immunol.* 81: 495–504.

Samter, M. and Beers, R. F. 1968. Intolerance to aspirin: clinical studies and considerations of its pathogenesis. *Ann. Int. Med.* 68: 975–983.

Sandine, W. E. and Daly, M. 1979. Milk intolerance. *J. Food Prot.* 42: 435–437.

Selner, J. C. and Staudenmayer, H. 1986. The relationship of the environment and food to allergic and psychiatric illness. In *Psychobiological Aspects of Allergic Disorders,* S. H. Young, J. M. Rubin, and H. R. Daman (Ed.), Praeger Publ., Westport, CT. p. 102–106.

Settipane, G. A., Chafee, F. H., Postman, I. M., Levine, M. I., Saker, J. H., Barrick, R. H., Nicholas, S. S., Schwartz, H. J., Honsinger, R. W., and Klein, D. E. 1976. Significance of tartrazine sensitivity in chronic urticaria of unknown etiology. *J. Allergy Clin. Immunol.* 57: 541–546.

Shakib, F., Brown, H. M., and Stanworth, D. R. 1984. Relevance of milk- and egg-specific IgG$_4$ in atopic eczema. *Int. Arch. Allergy Appl. Immunol.* 75: 107–112.

Shakib, F., Stanworth, D. R., Drew, R., and Catty, D. 1975. A quantitative study of the distribution of IgG subclasses in a group of normal human sera. *J. Immunol. Meth.* 8: 17–28.

Sheffer, A. L., Soter, N. A., McFadden, E. R., Jr., and Austen, K. F. 1983. Exercise-induced anaphylaxis: a distinct form of physical allergy. *J. Allergy Clin. Immunol.* 71: 311–316.

Shibasaki, M., Suzuki, S., Tajima, S., Nemoto, H., and Kuroume, T. 1980. Allergenicity of major component proteins of soybean. *Int. Arch. Allergy Appl. Immunol.* 61: 441–448.

Shibasaki, M., Suziki, S., Nemoto, H., and Kuroume, T.. 1979. Allergenicity and lymphocyte-stimulating property of rice protein. *J. Allergy Clin. Immunol.* 64: 259–265.

Simon, R. A. 1986. Adverse reactions to food additives. *N. Engl. Reg. Allergy Proc.* 7: 533–542.

Simon, R. A., Green, L., and Stevenson, D. D. 1982. The incidence of ingested metabisulfite sensitivity in an asthmatic population. *J. Allergy Clin. Immunol.* 69: 118.

Simoons, F. J. 1980. Age of onset of lactose malabsorption. *Pediatrics* 66: 646.

Sloan, A. E. and Powers, M. E. 1986. A perspective on popular perceptions of adverse reactions to foods. *J. Allergy Clin. Immunol.* 78: 127–139.

Solomons, N. W., Garcia-Ibanez, R., and Viteri, F. E. 1980. Hydrogen breath test of lactose absorption in adults: the application of physiological doses of whole cow's milk sources. *Am. J. Clin. Nutr.* 33: 545–554.

Spector, S. L., Wangaard, C. H., and Farr, R. S. 1979. Aspirin and concomitant idiosyncrasies in adult asthmatic patients. *J. Allergy Clin. Immunol.* 64: 500–506.

Speer, K. 1958. *The Management of Childhood Asthma.* Charles C. Thomas Publ., Springfield IL., p. 23.

Spies, J. R. 1977. Oilseed allergens, In *Immunological Aspects of Foods,* N. Catsimpoolas (Ed.). AVI Publishing, Westport, CT., p. 317–371.

Stare, F. J., Whelan, E. M., and Sheridan, M. 1980. Diet and hyperactivity: is there a relationship? *Pediatrics* 66: 521–525.

Stephenson, L. S. and Latham, M. C. 1974. Lactose intolerance and milk consumption: the relation of tolerance test to symptoms. *Am. J. Clin. Nutr.* 27: 296–303.

Stevenson, D. D., Simon, R. A., Lumry, W. R., and Mathison, D. A. 1986. Adverse reactions to tartrazine. *J. Allergy Clin. Immunol.* 78: 182–191.

Stevenson, D. D. and Simon, R. A. 1981. Sensitivity to ingested metabisulfites in asthmatic subjects. *J. Allergy Clin. Immunol.* 68: 26–32.

Strober, W. 1986. Gluten-sensitive enteropathy: a nonallergic immune hypersensitivity of the gastrointestinal tract. *J. Allergy Clin. Immunol.* 78: 202–211.

Swaisgood, H. E. 1985. Characteristics of edible fluids of animal origin:

milk. In *Food Chemistry,* 2nd ed., O. R. Fennema (Ed.). Marcel Dekker, New York, pp. 791–827.

Taylor, S. L. 1985. Food Allergies. *Food Technol.* 39(2): 98–105.

Taylor, S. L. 1986a. Immunologic and allergic properties of cows' milk proteins in humans. *J. Food Prot.* 49: 239–250.

Taylor, S. L. 1986b. Histamine food poisoning: toxicology and clinical aspects. *CRC Crit. Rev. Toxicol.* 17: 91–128.

Taylor, S. L. 1987. Allergic and sensitivity reactions to food components. In *Nutritional Toxicology,* Vol. II, J. N. Hathcock (Ed.). Academic Press, Orlando, FL, pp 173–198.

Taylor, S. L. 1988. Marine toxins of microbial origin. *Food Technol.* 42(3): 94–98.

Taylor, S. L., Guthertz, L. S., Leatherwood, M., Tillman, F., and Lieber, E. R. 1978. Histamine production by food-borne bacterial species. *J. Food Safety* 1: 173–187.

Taylor, S. L., Busse, W. W., Sachs, M. I., Parker, J. L., and Yunginger, J. W. 1981. Peanut oil is not allergenic to peanut-sensitive individuals. *J. Allergy Clin. Immunol.* 68: 373–375.

Taylor, S. L., Hui, J. Y., and Lyons, D. E. 1984. Toxicology of scombroid poisoning. In *Seafood Toxins,* E. P. Ragelis (Ed.). Amer. Chem. Soc., Washington, D.C., 417–430.

Taylor, S. L., Bush, R. K., and Busse, W. W. 1986a. Avoidance diets—how selective should we be? *N. Engl. Reg. Allergy Proc.* 7: 527–532.

Taylor, S. L., Higley, N. A., and Bush, R. K. 1986b. Sulfites in foods: uses, analytical methods, residues, fate, exposure assessment, metabolism, toxicity, and hypersensitivity. *Adv. Food Res.* 30: 1–76.

Taylor, S. L., Bush, R. K., and Busse, W. W. 1987a. Avoidance diets—how selective should they be? In *Food Allergy,* R. K. Chandra (Ed.). Nutrition Research Education Foundation, St. John's Newfoundland, 253–266.

Taylor, S. L., Lemanske, R. F., Jr., Bush, R. K., and Busse, W. W. 1987b. Chemistry of food allergens. In *Food Allergy,* R. K. Chandra (Ed.), Nutrition Research Education Foundation, St. John's Newfoundland, pp. 21–44.

Taylor, S. L., Bush, R. K., Selner, J. C., Nordlee, J. A., Wiener, M. C., Holden, K., Koepke, J. W., and Busse, W. W. 1988. Sensitivity of sulfited foods among sulfite-sensitive asthmatics. *J. Allergy Clin. Immunol.* 81: 1159–1167.

Thune, P. and Granholt, A. 1975. Provocation tests with antiphlogistica and food additives in recurrent urticaria. *Dermatologica* 151: 360–367.

Tuft, L. and Blumstein, G. I. 1946. Studies in food allergy. V. Antigenic relationships among members of fish family. *J. Allergy* 17: 329–339.

Van Toorenenbergen, A. W. and Aalberse, R. C. 1982. IgG$_4$ and release of histamine from human peripheral blood leukocytes. *Int. Arch. Allergy Appl. Immunol.* 67: 117–122.

Waring, N. P., Daul, C. B., deShazo, R. D., McCants, M. L., and Lehrer, S. B. 1980. Hypersensitivity reactions to ingested crustacea: clinical evaluation and diagnostic studies in shrimp-sensitive individuals. *J. Allergy Clin. Immunol.* 76: 440–445.

Wood, C. B. S. 1986. How common is food allergy? *Acta Paediatr. Scand.* 323: 76–83.

Wytock, D. H. and DiPalma, J. A. 1988. All yogurts are not created equal. *Am. J. Clin. Nutr.* 47: 454–457.

Yunginger, J. W., Sweeney, K. G., Sturner, W. Q., Giannandrea, L. A., Teigland, J. D., Bray, M., Benson, P. A. York, J. A., Biedrzycki, L., Squillace, D. L., and Helm, R. M. 1988. Fatal food-induced anaphylaxis. *JAMA* 260: 1450–1452.

Yunginger, J. W., Gauerke, M. B., Jones, R. T., Dahlberg, M. J. E., and Ackerman, S. J. 1983. Use of radioimmunoassay to determine the nature, quantity and source of allergenic contamination of sunflower butter. *J. Food. Prot.* 46: 625–628.

11

Role of Lipid Oxidation Products in Atherosclerosis

Paul B. Addis

University of Minnesota
St. Paul, Minnesota

Seok-Won Park*

Texas A&M University
College Station, Texas

INTRODUCTION

The past decade has seen the development of numerous important concepts related to coronary heart disease (CHD). Our primary focus is to explore the hypothesized link between lipid oxidation products, be they of dietary or in vivo origin, and atherosclerosis, an area of intense research activity. We will also briefly review some extremely interesting new findings in the areas of hypercholesterolemia and thrombosis/vascular spasm. Taken together, these new findings hold great promise for reducing the number of clinical cases of heart disease and other problems

---

Present affiliation: Bristol-Meyers U.S. Pharmaceutical and Nutritional Group, Evansville, Indiana.

related to atherosclerosis. The reader should consult Table 11.1 for a listing of abbreviations, symbols, and definitions used in this review.

Whereas study of the postulated link between diet and cancer is at an embryonic stage, research on the diet–CHD relationship is fairly mature, and it is our opinion that the fruits of this maturity are ripe for harvest. Because CHD risk factor intervention invariably involves dietary alteration, the potential implications to food product development and marketing will continue to be highly significant and will likely increase. Specific possibilities for "engineering" foods for purposes of producing favorable outcomes in CHD prevention will be discussed later.

As an aid to understanding atherosclerosis and CHD, it is helpful to arbitrarily divide CHD into three phases. The first phase, initiation of atherosclerosis (atherogenesis), is the least well-understood phase but begins in the endothelium of the vessel. Whatever the cause, atherogenesis sets into motion a complex series of pathological changes, which leads to phase 2, the familiar plaque accumulation that is the hallmark of atherosclerosis and is favored by elevated serum cholesterol (SC) (LDL). Phase 3 can be triggered by thrombosis and/or arterial spasm leading to a potentially fatal myocardial infarction (MI). The foregoing description differs significantly from the traditional view that atherosclerosis is simply a deposition of lipid in the vessel wall, the result of abnormally elevated SC. However, in recent years much evidence has accumulated that C deposition is merely a secondary process, preceded by a complex series of pathological changes involving the interplay of endothelial cells, macrophages, platelets, growth factors, chemotactic agents, ASMCS, lipoproteins, and foam cells, and culminating in either spasm- or thrombus-induced MI.

A great deal of evidence suggests that LOPS both initiate and promote atherosclerosis and that one group of LOPS—COPS—are far more atherogenic than C itself. Whether *dietary* or in vivo forms of LOPS (or both) are involved is not yet clear. Nevertheless, these findings are extremely interesting in that they suggest that better inhibition of rancidity may help to lessen the degree to which consumers are exposed to atherogenic chemicals. Where higher levels of antioxidants are employed, the in vivo production of LOPS might also be reduced. Furthermore, recent findings have revealed surprising and potentially very exciting findings, which suggest that increasing the ω-3/ω-6 ratio may reduce the risk of thrombosis and/or spasm, even after atherosclerosis has affected the artery substantially. It is obvious that potentially outstanding opportunities for reducing CHD prevalence lie ahead!

TABLE 11.1 Definitions, Symbols, and Abbreviations Used

Abbreviation/Symbol	Definition
ADI	Average daily intake
ASMCS	Arterial smooth muscle cells
BHA, BHT, PG	Antioxidants: Buylated hydroxy anisole, butylated hydroxy toluene, propyl gallate
C	Cholesterol[a] (Cholest-5-ene-3β-ol)[b]
CHD	Coronary heart disease
COPS	Cholesterol oxidation products
α-epoxide	α-epoxide[a] (5,6α-epoxy-5α-cholestan-3β-ol)
β-epoxide	β-epoxide[a](5,6β-epoxy-5β-cholestan-3β-ol)
7α-OH	7α-hydroxycholesterol[a] (cholest-5-ene-3β, 7β-diol)[b]
7β-OH	7β-hydroxycholesterol[a] (choleste-5-ene-3β,7β-diol)[b]
7-keto	7-ketocholesterol[a] (3β-hydroxycholeste-5-en-7-one)[b]
25-OH	25-hydroxycholesterol[a] (cholest-5-ene-3β, 25 diol)[b]
triol	cholestane-triol[a] (5α-cholestane-3β,5α,6β-triol)[b]
DFO	Desferrioxamine (Fe chelator)
DHA	Docosahexaneoic acid
EPA	Eicosapentaenoic acid
FAHP	Fatty acid hydroperoxide
FH	Familial hypercholesterolemia
GLC	Gas-liquid chromatography
HDL, LDL, VLDL	High, low, very low density lipoproteins
HMGCoAR	3-hydroxy 3-methylglutary coenzyme A reductase
HPLC	High performance liquid chromatography
LAHP	Linoleic acid hydroperoxide
LOPS	Lipid oxidation products
MA	Malonaldehyde (malondialdehyde)
MS	Mass spectroscopy
O_2^-	Superoxide anion radical
P/S	Polyunsaturated/saturated ratio
PDGF	Platelet-derived growth factor
PUFAS	Polyunsaturated fatty acids
MI	Myocardial infarction (heart attack)
SC	Serum cholesterol
SEM	Scanning electron microscopy
SOD	Superoxide dismutase
TEM	Transmission electron microscopy
TBARS	Thiobarbituric acid reactive substances
TMS	Trimethyl silyl (derivatives formed with COPS)
WOF	Warmed-over flavor (rancidity occurring after meat is cooked)

[a]Common name.
[b]Systematic name from IUPAC-IUB 1967 revised.

ATHEROSCLEROSIS

Literature on atherosclerosis is dominated by two compeling hypotheses, the "lipid hypothesis" and the "response-to-injury hypothesis." The lipid hypothesis suggests that atherosclerosis is caused by hypercholestero-lemia-induced deposition of lipid in the vessel wall. C plays a pivotal role in the lipid hypothesis, whereas oxidized lipids do not. In contrast, LOPS easily fit into the response-to-injury hypothesis because they may in fact be the injurious agents. Oxidation products may well be more important than C itself as a dietary component. In this review we attempt to establish a link between LOPS and the "injury" hypothesis; however, the ultimate acceptance of the injury hypothesis is not dependent on the acceptance of LOPS as bona fide atherogenic agents.

Both hypotheses have received a great deal of experimental support over the past 70 years, and a current view of atherosclerosis must include the key elements of both (Moore, 1985). The strength of the response-to-injury hypothesis lies in its ability to explain phase 1, especially the in-jurious initiation step, as well as subsequent changes which are conducive to preparing the artery to accept large quantities of lipid and to deposit plaque. The "injury" hypothesis also does well with respect to explaining pathological details of phase 2. The lipid hypothesis offers excellent elu-cidation of the well-established relationship between high SC and ac-celerated atherosclerosis.

Lipid Hypothesis

Early support for the lipid hypothesis came from the publication by Anitschow (1913) of his studies of feeding C dissolved in vegetable oil to rabbits. The observation of a high frequency of atherosclerotic lesions in cholesterol-fed rabbits compared to controls led to the "obvious" conclu-sion that C was atherogenic. Anitschow's early research has been "corro-borated" countless times. Later researchers began to measure SC and found extremely high values in C-fed rabbits. These results and direct studies in humans challenged with high levels of dietary fat and C strengthened the lipid hypothesis. The impossibility of reviewing the vast CHD literature is obvious; therefore, only two other "rabbit" studies will be reviewed, which support the lipid hypothesis.

Duff et al. (1957) employed, as a C diet, 93 g of rabbit food coated with 6 g corn oil and 1 g powdered C. Control rabbits received food coated with corn oil without C. Atherosclerotic lesions were seen as early as 16 hr after commencement of C feeding, but this response varied greatly among rabbits. Some rabbits resisted lesion development after 30 days on the C diet. The study relied heavily on sudanophilic staining to discern patterns of lesion development.

A different approach was used by Langner and Bement (1985), who fed rabbits a 2% C diet for 90 days, sacrificed nine animals and fed the remaining seven a low C diet for 7 months to determine whether lesion regression occurred. The C diet was prepared by dissolving C in chloroform, absorbing it onto feed and allowing it to air dry. SC varied from 30 mg/100 mL in control rabbits to 2624 mg/100 mL in C-fed rabbits, and, as expected, lesions were more numerous in C-fed animals. Lesion regression was found not to occur in spite of the lengthy time on the control diet.

It is not particularly difficult to see how the popularity of the lipid hypothesis came about. Simply feed large doses of C to rabbits and permit hypercholesterolemia to induce sudanophilic lesions in the artery. It mattered little to researchers whether C was angiotoxic or hypercholesterolemic (or both). Dietary C had become inextricably linked to atherosclerosis.

However, not all researchers accept the lipid hypothesis in its entirety, in particular the central role played by C and also the applicability of the results of rabbit-feeding studies to humans. Neither Duff et al. (1957) nor Langner and Bement (1985) nor any other studies we are aware of, except that of Higley et al (1986) to be reviewed later, were concerned with the issue of purity of C and its stability during the experiment. In fact, both reports included descriptions of feed preparation which practically assured the existence of significant levels of COPS, a procedure which is typical. Taylor et al. (1979) were among the first laboratories to call for a reinterpretation of C feeding studies based on findings by them and other groups that: (1)USP-grade C was commonly contaminated with COPS; (2) storage of C in the typical manner caused further COPS formation; (3) C freed of COPS was not atherogenic or angiotoxic in spite of being able to induce hypercholesterolemia; and (4) each individual COP and COPS mixture were angiotoxic and atherogenic. These findings have stimulated a great deal of interest and several pertinent reviews are recommended to the reader: Smith (1981); Addis et al. (1983); Finocchiaro and Richardson (1983); Addis (1986); and Smith (1987). The prevailing opinion is that COPS have one or more of the following biological activities (with C exhibiting minimal activity or a complete absence of the stated activity): atherogenicity, angiotoxicity, cytotoxicity, mutagenicity, and inhibition of a number of enzymes, most notably HMGCoAR. The angiotoxic and cytotoxic properties of COPS could explain their role as initiators of atherosclerotic lesions if the "injury" hypothesis is accepted. Endothelial cell damage could set into motion the complex series of pathological changes leading ultimately to plaque, wall thickening, and lumen narrowing.

The reader should consult the reviews cited in the foregoing paragraph to access the early articles related to the COPS–atherosclerosis connection. Several recent studies have provided further support to the concept that COPS are initiators of atherosclerosis, whereas C is involved only in plaque deposition (phase 2). Earlier research had indicated that of all COPS, 25-OH and triol were the most atherogenic. Peng et al. (1985a) noted similar patterns in a study of the effects of COPS on the uptake of C by ASMCS incubated in a various COPS/C media. Triol at 100 μg/mL reduced uptake of C to 10% of control values. Also, α-epoxide and 25-OH reduced C uptake by up to 60%. The 7-oxy derivatives were less potent but displayed significant inhibition. COPS also inhibited C synthesis by ASMCS. These results emphasize the important role that C has in the health of cells. Thus, the angiotoxic effects of COPS could be in part due to their ability to render cells "C-starved" by a combination of inhibiting C uptake from exogenous sources and inhibiting cellular biosynthesis of C.

To better visualize the cytotoxic effects at the cellular level, a SEM study was conducted by Peng et al (1985a). Triol and 25-OH were given intravenously at 2.5 mg/kg body weight to male New Zealand rabbits. Compared to control rabbits (injected with vehicle only), SEM revealed luminal surface lesions resembling balloon-like protrusions and crater-like defects in treated rabbits after only 24 hours. This study is illustrative of the acute response of the artery to COPS and emphasizes their "initiation" role in atherosclerosis. Peng et al. (1985a) also noted areas of desquamated endothelium and numerous platelets, erythrocytes, and leukocytes adhering to the areas of endothelial injury. Such endothelial alterations are entirely consistent with the earliest signs of atherosclerosis (Ross, 1986) to be discussed later.

If dietary COPS are to be considered as bona fide risk factors for atherosclerosis, it must be shown that COPS are absorbed, distributed, and assimilated via lipoproteins in humans. The authors are unaware of good, quantitative studies in humans on COPS absorption. In the rabbit, Peng et al. (1987) have demonstrated the rapid absorption of COPS. The distribution of absorbed COPS was interesting and perhaps significant in that HDL displayed little affinity for COPS, whereas LDL and VLDL displayed high affinity for 25-OH. Triol and the 7-oxy derivatives were more selectively transported in VLDL. The findings were consistent with earlier research on squirrel monkeys (Peng et al., 1982).

Primarily because it is exquisitely sensitive to dietary C and the development of atherosclerosis, the rabbit is popular as a model for human CHD. In this case, popularity does not equate to appropriateness. Therefore, the search is ongoing to find more appropriate but still relatively inexpensive models. Matthias et al. (1987) employed rats, a species resistant to both atherosclerosis and arteriosclerosis. Male Wistar rats (n = 86) were used in a series of experiments in which triol and C were administered via a gastric tube in 0.75 mL olive oil. The authors induced hypertension by subcutaneous injection of angiotension II. Variations were made in dosage, frequency of application, and duration. Triol consistently produced cellular damage to aortic endothelial and ASMCS. C administered at the same levels did not elicit cytotoxic effects. Simultaneous administration of C plus triol showed no potentiation effect, but angiotension II, by inducing hypertension, exacerbated the atherogenesis seen in the medial layer of the artery (Matthias et al., 1987).

The White Carneau pigeon is another model for atherosclerosis deemed appropriate by some researchers and has been the subject of "low-level" triol-feeding studies by Jacobson et al. (1985). Either 0.05% pure C or 0.05% pure C plus "traces" of triol (0.3% of C or 0.16 mg triol plus 51.9 mg C per mL olive oil) was given by gavage. No differences were seen between treated and control pigeons for aortic total C and C ester, but triol-treated birds displayed 42% greater aortic calcium accumulation (P < 0.02) and 87% greater lumenal stenosis (P < 0.01) than control birds. Jacobson et al. (1985) claimed that their triol levels were representative of the ADI, but such data have not yet been collected (Addis, 1986). Nevertheless, Jacobson et al. (1985) deserve commendation for using a C level which was far closer to the human ADI than do most researchers and also showing similar restraint in the triol levels they employed.

Cultured porcine vascular endothelial cells were used by Hennig and Boissonneault (1987) to compare the influence on barrier function of C and triol. C had no effect on albumin transfer, but exposure to 20 µM triol resulted in maximum albumin transfer. Triol induced albumin transfer in as few as 2 hr, but 24 hr produced vivid morphological alterations in the endothelium (Henning and Boissonneault, 1987).

Solid epidemiological data are needed to better elucidate the possible role of COPS vis-a-vis C in human atherosclerosis. Unfortunately, epidemiological evidence is practically nil because of limited reliable data on COPS in foodstuffs, in turn the result of inadequate methodology (Addis, 1986). One modest population study has been published, however, which provided an interesting finding possibly related to human CHD. Jacobson (1987) noted that Indian immigrants to London and Trinidad experience a 1.5- to 2.0-fold higher rate of MI, which cannot be adequately explained by risk factors associated with these two populations (Miller et al., 1988). Neither group consumes much saturated fat and C, nor are they heavy users of tobacco or experience hypertension and SC (and LDL) at abnormally high levels. However, both populations frequently employ a clarified butter-oil product, "ghee," in cooking. Ghee is stored up to several months at ambient temperature and exposed to light at least part of the time. Jacobson (1987) noted substantial quantities of COPS (12.3% of sterols) in ghee. Fresh butter COPS could not be detected by the same methods. The author concluded that COPS could provide a logical explanation for the high rates of CHD observed. Unfortunately, none of the COPS HPLC peaks were confirmed by MS, but it does seem to be safe to assume that some COPS are present in ghee subject to lengthy storage. The results of the study by Jacobson (1987) are intriguing, but far more research on levels of COPS in commonly consumed foodstuffs will be required to permit adequate epidemiological research to be conducted.

The studies of COPS raise significant questions about the validity of the lipid hypothesis as well as the importance of pure dietary C in human CHD. In recent years there has developed a parallel line of evidence against the lipid hypothesis. Several studies of FAHPS and either atherogenesis in rabbits or factors related to CHD in humans have been conducted by Yagi and coworkers. Yagi's findings were reviewed recently by Addis (1986), who noted that by using the TBARS assay it was found that serum lipid peroxide levels increased with age, the development of diabetes, and diabetes-induced angiopathy. A series of studies on atherogenic effects in the rabbit by Yagi and colleagues suggested a possible role for LAHP as an inducer of atherosclerosis in a manner somewhat analogous to COPS. Intravenous adminstration of LAHP produced lesions which are very similar to those seen during early-stage athersclerosis.

Sasaguri et al. (1984) provided TEM evidence that cultured human endothelial cells were damaged after only 3 hr exposure to 1.0 nmol/mL LAHP. Nishigaki et al. (1984) were able to accelerate LDL uptake by cultured ASMCS by 3–6 nmol/mL LAHP, suggesting that like COPS, FAHPS can promote plaque accumulation as well as be an initiator of atherosclerosis. Yagi et al. (1987) reported that both ASMCS and macrophages are stimulated to form lipid-laden cells by LAHP and LDL. Studies on humans consuming thermally oxidized soya bean oil (compared to fresh oil) demonstrated an elevation of lipid peroxides in chylomicrons (Naruszewicz et al., 1987). Administration of the peroxide-rich chylomicrons to mice resulted in more rapid uptake by macrophages than chylomicrons obtained from humans after ingestion of fresh oil (which resulted in no elevation of chylomicron peroxides). Yagi et al. (1981) noted the rapid assimulation into aortal tissue of LAHP injected via ear vein into rabbits and damage to intima. Linoleate or secondary degradation products of LAHP have little or no effect on endothelium or thoracic aorta. However, LAHP causes marked damage to endothelial cells, including holes in many cells and denucleation of some. Subendothelial fibrous tissue was exposed in some areas (Yagi, 1980). LAHP also inhibits prostacyclin synthesis by the artery, promoting atherosclerosis (Sasaguri et al., 1985). In three reviews (Yagi, 1986; 1987; 1988) Yagi clearly stated the opinion that serum lipid peroxides, whether from dietary or in vivo sources, are important in the pathogenesis of atherosclerosis. An interesting study in the rabbit (Thiery and Seidel, 1987) appears to support this contention. In their study, fish oil actually enhanced C-induced atherosclerosis and elevated serum peroxides. It was not determined whether the fish oil contained peroxides or accelerated in vivo oxidation but the unusual finding of fish oils apparently accelerating, rather than inhibiting, atherosclerosis stresses the importance of understanding the role of LOPS in this disease.

Research reviewed on both COPS and FAHPS provide a compelling amount of evidence that these angiotoxic chemicals can both initiate and promote atherosclerosis. It is vital that carefully controlled absorption and lipoprotein distribution studies be done on human subjects with small quantities of FAHPS and COPS. This appears to be the missing link in an otherwise complete scenario implicating COPS and FAHP in atherogenesis.

Scientific literature suggests that COPS (and FAHPS) are far more atherogenic than C itself. However, not all researchers who have compared COPS with C agreed that COPS are atherogenic. Higley et al. (1986) studied the comparative atherogenic effects of COPS and C in rabbits and stimulated a great deal of controversy by publishing results contradicting most other reports. Therefore, a detailed inquiry seems appropriate. Three treatments were used to study subchronic effects of feeding C, COPS, or a mixture of COPS and C. To prepare COPS, C was dissolved in toluene and refluxed under a stream of dry air at 110°C for 64 hr. Research on C. autoxidation predicts a poor yield of triol and 25-OH by this technique with a rich yield of 7-oxy COPS and epoxides (Smith, 1981), and the analysis by HPLC of the three feeds confirmed this fact. Precautions were taken to prevent further oxidation of lipids in the feed during storage. The feed was prepared by mixing the ration with the C and/or COPS mixture dissolved in heated corn oil in a food processor. Feed was prepared weekly and packaged in daily allotments in plastic pouches sealed under nitrogen. Pouches were stored in anaerobic jars under nitrogen at −15°C. To our knowledge, no other researchers have employed such careful techniques to prevent oxidation during storage. The results of HPLC analysis indicated that the pure C in the feed exceeded 99.9% purity with respect to other sterol compounds. The COPS group contained only 0.06% C. The mixed group was somewhat intermediate in most of the compounds present.

The key findings concerning arterial lesion quantification may be summarized as follows (Higley et al., 1986): The control group of four animals had the fewest gross and histochemically detected lesions. The severity of the lesions was also the least in this group. What was unusual about the study was the finding of the greatest number of gross and histochemical lesions and the most severe (grade C) lesions in the C group and the finding that COPS caused the least number of gross lesions and also being rated quite low in terms of most severe (C grade) lesions. The COPS rabbits had only one-third as many of these as the C group and only one more than the mixture group. Calcium staining in the arterial lesions was found to be the most prevalent in the C-fed group and the least prevalent in COPS groups.

Higley et al. (1986) interpreted their findings to indicate that C is atherogenic to rabbits and that COPS appear not to be as atherogenic as pure C. The authors concluded that although the total number of lesions was equivalent for the three treated groups, the severity of the atherogenic lesions was clearly greater in the C-fed animals. Higley et al. (1986) claimed the dissimilarity between their results and those of earlier studies was because the earlier studies' COPS preparations containing C (as much as 38%) as well as COPS, confounding the issue. (This was clearly not the case in the study conducted by Jacobsen et al., 1985.) The authors concluded that C appeared to be much more atherogenic to rabbits than COPS or mixtures of C and COPS. They also concluded that the focus of attention should remain on C rather than COPS " in relation to human atherogenesis and dietary factors."

In spite of the fact that the work by Higley et al. (1986) was carefully done in many respects, other workers in the field including us have interpretations of the data which significantly differ from theirs. Higley et al (1986) did not rely upon the use of MS to identify with certainty the chromatographic peaks they measured. Therefore, we cannot be absolutely sure that the chromatographic peaks were identified correctly in all cases (Addis, 1986). Even the use of cochromatography of standards, and perfect amplification of unknown but suspected peaks with such standards, does not rule out misidentification. Also, as the authors themselves point out, "the composition of the COPS mixture may be a critical factor." The COPS mixture used was particularly rich in the epoxides, 7-hydroperoxide of C and the 7-oxy COPS. Studies which have demonstrated the atherogenicity of mixtures of COPS have always included generous amounts of triol and/or 25-OH (Taylor et al. 1979; Addis, 1986), and indeed it is probably safe to say that most researchers recognize triol and 25-OH to the most potent atherogenic forms of COPS known at this time (Peng et al., 1985b). A key statement of Higley et al. (1986) is "although the COPS group had more A-type lesions than the C group, the likelihood of observing smooth muscle cell egration into the intima" is greatest in the C and C/COPS groups. It would appear that in fact the authors measured the well-known effect of diet-induced hypercholesterolemia producing a rapid conversion of A-type lesions to more advanced lesions, a fact which would have been known had they determined serum C. Again, consider the relative roles of C and COPS as articulated in so many earlier studies (Addis, 1986). The prevalent view is that COPS act as initiators of atherosclerosis, not so much as "promoters," a role in which dietary C is clearly involved in the rabbit. Therefore, it is widely recognized that LDL is important in conversion of macrophages and ASMCS into foam cells and that this one of the hallmarks of atherosclerosis (Ross, 1986). However, this could be viewed as the "promotion phase" of atherosclerosis (phase 2), not the initiating phase. Unfortunately, Higley et al. (1986) did not assay plasma C levels. It is widely recognized that COPS exert their atherogenic effects in the absence of elevating SC. In contrast, COPS researchers have been practically unanimous in their agreement that the earlier stages of atherosclerosis were not caused by C from LDL but rather by some sort of injurious (angiotoxic) substance, possibly COPS. The very early stages of atherosclerosis (Ross, 1986) were not studied by Higley et al. (1986), who began histochemical assessment after an 11-wk dietary treatment, too late to detect early changes related to atherogenesis. The very high C levels in the C-group (35 × ADI) ensured rapid maturation of the lesions in that group.

It would appear that Higley et al. (1986) suggest two important things, one of which was agreed upon prior to the publication of this study. The primary role, if any, of dietary COPS in atherosclerosis occurs very *early* in the lesion formation phase. Pure C is important as a factor which converts macrophages and ASMCS into foam cells and therefore furthers the atherosclerosis process which was begun by the earlier injury. It would appear that Higley et al. (1986) missed most of the early angiotoxicity phase as the endothelial layer of the artery was not studied. The other main contribution of this paper would suggest that in the absence of significant quantities of triol and 25-OH, angiotoxicity may be less. These are important possibilities which should be explored further. Another factor which may have been important was the possible existence of FAHPS in the rabbit feed used, although this measurement was not done.

It is obvious that much further research will be required to delineate the potential effects of dietary LOPS as factors stimulating atherosclerosis.

Also obvious is the need to modify the lipid hypothesis to account for the role of COPS vis-à-vis C in atherosclerosis.

Response-to-Injury Hypothesis

An "injury" to the endothelium is the initiating event in atherogenesis, according to the "response-to-injury" hypothesis (Ross, 1986). Although much more research is needed on the agents responsible for endothelial injury, the detailed pathology of early atherosclerosis is yielding answers to careful investigators, and along with the answers comes the improved possibility of favorably altering the course of the disease.

Temporal pathological details have been carefully recorded by Faggiotto et al. (1984) and Faggiotto and Ross (1984). These experiments employed 14 pigtail monkeys (*Macaca nemestrina*), 3 to 5 years of age. Four controls and 10 treated monkeys were fed control and atherogenic diets, respectively (Table 11.2). The composition of the two diets is revealing and illustrates the difficulty involved in attempting to differentiate between C and COPS as the atherogenic factor involved. The atherogenic diet was somewhat higher in total energy content, percentage of energy from fat

TABLE 11.2 Partial Summary of Atherogenic and Control Diets Fed to Monkeys

Characteristic	Atherogenic $n = 10$[a]	Control $n = 4$[a]
Energy, %		
Protein	18	22
Carbohydrate	40	49
Fat	42	29
kcal/100 g diet	450	362
Cholesterol, mg/100 g	500[b]	18
Cholesterol, mg/kcal	1.11	0.05
Dried egg yolk, %	5.2	0.37
Lard, %	12	7
Tallow, %	3	3

[a]Number of animals on each diet. Animals were selected from a population of 70 monkeys; all 14 were shown to be "responders" to a high cholesterol diet.
[b]Cholesterol was supplemented to raise levels to 500 mg/100g.
Source: Modified from Faggiotto et al. (1984).

and much higher in C, lard, and, significantly, dried egg yolks (Table 11.2). The authors of these studies were not attempting to determine the relative atherogenic potency of COPS vs C. However, there can be little doubt that the powdered eggs contributed significant quantities of COPS to the atherogenic diet (Tsai and Hudson, 1984; Missler et al., 1985; Nourooz-Zadeh and Appelqvist, 1987; Sander et al., 1988a,b,c). Faggiotto et al. (1984) measured SC, noting a three- to fivefold higher level in monkeys on the atherogenic diet than controls. Serum COPS were not determined but were undoubtedly higher in treated monkeys (Peng et al., 1982; 1987).

The study by Faggiotto et al. (1984) provides a fascinating account of the step-by-step pathological processes involved in the development of a mature atheromatous plaque as revealed by TEM, SEM, and histochemistry. After only 12 days of hypercholesterolemia, adherence of monocytes to the endothelium was noted. Next, monocytes exhibited a subendothelial migration, accumulated lipid, and became lipid-laden macrophages (foam cells). After 2 months, foam cells were sufficiently numerous to form fatty streaks, which were the likely causes of disturbances seen in the overlying endothelium at that time. The discontinuity in the endothelium leads to accelerated pathological changes, beginning with the attachment of numerous monocytes, continuing with monocytes adding to fatty streaks in the intima, the appearance of lipid-laden ASMCS (2 to 3 months), leading ultimately to endothelial denudation, exposure of foam cells to the circulation, and their egress into the blood.

After 4 months, macrophages and platelets adhere to the denuded artery to form a mural thrombus. Secretion of a potent mitogen or growth factor, either derived from platelets (PDGF) or local cells of the arterial wall (ASMCS or macrophages), stimulates proliferation of ASMCS which, together with their conversion to foam cells (by LDL), leads to arterial (intimal) wall thickening, the hallmark of atherosclerosis (Nilsson, 1986). Wall thickening is also directly proportional to lumen stenosis.

The research of Faggiotto et al. (1984) and Faggiotto and Ross (1984) emphasize the tremendous complexity of the atherosclerotic process. A logical question to address at this point is, why does ASMC proliferation occur in the intima because ASMCS are normally a medial component. The answer may lie in PDGF (Ross, 1986). PDGF is a cationic protein (28,000–32,000 daltons) stored in alpha granules of platelets and exhibiting a high affinity to ASMCS. PDGF is also a chemoattractant, presumably allowing PDGF to bind to sites of endothelial injury and recruit ASMCS from the media into the intima (Ross, 1986). Therein may lie the answer to the curious phenomenon of medial-derived ASMCS ultimately causing intimal thickening.

Combined "Lipid" and "Injury" Hypotheses

Discussions of the relative merits of the "injury" and "lipid" hypotheses have been published recently (Moore, 1985; Nilsson, 1986). Still unclear is the precise role of platelets in the plaque-initiation process, although much evidence suggests that plaques grow by the accretion of thrombus material. Because monocytes appear to participate in the earliest stage, atherogenesis could be viewed as an inflammation rather than a thrombogenic event (Nilsson, 1986).

It should be apparent from the discussion of FAHPS and COPS as well as the "injury" hypothesis that these avenues of research have much to offer each other. The literature includes numerous studies, which suggested that the very first step in atherosclerosis, endothelial injury, could be caused by dietary LOPS (Yagi, 1980; Yagi et al., 1981; Peng et al., 1985a,b; Addis, 1986).

Evidence favoring the lipid hypothesis, though most likely flawed because of COPS contamination of C used in such studies, is nevertheless very strong as it pertains to the postinitiation phase. Moore (1985) concludes, and we concur, that elements of both the "lipid" and "injury" hypotheses are necessary for even a partial explanation of the complex nature of atherosclerosis. Certainly, it would be unwise to discard all elements of the lipid hypothesis should dietary LOPS be proven to play a pivotal role in atherogenesis. Also, even if dietary LOPS are ultimately proven to be unimportant in atherogenesis, it would not detract significantly from the attractiveness of the "injury" hypothesis.

It seems likely that LOPS may play a key role in initiating atherosclerosis by injuring the endothelium or causing an inflammation in it. LOPS may also act to promote atherosclerosis by facilitating the binding of LDL to ASMCS. The role of pure C would appear to be limited to the second phase of atherosclerosis as LDL, using C, stimulates foam cell formation. However, the broader issue of determining the role of dietary C in SC and plaque accumulation, often a confused issue, will be dealt with later.

ROLE OF OXIDIZED LIPIDS

Several possibilities exist for LOPS to become involved in arterial injury and atherosclerosis. The three most obvious sources of LOPS are dietary, in vivo metabolism, and pathological production (i.e., via superoxide anion radical production). The general types of compounds which could be involved in endothelial damage are aldehydes (MA), FAHPS, and COPS. Occurrence in food products of MA and COPS has been reviewed by Addis et al. (1983) and Addis (1986). In vivo production of MA and other aldehydes will be discussed later. We wish to report primarily the most recent data on COPS in this review. Numerous reports exist in which the common occurrence of rancidity in foods (Addis, 1986) assures us that the diet includes plentiful supplies of FAHPS. However, the lack of reliable methodology limits what can be said about specific quantities of FAHPS, including LAHP, reported to be atherogenic by Yagi (1980). Nevertheless, French fries and foods fried in vegetable oils are a large source of FAHPS (Carlson and Tabacchi, 1986) and adverse effects of heated oils are well established (Alexander et al., 1987).

Not all reports on COPS in foods can be accepted because of severe methodological limitations (Addis, 1986). Improved methods developed since 1980 have greatly aided the analysis of COPS in the presence of interfering substances like triglycerides, C, and phospholipids (Addis, 1986). Key considerations include the use of high-resolution procedures (HPLC or GLC), cold rather than hot saponification and the confirmation of all suspected chromatographic peaks by a two-step procedure: (1) co-chromatography with a known COP standard; and (2) MS confirmation (Addis, 1986). Any time an investigator wishes to report that a food contains COPS at significant levels, MS should be done to confirm the findings. Our experience has included instances where cochromatography with a known standard produced a perfect amplification of the chromatographic peak, but MS subsequently did not confirm the identical nature of the COP standard and the suspected COP.

COPS in food products reported in earlier but reliable studies included the following foods: heated tallow, food fried in tallow in fast food restaurants, powdered eggs, and dried liver and brain (Park and Addis, 1985a; 1986a,b). In this report, only those papers published subsequent to Addis (1986) will be reviewed. We will largely ignore FAHPS and MA and other aldehydes for reasons stated earlier but with the understanding that they are ubiquitous in our food supply (Addis et al., 1983; Csallany et al., 1984; Addis, 1986).

COPS in Foods: Recent Findings

Park and Addis (1987) investigated the occurrence of COPS in broiled beef steaks and precooked beef and turkey products. Broiling longissimus muscle steaks to internal temperatures of 60 and 80°C produced small quantities of what was suspected to be, based on retention times, 7α-OH and 7-keto, two COPS of very low atherogenic potential. Because of the low levels of the suspected COPS, confirmation by GC-MS was not attempted. Our opinion is that freshly broiled steak probably possesses very little if any atherogenic potential from COPS.

Park and Addis (1987) also studied the role of WOF lipid oxidation on COPS levels in meat which was comminuted, cooked, and stored at 4°C. Beef and turkey were compared. WOF was followed by TBARS analysis (Rethwill et al., 1981), which, along with COPS, was determined at 0, 3, and 8 days after cooking. The C-7 COPS and α- and β-epoxide were noted at 3 and 8 days (confirmed by GC-MS), whereas TBARS were detected at 0 days and increased thereafter. COPS (total) increased with increasing TBARS but not in a linear fashion. 7-Keto was the predominant COP formed, with 7α, 7β, and the epoxides following in decreasing order. WOF involves oxidation of phospholipids and triglycerides, but the highly polyunsaturated phospholipids appear to be most closely involved (Pearson et al., 1977). Park and Addis (1987) suggested that as WOF autoxidation of phospholipids proceeds, the C component of phospholipid-rich muscle membranes may be attacked by free radicals produced. Consistent with this idea is the fact that turkey developed higher of both COPS and TBARS than beef and has higher levels of polyunsaturated membrane lipids (Allen and Foegeding, 1981). These results are not definitive and much more research is needed in the area of WOF and potentially atherogenic LOPS. Consider, for example, FAHPS levels in such products. Because of the increasing popularity of convenience products containing precooked meat, a high priority should be given to this area of research. Such efforts will also yield numerous benefits with respect to quality and nutrient content of convenience products because both of these important characteristics are adversely affected by lipid oxidation.

Eggs and egg products have been targeted by the medical profession for some time, primarily due to the high yolk C content and the mistaken perception that yolk lipids are highly saturated. Ironically, a desirable characteristic of yolk—a relatively high P/S ratio—is an undesirable characteristic with regard to the potential for C oxidation in processed eggs and, along with the high iron and C contents of yolk, may explain the proclivity of spray-dried eggs to develop significant COPS levels.

Morgan and Armstrong (1987) determined the α- and β-epoxide content of eggs as a function of operating parameters, proxidants, and antioxidants. Lack of MS confirmation and the limitation of the results to the epoxides limit the usefulness of their data, but significant were the findings that direct heating plus H_2O_2 addition to the eggs were required to oxidize C during drying (H_2O_2 is used in the removal of sugar prior to drying). Higher outlet temperatures were reported to generate higher epoxide levels (Morgan and Armstrong, 1987), in agreement with Tsai and Hudson (1985).

BHA, BHT, and PG were added to liquid yolk prior to drying. All three were effective at reducing but not eliminating epoxides (Morgan and Armstrong, 1987). Epoxides increased greatly during storage in H_2O_2-treated spray-dried yolk, even with 87 ppm BHT present. The control treatment (absence of H_2O_2) showed essentially no increase from 0 to 4 months. Sander et al., (1988a) noted that α- and β-epoxide levels in nine powdered egg products reached levels as high as 111 and 46 ppm, respectively. Little if any triol and 25-OH could be detected.

The results of much more research would suggest that powdered eggs represent one of the most concentrated sources of COPS in the human diet (Tsai and Hudson, 1985; Missler et al., 1985; Naber and Biggert, 1985; Sander et al., 1988a). The toxicological significance, if any, is unknown; we don't even know that powdered egg COPS are absorbed by humans. Obviously, studies on toxicology of dietary powdered eggs in laboratory animals and absorption studies in humans are urgently needed.

Much more significant than powdered eggs, in terms of human consumption, are fresh or freshly cooked eggs and products derived from them; yet, no research employing modern methodology on COPS content of fresh eggs had been reported prior to 1987. Nourooz-Zadeh and Appelqvist (1987), employing a modification of the TMS-derivatization capillary GLC method of Park and Addis (1985b), were unable to detect COPS in fresh eggs (0.2 ppm detection limit). COPS were noted in spray-dried egg yolk, however, reaching 12 ppm in some samples.

A more complete study of the fresh egg has been completed by Perren et al. (1989), who, in contrast to Nourooz-Zadeh and Appelqvist (1987), reported fairly consistent and moderate levels of COPS in fresh eggs. The authors also noted that refrigerated eggs developed increasingly higher levels up to 4 wk storage followed by, surprisingly, a decline in COPS levels! Because of the recent trend to hard-cook eggs and sell them through vending machines, a procedure involving possibly a 4-wk shelf-life, the results of Perren et al. (1989) need further verification and study.

Dairy products, containing variable but significant C levels and a highly saturated fat, have been implicated in CHD. Interestingly, from the standpoint of C oxidation, dairy products would appear to be more favorably situated than eggs, with little PUFA, frequently low C levels and low contents of iron and, usually, low levels of other prooxidants. However, spray-dried dairy products experience conditions similar to powdered eggs and, therefore, may experience C oxidation. Nourooz-Zadeh and Appelqvist (1988) assayed cream-, whole milk-, and skim milk-powders and noted that "high heat" conditions produced very low levels of COPS. Storage (11 to 37 months) increased COPS to substantially higher levels, reaching as high as 77.9 ppm total COPS in one sample stored 34 months, including 2.5 ppm triol and 0.6 ppm 25-OH.

Very recent studies by Sander et al. (1988a) have reported COPS levels in a wide variety of foods including dairy products. The capillary GLC technique developed by us (Park and Addis, 1985b) was employed in these studies. Fresh dairy products, including sour cream, butter, cottage cheese, evaporated milk, ice cream, yogurt, and whole milk, displayed few if any COPS, and if they did the levels were very low. A cream cheese showed 9 ppm α-epoxide and 3 ppm 7-keto, both confirmed with MS, but no other peaks.

Sander et al. (1988b) studied effects of processing stage and storage condition on COPS levels in fresh butter and cheddar cheese. For both products, only a few COPS were noted and those were at very low levels. Processing and storage appeared to have no effect on levels of COPS seen, even after storage of 6 months for butter and 7 months for cheddar. However, adverse storage conditions, such as exposing cheddar to light or holding butter oil at 110°C, resulted in large increases in COPS levels (Sander et al., 1988c). Sander et al. (1988a) found that dehydrated chicken, turkey, and beef displayed 0 to 43 ppm, and powdered cheeses contained 0 to 17 ppm total COPS.

The foregoing studies clearly document the relatively frequent occurrence of COPS in our food supply. Although COPS are fairly common, the quantities of triol and 25-OH would appear to be small, and much of our C-containing foods are free of COPS (Park and Addis, 1985a; 1987; Sander et al., 1988b). However, on this specific point, much more research is needed. The 7-oxy COPS are fairly commonly seen and, although they may be only weakly atherogenic, other types of cytotoxic properties could be possessed by the 7-oxy compounds (Higley and Taylor, 1984). The two remaining COPS, the epoxides, are more highly atherogenic than the 7-oxy COPS but far less so than triol or 25-OH (Smith and Johnson, 1988). However, the epoxides are also weakly mutagenic (Sevanian and Peterson, 1986) and conceivably could be hydrolyzed to triol (Smith and Johnson, 1988).

To effectively evaluate the atherogenic potential of LOPS will require a tremendous effort at a high cost but we believe that the research must be done. As stated earlier, human absorption studies must be promptly done. If absorption is seen, a series of toxicology studies should be conducted. One approach would be to feed to rabbits human foods with realistic levels of fat, C, and LOPS present. An approach somewhat similar to that taken by Higley et al. (1986) could be done except that COPS and FAHPS would be produced by food lipid autoxidation and atherogenesis would be monitored starting at a very early stage. Under these conditions, negative findings would strongly suggest that LOPS do not initiate atherosclerosis in humans because the rabbit is a very susceptible animal with regard to atherosclerosis.

If positive results are seen in the rabbit, similar work could be conducted on monkeys and pigs, animals with physiologies similar to that of the human.

At the same time, much emphasis must be placed on prevention of lipid autooxidation in foods (Addis, 1986).

In vivo Oxidation and Modified LDL

If we were certain that dietary COPS and FAHPS played no role in atherosclerosis, that they are not absorbed, there would remain the interesting findings of these compounds in human serum lipoproteins. Gray et al. (1971) reported high levels (3250 µg/100 mL serum) of α-epoxide in hypercholesterolemics and much lower levels in controls. Recently, the senior author's laboratory has developed methodology to quantify several COPS in the plasma lipoproteins of humans and have noted in some samples relatively high levels of COPS (Emanuel et al., 1988). Earlier, Yagi's work on lipid peroxides in lipoproteins was reviewed by Addis (1986). The significance and the sources of these highly active compounds are uncertain at this time but will undoubtedly be the subject of much future research. One potentially very important area where LOPS may be affecting atherosclerosis is through oxidized LDL or "m-LDL." An excellent review of m-LDL has been published (Jurgens et al., 1987).

It is extremely well established that LDL plays a pivotal role in atherosclerosis, primarily by promoting the accumulation of lipid in the lesion. ASMCS and macrophages bind LDL via the LDL receptor and internalize it by endocytosis. Foam cells are lipid-laden cells derived from macrophages and ASMCS but the macrophages don't recognize specific native LDL. However, m-LDL is internalized by macrophages via receptor-mediated pathways. Chait et al. (1980) showed that PDGF stimulates increased availability of LDL receptors on ASMCS. Henriksen et al. (1981) demonstrated the modification of human LDL with cultured rabbit endothelial cells, noting a distinct increase in density of "m-LDL" and a three- to fourfold increase in uptake and degradation of m-LDL by murine macrophages. It appears that a scavenger receptor is involved which recognizes only the m-LDL. The same authors (1983) showed the production of m-LDL by human endothelial cells. Therefore, m-LDL may be an important participant in atherosclerosis.

Excellent evidence exists that lipid oxidation by endothelial cells and ASMCS is responsible for LDL modification (Morel et al., 1983; Esterbauer et al., 1987). Chait et al. (1986) showed that superoxide radical anion (O_2^-) was able to modify LDL. Modification involves increases in both lipid TBARS and electrophoretic mobility (Table 11.3), the latter effect caused by aldehydic reactions with basic groups on the protein, promoting a more intense net negative charge. LDL modification was inhibited by SOD, BHT, and DFO, in all three cases suggesting a free radical mechanism for LDL modification (Table 11.4). Hiramatsu et al., (1987) confirmed the findings of Chait et al. (1986) and demonstrated that optimal LDL oxidation required mononuclear cells present in addition to O_2^-. Hiramatsu et al. (1987) also suggested two mechanisms whereby m-LDL could promote atherosclerosis-cytotoxicity of m-LDL and its facilitated uptake via the scavenger receptor.

Evidence for the cytotoxicity of m-LDL has been reported by Chan and Pollard (1981), Hessler et al. (1983), and Bernheimer et al. (1987). Evidence for the increased uptake of m-LDL, in addition to the studies cited earlier, include the research of Quinn et al. (1987) and Mazzone et al. (1987). Parthasarathy et al. (1987) proved that recognition of m-LDL by the receptor is based on nonlipid portions of the molecule. The possible pathophysiological role of O_2^- in m-LDL formation includes the fact that activation of monocytes involves the production of O_2^- and the fact that Chait et al. (1986) demonstrated that ASMCS have similar capabilities.

TABLE 11.3 Cellular Modification of LDL by ASMCS and Mononuclear Cells

Cells		TBARS	Electrophoretic mobility
		LDL modification	
ASMCS	−Fe	1.0	1.1
	+Fe	30.5	3.6
Mononuclear	−Fe	0.6	1.0
	+Fe	52.3	4.4

Source: Modified from Chait et al. (1986).

TABLE 11.4 Inhibition of LDL Modification by Free Radical Inhibitors

Inhibitor	Inhibition of TBARS (%)	
	ASMCS	Mononuclear
SOD	94	87
BHT	99	100
DFO	100	74

Source: Modified from Chait et al. (1986).

LIPOPROTEINS AND DIET

Native molecules such as LDL and HDL are recognized to be extremely important in atherosclerosis. The foregoing discussion emphasizes the role of LDL in the plaque phase (phase 2). Diet is an important determinant of LDL and HDL levels. Although the primary focus of this review has been phase 1—initiation of atherosclerosis—a major part of the available CHD literature has been on dietary effects on SC and LDL. Indeed, this is a critical aspect, if not the most critical aspect, of CHD. However, we have attempted to challenge the reader to consider more thoroughly the possible opportunities to influence CHD prevalence by considering phase 1 (and even phase 3), subjects which in our opinion are not usually given adequate attention. Because CHD obviously depends on all three phases, and because some truly revolutionary findings are occurring in phases 2 and 3, a brief update on both hypercholesterolemia and thrombosis/spasm will be presented.

Hypercholesterolemia: FH and Diet-Related

FH, characterized by elevated SC and early MI, is an autosomal dominant trait. Two clinical forms exist: the more severe homozygous and less severe heterozygous. Brown and Goldstein (1986), in an excellent review, outlined the important research leading to their dramatic discovery of LDL receptors and the finding that a lack of liver LDL receptors, and the inability to clear LDL from the circulation, results in homozygous FH. Heterozygous FH results from a reduction in the number of receptors.

Evidence is presented by Brown and Goldstein (1986) that a high saturated fat diet in the normal population represses receptor synthesis and reduces clearing of LDL. Foam cell production would be facilitated under such conditions. The LDL receptor findings explain the well-known effect of increasing SC as dietary saturated fat increases. However, recently some exciting new concepts have developed which are likely to alter some traditional ideas on diet and SC. These results will be reviewed briefly, and the reader is urged to consult the original references.

In terms of SC, long-held theories included the concepts that dietary saturated, monounsaturated, and polyunsaturated fats had the following effects: elevate, no effect, and lower. However, Mattson and Grundy (1985) reported that a monounsaturated fatty acid (oleic) was as effective as polyunsaturated (linoleic) in lowering SC and LDL in normotriglyceridemic patients. Subsequently, Grundy (1986) compared a high monounsaturated and a low fat (high carbohydrate) diet to one high in saturated fat. Again, SC and LDL were lowered by monounsaturates at least as effectively as the low fat diet. These results suggest that high monounsaturated fat diets be used more extensively in the management of hypercholesterolemia because of several advantages over vegetable oil polyunsaturates including: (1) much slower rate of oxidation; (2) less thrombogenesis and/or spasm (compared to linoleate); and (3) less tendency to reduce HDL. Also, compared to a low fat, high carbohydrate diet, monounsaturates do not raise serum triglycerides and probably result in greater palatability for the patient (Grundy, 1986).

Although there is general agreement that saturated fat raises SC and LDL, very recent research demonstrates that saturated fats are heterogeneous with respect to their effects on SC. Bonanome and Grundy (1988) noted that stearic acid actually lowered SC in men and did so equivalent to or slightly more extensively than oleic acid. Interestingly, both stearate and oleate are major fatty acids in beef and beef fat.

Dietary Cholesterol

Also in a rapid state of change, and equally controversial, are recommendations concerning dietary C. Naturally, the following remarks will be brief and refer only to native C; our earlier-stated concerns about dietary COPS are clear enough! Consulting the original literature will be important in gaining a complete understanding of this complex area.

Does dietary C raise SC? Is dietary C related to CHD? The answer to the second question, by Oliver (1981), appears to be, probably not, because according to him the epidemiological evidence for a dietary C–CHD relationship "is weak." The first question is extremely controversial. At very high levels of C intake (>1000 mg per day) most individuals respond by increasing SC because a "nonphysiological" dose overburdens the three compensation mechanisms: decreased synthesis and absorption of C and increased excretion via bile salt synthesis. At more reasonable intakes (500 mg) or even at comparisons of 250 vs 800, most individuals compensate for increased dietary C by decreasing absorption and synthesis and increasing excretion, thereby maintaining homeostasis of SC (McNamara, 1987; McNamara et al., 1987). However, in approximately 33% of the population, homeostasis is not maintained and SC rises. Such individuals are called "responders" because they respond to dietary C. Although many responders are moderate in degree of response, prompting much debate, some respond markedly and will therefore probably experience an increased risk of CHD. In nonresponders, the result are much different. Ginsberg et al. (1981) noted that no differences occurred for SC, triglycerides, or LDL, or apoprotein B in VLDL and LDL between 150 mg C and 500 mg C/1000 kcal energy intakes.

A recent article by Edington et al. (1987) appears to provide some key answers about dietary C and SC, including responders, and would suggest that by following three commonly prescribed recommendations—lowering saturated (and raising polyunsaturated and/or monounsaturated) fatty acid intakes, decreasing total fat intake, and raising consumption levels for fiber—even "responders" and hyperlipidemics need not be concerned with C intake. A 24-wk trial was conducted using healthy subjects (n = 135; 27 men, 108 women) and hyperlipidemia patients (n = 33; 20 men, 13 women). Reduced fat diets (26% of kcal for patients, 35% for healthy volunteers), including two eggs per week, were employed for the first 8 wk of this study. These low fat diets were continued throughout the 24-wk experiment, but during the last 16 wk, the participants ate either two or seven eggs per week. After 4 wk a small (<1%) but significant increase in SC was noted in the healthy volunteers but not in hyperlipidemics. These differences were not significant for SC and LDL after 8 wk. Edington et al. (1987) concluded that the "responders" phenomenon is a short-term effect and should not form the basis for dietary recommendations and, further, that by following the prudent dietary guidelines outlined earlier, dietary C becomes unimportant as a factor influencing SC.

Dietary guidelines were the subject of an interesting review by Truswell (1987), who noted that of the published guidelines from 14 countries, only the U.S. guidelines refer to dietary C. Given the great confusion that exists among consumers (dietary C and SC, fat and C) and the results of Edington et al. (1987), it may be that omitting recommendations on dietary C may be a good idea. Before this is done it is important to have a better idea of both the levels and toxicity of COPS in foods as well as further efforts to reduce COPS levels in the food supply. The potential damage to blood vessels which can be inflicted by COPS does not depend upon or cause an elevation in SC.

These are important considerations for all food products of animal origin and the industries which produce and process them. Such animal products are largely flexible with respect to fat levels, and many can be redesigned to achieve more favorable balances with respect to fatty acid contents. Protection of lipids from autoxidation is also an attainable goal. However, the removal of C from these products is difficult from a technical standpoint and therefore extremely expensive, and is simply not necessary, especially if oxidation protection can be provided.

THROMBOSIS AND SPASM

Neither arterial injury nor atherosclerosis is able to cause a heart attack. MIs result from either one or both of coronary thrombosis and arterial spasms. Obviously, the more atherosclerotic (occluded) is the lumen, the more likely is the occurrence of severe damage to the heart by thrombosis and/or spasms. And, as was discussed earlier, thrombogenesis is the result of platelet activity in the injured artery. For these reasons, much research interest has surrounded the reports of favorable effects of ω-3 fatty acids on CHD in general and on thrombosis/spasm in particular. The possibility of preventing sudden death or MI in patients with extemsively occluded arteries with dietary ω-3 fatty acids is an intriguing one, for the principal benefit of fish oils appears to be in the area of influencing eicosanoid synthesis, thereby reducing platelet aggregation and arterial spasm.

Recent key references include Glomset (1985); Kromhout et al. (1985); Phillipson et al. (1985); and Lands (1986). At issue is really more than the ω-3 content of the diet but rather the ω-3/ω-6 ratio, and it's interesting to note that in a review Kinsella (1981) cautioned against potential detrimental effects of over consumption of ω-6 PUFAS including tissue peroxidation and upsetting "prostaglandin homeostasis."

Five properties are commonly attributed to fish oil ω-3 fatty acids (EPA, DHA). These include reduced serum triglycerides, platelet aggregation, and arterial spasm—all well accepted—and reduction in blood pressure and SC, not as well accepted. However, the benefits of increases in EPA and DHA (as well as reduced intake of ω-6 oils) may extend to much earlier in CHD pathology than previously recognized. In two excellent reviews, Leaf and Weber (1987, 1988) discussed the substantial evidence that some of the early steps in atherosclerosis may be interrupted by EPA and DHA intakes. These authors list at least eight potential antiatheromatous effects of ω-3 fatty acids. Recalling our earlier discussion of Ross's (1984) description of atherosclerosis, the delaying or interrupting of atherosclerosis is apparently possible by reducing the aggregation of platelets, thereby preventing the effects of PDGF, which acts both as a chemotactic agent and proliferation factor.

Interrupting the activity of platelets in early atherosclerosis as well as preventing thrombogenesis and spasm in late atherosclerosis could conceivably form an effective preventive strategy designed to delay symptomatic CHD. Current research interests in the incorporation of EPA and DHA into foods not normally known to contain them stem primarily from the foregoing considerations.

Many other dietary improvements are possible by altering food ingredients, substituting more acceptable ingredients for less acceptable ones, and literally engineering food with the prevention of CHD and other chronic diseases in mind. Fig. 11.1 illustrates some of the many possible approaches.

CONCLUSIONS

Our primary objective has been to review evidence linking LOPS to atherosclerosis and CHD in a manner which stimulates new avenues of thought and research. We also have provided a brief summary of important recent findings which are challenging the way researchers and clinicians view fats and cholesterol in the human diet. Several conclusions will be developed, including a series of questions.

1.   As it pertains to human atherosclerosis, a great deal of evidence indicates that pure C is neither angiotoxic nor hypercholesterolemic and therefore cannot either initiate or promote atherosclerosis and CHD.

2.   The predominant evidence suggests an important role in initiating atherosclerosis for both dietary COPS and FAHPS and a significant role for FAHPS in promoting atherosclerosis, but absorption studies in humans are urgently needed to eliminate ambiguities.

3.   As a corollary to (1) and (2), future research should focus on protecting food lipids from oxidation, not removing C from food.

4.   Earlier recommendations to the public concerning fat and C intake need extensive revision. C limitations are not necessary and serve only to

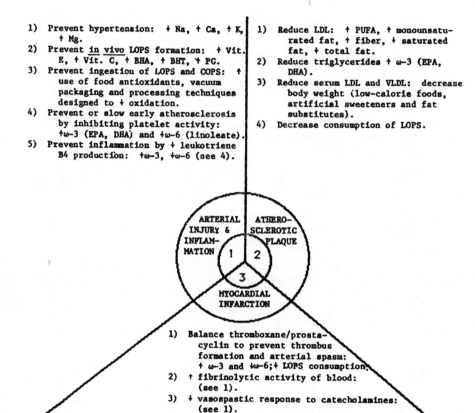

1) Prevent hypertension: + Na, + Ca, + K, + Mg.
2) Prevent <u>in vivo</u> LOPS formation: + Vit. E, + Vit. C, + BHA, + BHT, + PG.
3) Prevent ingestion of LOPS and COPS: + use of food antioxidants, vacuum packaging and processing techniques designed to + oxidation.
4) Prevent or slow early atherosclerosis by inhibiting platelet activity: +ω-3 (EPA, DHA) and +ω-6 (linoleate).
5) Prevent inflammation by + leukotriene B4 production: +ω-3, +ω-6 (see 4).

1) Reduce LDL: + PUFA, + monounsaturated fat, + fiber, + saturated fat, + total fat.
2) Reduce triglycerides + ω-3 (EPA, DHA).
3) Reduce serum LDL and VLDL: decrease body weight (low-calorie foods, artificial sweeteners and fat substitutes).
4) Decrease consumption of LOPS.

ARTERIAL INJURY & INFLAMMATION

ATHEROSCLEROTIC PLAQUE

1 2

3

MYOCARDIAL INFARCTION

1) Balance thromboxane/prostacyclin to prevent thrombus formation and arterial spasm: + ω-3 and +ω-6;+ LOPS consumption.
2) + fibrinolytic activity of blood: (see 1).
3) + vasospastic response to catecholamines: (see 1).
4) If MI occurs, minimize infarct size, acute arrhythmias and sudden death: (see 1).

FIG. 11.1 Speculations on potential dietary interventions for prevention of CHD.

confuse. Recommendations to the public should result in increased intake of ω-3 (linolenate, EPA, DHA) and monosaturated (ω-9) and reduced intake of ω-6 (linoleate). More emphasis should be placed on limiting short chain fatty acid intake. The public should be educated about the possible toxicity of consuming rancid foods and how to recognize rancidity organoleptically.

5. Many opportunities exist to improve foods by engineering them to possess a more favorable lipid and carbohydrate composition, but these efforts must be accompanied by increased vigilance against lipid oxidation.

6. Future research should focus on answering the following questions:

a. What is the cellular mechanism of injury to the endothelium that initiates atherosclerosis?

b. What is the relative importance of dietary vs. in vivo produced LOPS, if any, in atherosclerosis?

c. Is it possible to prevent or significantly delay human arterial endothelial injury by either protecting foods against lipid oxidation or increasing intake of antioxidants?

d. How quickly and efficiently are COPS and FAHPS absorbed into the circulation in humans, and what pattern exists with respect to absorbed LOPS distribution among chylomicrons, VLDL, LDL and HDL?

e. Do α- and β-epoxide experience hyrolysis to triol in the stomach, and, if so, how much triol is absorbed?

f. How effective is soluble fiber in reducing levels of serum LOPS in humans?

g. How atherogenic are LOPS in rabbits and monkeys at realistic intake levels of fat, fiber, C and LOPS?

h. How good is the agreement among the numerous methods used for COPS analysis in foods? Should researchers move toward selecting a single method, using it in all labs and conducting interlaboratory comparisons?

It is obvious that much research needs to be conducted to answer the foregoing questions, but the authors have been encouraged by the increased number of researchers involved in LOPS-atherosclerosis research, the available methodology, and the spirit of excitement and cooperation existing in this field of research.

ACKNOWLEDGEMENTS

Published as contribution No. 15,329 of the series of the Minnesota Agricultural Experiment Station on research conducted under Project 23, supported by funds from Carnation, American Meat Institute, and Southeast Poultry and Egg Association.

REFERENCES

Addis, P. B., Csallany, A. S., and Kindom, S. E. 1983. Some lipid oxidation products as xenobiotics. *Xenobiotics in Foods and Feeds.* (Ed.) Finley, J. W. and Schwass, D. E. ACS Symposium Series, No. 234. p. 85–98. American Chemical Society, Washington, DC.

Addis, P. B. 1986. Occurrence of lipid oxidation products in foods. *Food Chem. Toxic.* 24: 1021.

Alexander, J. C., Valli, V. E., and Chanin, B. E. 1987. Biological observations from feeding heated corn oil and heated peanut oil to rats. *J. Toxicol. Environ. Hlth.* 21: 295.

Allen, C. E. and Foegeding, E. A. 1981. Some lipid characteristics and interactions in muscle foods—a review. *Food Technol.* 35: 253.

Anitschow, N. 1913. Über die Veränderungen der Kaninchenaorta bei experimenteller Cholesterinsteatose. *Beitr. Path. Anat. Allg. Path.* 56: 379.

Bernheimer, A. W., Robinson, W. G., Linder, R., Mullins, D., Yip, Y. K., Cooper, N. S., Seidman, I., and Uwajima, T. 1987. Toxicity of enzymically-oxidized low-density lipoprotein. *Biochem. Biophys. Res. Comm.* 148: 260.

Bonanome, A. and Grundy, S. M. 1988. Effect of dietary stearic acid on plasma cholesterol and lipoprotein levels. *New Engl. J. Med.* 318: 1244.

Brown, M. S. and Goldstein, J. L. 1986. A receptor-mediated pathway for cholesterol homeostasis. *Science* 232: 34.

Carlson, B. L. and Tabacchi, M. H. 1986. Frying oil deterioration and vitamin loss during foodservice operation. *J. Food Sci.* 51: 218.

Chait, A., Ross, R., Albers, J. J., and Bierman, E. L. 1980. Platelet-derived growth factor stimulates activity of low density lipoprotein receptors. *Proc. Natl. Acad. Sci.* 77: 4084.

Chait, A., Heinecke, J. W., Hiramatsu, K., Baker, L., and Rosen, J. 1986. Superoxide-mediated modification of LDL by cells of the arterial wall. *Atherosclerosis* 7: 491.

Chan, S. Y. and Pollard, M. 1981. Characterization of a very-low-density lipoprotein (VLDL)-associated cytotoxic factor. *Brit. J. Cancer.* 44: 410.

Csallany, A. S., Guan, M. D., Manwaring, J. D., and Addis, P. B. 1984. Free malonaldehyde determination in tissues by high-performance liquid chromatography. *Anal. Biochem.* 142: 277.

Duff, G. L., McMillan, G. C., and Ritchie, A. C. 1957. The morphology of early atherosclerotic lesions of the aorta demonstrated by the surface technique in rabbits fed cholesterol. *Am. J. Path.* 33: 845.

Edington, J., Geekie, M., Carter, R., Benfield, L., Fisher, K., Ball, M., and Mann, J. 1987. Effect of dietary cholesterol on plasma cholesterol concentration in subjects following reduced fat, high fibre diet. *Brit. Med. J.* 294: 333.

Emanuel, H. A., Addis, P. B., Bergmann, S. D., and Zavoral, J. H. 1988. Capillary GC quantification of cholesterol oxidation products in human plasma lipoproteints. *Free Rad. Biol. Med.* (In press.)

Esterbauer, H., Jurgens, G., Quehenberger, O., and Koller, E. 1987. Autoxidation of human low density lipoprotein: Loss of polyunsaturated fatty acids and vitamin E and generation of aldehydes. *J. Lipid Res.* 28: 495.

Faggiotto, A., Ross, R., and Harker, L. 1984. Studies of hypercholesterolemia in the nonhuman primate: I. Change that lead to fatty streak formation. *Arteriosclerosis* 4: 323.

Faggiotto, A. and Ross, R. 1984. Studies of hypercholesterolemia in the nonhuman primate: II. Fatty streak conversion to fibrous plaque. *Arteriosclerosis* 4: 341.

Finocchiaro, E. T. and Richardson, T. 1983. Sterol oxides in foodstuffs: A review. *J. Food Prot.* 46: 917.

Ginsberg, H., Le, N-A., Mays, C., Gibson, J., and Brown, W. V. 1981. Lipoprotein metabolism in nonresponders to increased dietary cholesterol. *Arteriosclerosis* 1: 463.

Glomset, J. A. 1985. Fish, fatty acids, and human health. *New Engl. J. Med.* 312: 1253.

Gray, M. F., Lawrie, T. D. V., and Brooks, C. J. W. 1971. Isolation and identification of cholesterol α-oxide and other minor sterols in human serum. *Lipids* 6: 836.

Grundy, S. M. 1986. Comparison of monounsaturated fatty acids and carbohydrates for lowering plasma cholesterol. *New Engl. J. Med.* 314: 745.

Hennig, G. and Boissonneault, G. A. 1987. Cholestan-3β, 5α, 6β-triol decreases barrier function of cultured endothelial cell monolayers. *Atherosclerosis* 68: 255.

Henriksen, T., Mahoney, E. M., and Steinberg, D. 1981. Enhanced macrophage degradation of low density lipoprotein previously incubated with cultured endothelial cells: Recognition by receptors for acetylated low density lipoproteins. *Proc. Natl. Acad. Sci. USA* 18: 6499.

Henriksen, T., Mahoney, E. M., and Steinberg, D. 1983. Enhanced macrophage degradation of biologically modified low density lipoprotein. *Arteriosclerosis* 3: 149.

Hessler, J. R., Morel, D. W., Lewis, J., and Chisolm, G. M. 1983. Lipoprotein oxidation and lipoprotein-induced cytotoxicity. *Arteriosclerosis* 3: 215.

Higley, N. A. and Taylor, S. L. 1984. The steatotic and cytotoxic effects of cholesterol oxides in cultured cells. *Food Chem. Toxicol.* 22: 983.

Higley, N. A., Beery, J. T., Taylor, S. L., Porter, J. W., Dziuba, J. A., and Lalich, J. J. 1986. Comparative atherogenic effects of cholesterol and cholesterol oxides. *Atherosclerosis* 62: 91.

Hiramatsu, K., Rosen, H., Heinecke, J. W., Wolfbauer, G., and Chait, A. 1987. Superoxide initiates oxidation of low density lipoprotein by human monocytes. *Arteriosclerosis* 7: 55.

Jacobson, M. S. 1987. Cholesterol oxides in Indian ghee: possible cause of unexplained high risk of atherosclerosis in Indian immigrant populations. *Lancet* 2(8560): 656.

Jacobson, M. S., Price, M. G., Shamoo, A. E., and Heald, F. P. 1985. Atherogenesis in White Carneau pigeons: effect of low-level cholestanetriol feeding. *Atherosclerosis* 57: 209.

Jurgens, G., Hoff, H. F., Chisolm, G. M. III, and Esterbauer, H. 1987. Modification of human serum low density lipoprotein by oxidation—characterization and pathophysiological implications. *Chem. Phys. Lipids* 45: 315.

Kinsella, J. E. 1981. Dietary fat and prostaglandins: Possible beneficial relationships between food processing and public health. *Food Technol.* 35: 89.

Kromhout, D., Bosschieter, E. B., and Coulander, C. D. L. 1985. The inverse relationship between fish consumption and 20-year mortality from coronary heart disease. *New Engl. J. Med.* 312: 1205.

Lands, 1986.

Langner, R. O. and Bement, C. L. 1985. Lesion regression and protein synthesis in rabbits after removal of dietary cholesterol. *Arteriosclerosis* 5: 74.

Leaf, A. and Weber, P. C. 1987. A new era for science in nutrition. *Am. J. Clin. Nutr.* 45: 1048.

Leaf, A. and Weber, P. C. 1988. Cardiovascular effects of n-3 fatty acids. *New Engl. J. Med.* 318: 549.

Matthias, D., Becker, C. H., Godicke, W., Schmidt, R., and Ponsold, K. 1987. Action of cholestane-3β, 5α, 6β-triol on rats with particular reference to the aorta. *Atherosclerosis* 63: 115.

Mattson, F. H. and Grundy, S. M. 1985. Comparison of effects of dietary saturated, monounsaturated, and polyunsaturated fatty acids on plasma lipids and lipoproteins in man. *J. Lipid Res.* 26: 194.

Mazzone, T., Lopez, C., and Bergstraesser, L. 1987. Modification of very low density lipoproteins leads to macrophage scavenger receptor uptake and cholesteryl ester deposition. *Arteriosclerosis* 7: 191.

McNamara, D. J. 1987. Effects of fat-modified diets on cholesterol and lipoprotein metabolism. *Ann. Rev. Nutr.* 7: 273.

McNamara, D. J., Kolb, R., Parker, T. S., Samuel, P., Brown, C. D., and Ahrens, E. H., Jr. 1987. Heterogeneity of cholesterol homeostasis in man—response to changes in dietary fat quality and cholesterol quantity. *J. Clin. Invst.* 79: 1729.

Miller, G. J., Kotecha, S., Wilkinson, W. H., Wilkes, H. Stirling, Y., Sanders, T. A. B., Broadhurst, A., Allison, J., and Meade, T. W. 1988. Dietary and other characteristics relevant for coronary heart disease in men of Indian, West Indian and European descent in London. *Atherosclerosis* 70: 63.

Missler, S. R., Wasilchuk, B. A., and Merritt, C., Jr. 1985. Separation and identification of cholesterol oxidation products in dried egg preparations. *J. Food Sci.* 50: 595.

Moore, S. 1985. Pathogenesis of atherosclerosis. *Metabolism* 34: 13.

Morel, D. W., DiCorleto, P. E., and Chisolm, G. M. 1984. Endothelial and smooth muscle cells alter low density lipoprotein in vitro by free radical oxidation. *Arteriosclerosis* 4: 357.

Morgan, J. N. and Armstrong, D. J. 1987. Formation of cholesterol-5,6-epoxides during spray-drying of egg yolk. *J. Food Sci.* 52: 1224.

Naber, E. C. and Biggert, M. D. 1985. Analysis for and generation cholesterol oxidation products in egg yolk by heat treatment. *Poul Sci.* 64: 341.

Naruszewicz, M., Wozny, E., Mirkiewicz, E., Nowicka, G., and Szostak, W.

B. 1987. The effect of thermally oxidized soya bean oil on metabolism of chylomicrons. Increased uptake and degradation of oxidized chylomicrons in cultured mouse macrophages. *Atherosclerosis* 66: 45.

Nilsson, J. 1986. Growth factors and the pathogenesis of atherosclerosis. *Atherosclerosis* 62: 185.

Nishigaki, I., Hagihara, M., Maseki, M., Tomoda, Y., Nagayama, K., Nakashima, T., and Yagi, K. 1984. Effect of linoleic acid hydroperoxide on uptake of low density lipoprotein by cultured smooth muscle cells from rabbit aorta. *Biochem. Intl.* 8: 501.

Nourooz-Zadeh, J. and Appelqvist, L. A. 1987. Cholesterol oxides in Swedish foods and food ingredients: Fresh eggs and egg products. *J. Food Sci.* 52: 57.

Nourooz-Zadeh, J. and Appelqvist, L. A. 1988. Cholesterol oxides in Swedish foods and food ingredients: Milk powder products. *J. Food Sci.* 53: 74.

Oliver, M. F. 1981. Diet and coronary heart disease. *Brti. Med. Bull.* 37: 49.

Park, S. W. and Addis, P. B. 1985a. HPLC determination of C-7 oxidized cholesterol derivatives in foods. *J. Food Sci.* 50: 1437.

Park, S. W. and Addis, P. B. 1985b. Capillary column gas-liquid chromatographic resolution of oxidized cholesterol derivatives. *Anal. Biochem.* 149: 275.

Park, S. W. and Addis, P. B. 1986a. Identification and quantitative estimation of oxidized cholesterol derivatives in heated tallow. *J. Agric. Food Chem.* 34: 653.

Park, S. W. and Addis, P. B. 1986b. Further investigation of oxidized cholesterol derivatives in heated fats. *J. Food Sci.* 51: 1380.

Park, S. W. and Addis, P. B. 1987. Cholesterol oxidation products in some muscle foods. *J. Food Sci.* 52: 1504.

Parthasarathy, S., Fong, L. G., Otero, D., and Steinberg, D. 1987. Recognition of solubilized apoproteins from delipidated, oxidized low density lipoprotein (LDL) by the acetyl-LDL receptor. *Proc. Natl. Acad. Sci.* 84: 537.

Pearson, A. M., Love, J. D., and Shorland, F. B. 1977. Warmed-over flavor in meat, poultry, and fish. *Adv. Food Res.* 23: 2.

Peng, S. K., Taylor, C. B., Huang, W. Y., Hill, J. C., and Mikkelson, B. 1982. Distribution of 25-hydroxycholesterol in plasma lipoproteins and its role in atherogenesis. *Atherosclerosis* 41: 395.

Peng, S. K., Morin, R. J., Tham, P., and Taylor, C. B. 1985a. Effects of oxy-generated derivatives of cholesterol on cholesterol uptake by cultured aortic smooth muscle cells. *Artery* 13: 144.

Peng, S. K., Taylor, C. B., Hill, J. C., and Morin, R. J. 1985b. Cholesterol oxidation derivatives and arterial endothelial damage. *Atherosclerosis* 54: 121.

Peng, S. K., Phillips, G. A., Guang-Zhi, X., and Morin, R. J. 1987. Transport of cholesterol autoxidation products in rabbit lipoproteins. *Atherosclerosis* 64: 1.

Perren et al. 1989.

Phillipson, B. E., Rothrock, D. W., Connor, W. E., Harris, W. S., and Illingworth, D. R. 1985. Reduction of plasma lipids, lipoproteins, and apoproteins by dietary fish oils in patients with hypertriglyceridemia. *New Engl. J. Med.* 312: 1210.

Quinn, M. T., Parthasarathy, S., Fong L. G., and Steinberg, D. 1987. Oxidatively modified low density lipoproteins: A potential role in recruitment and retention of monocyte/macrophages during atherogenesis. *Proc. Natl. Acad. Sci.* 984: 2995.

Rethwill, C. E., Bruin, T. K., Waibel, P. E., and Addis, P. B. 1981. Influence of dietary fat source and vitamin E on market stability of turkeys. *Poul. Sci.* 60: 2466.

Ross, R. 1986. The pathogenesis of atherosclerosis - an update. *New Engl. J. Med.* 314: 488.

Sander, B. D., Addis, P. B., Park, S. W., and Smith, D. E. 1988a. Quantification of cholesterol oxidation products in a variety of foods. *J. Food Prot.* (In press.)

Sander, B. D., Smith, D. E., and Addis, P. B. 1988b. Effects of processing stage and storage conditions on levels of cholesterol oxidation products in butter and cheddar cheese. *J. Dairy Sci.* (In press.)

Sander, B. D., Smith, D. E., Addis, P. B., and Park, S. W. 1988c. Effects of prolonged and adverse storage conditions on levels of cholesterol oxidation products in dairy products. *J. Food Sci.* (In press.)

Sasaguri, Y., Nakashima, T., Morimatsu, M., and Yagi, K. 1984. Injury to cultured endothelial cells from human umbilical vein by linoleic acid hydroperoxide. *J. Appl. Bioch.* 6: 144.

Sasaguri, Y., Morimatsu, M., Nakashima, T., Tokunaga, O., and Yagi, K. 1985. Difference in the inhibitory effect of linoleic acid hydroperoxide on prostacyclin biosynthesis between cultured endothelial cells from human umbilical cord vein and cultured smooth muscle cells from rabbit aorta. *Biochem. Intl.* 11: 517.

Sevanian, A. and Peterson, A. R. 1986. The cytotoxicity and mutagenic properties of cholesterol oxidation products. *Fd. Chem. Toxic.* 24: 1103.

Smith, L. L. 1981. "Cholesterol Autoxidation." Plenum Press. New York and London.

Smith, L. L. 1987. Cholesterol autoxidation. *Chem. Phys. Lipids* 44: 87.

Smith, L. L. and Johnson, B. H. 1987. Biological activities of oxysterols. Free Radical Biol. Med. (In press.)

Steinbrecher, U. P. 1987. Oxidation of human low density lipoprotein results in derivatization of lysine residues of apolipoprotein B by lipid peroxide decomposition products. *J. Biol. Chem.* 262: 3603.

Taylor, C. B., Peng, S. K., Werthessen, N. T., Tham, P., and Lee, K. T. 1979. Spontaneously occurring angiotoxic derivatives of cholesterol. Am. J. Clin. Nutr. 32: 40.

Thiery, J. and Seidel, D. 1987. Fish oil feeding results in an enhancement of cholesterol-induced atherosclerosis in rabbits. Atherosclerosis. 63: 53.

Truswell, A. S. 1987. Evolution of dietary recommendations, goals, and guidelines. *Am. J. Clin. Nutr.* 45: 1060.

Tsai, L. S. and Hudson, C. A. 1984. Cholesterol oxides in commercial dry egg products: Isolation and identification. J. Food Sci, 49: 1245.

Yagi, K. 1980. Toxicity of lipid peroxides in processed foods. Biochem. Rev. 50: 42.

Yagi, K. 1986. A biochemical approach to atherosclerosis. *Trends Biochem. Sci.* 11: 18.

Yagi, K. 1987. Lipid peroxides and human diseases. *Chem. Phys. Lipids* 43: 337.

Yagi, K. 1988. Lipid peroxides in atherosclerosis. *The Role of Oxygen in Chemistry and Biochemistry.* (Ed.) Ando, W. and Moro-oka p. 383–390. Elsevier Science Pub. B.V. Amsterdam.

Yagi, K., Inagaki, T., Sasaguri, Y., Nakano, R., and Nakashima, T. 1987. Formation of lipid-laden cells from cultured aortic smooth muscle cells and macrophages by linoleic acid hydroperoxide and low density lipoprotein. *J. Clin. Biochem. Nutr.* 3: 87.

Yagi, K., Ohkawa, H., Ohishi, N., Yamashita, M., and Nakashima, T. 1981. Lesion of aortic intima caused by intravenous administration of linoleic acid hydroperoxide. *J. Appl. Biochem.* 3: 58.

12

Toxicological and Pharmacological Interactions as Influenced by Diet and Nutrition

Wayne R. Bidlack and John F. Riebow
University of Southern California School of Medicine
Los Angeles, California

INTRODUCTION

The role of nutrition in health has been accepted in both the prevention of disease as well as in the treatment of many disease states. Although malnutrition is still a major problem in other areas of the world, the majority of people in the United States are considered not to be at risk for nutritional deficiency diseases. What this means to the human organism is that nutrients necessary for cell function, growth, and development are present in sufficient amounts to allow the individual to reach their genetic potential.

Each of us is exposed to a variety of xenobiotic agents each day. (The term xenobiotic simply refers to any foreign substance.) Xenobiotics include beneficial compounds such as nutrients or therapeutic agents, non-harmful compounds that may play no biological role, or potentially harmful compounds, such as naturally occurring food chemical components (some of which are toxic) and manmade chemicals including agricultural chemicals (pesticides, herbicides, and fungicide residues) and food additives. Frequently, considerations of xenobiotic exposure are focused solely on accidental intake from food and water contamination, while a much larger portion of the population knowingly expose themselves to clearly identified toxic agents, specifically ethanol and nicotine.

If the xenobiotic is taken as part of a therapeutic regimen to counter a disease or its symptoms, the evaluation of the effect is termed pharmacology. The study of pharmacology is concerned with drug (chemical substances that are of therapeutic value) absorption, distribution, biotransformations, and elimination, physical and chemical properties of drugs including their biochemical and physiological effects, mechanism of drug action, and therapeutic and potential adverse action of drugs.

Evaluation of the toxic effects of xenobiotic exposure is the science of toxicology. Initially, toxicology served as the branch of pharmacology which was concerned with the potential adverse effects of drug action. However, today the field of toxicology has grown into its own specialty area concerned with the potential toxic action of any chemical substance present in the environment upon living organisms. Such toxicants can be naturally occurring substances as well as a variety of chemicals in common use in the chemical, agricultural, and food industries. The principles of toxicology are closely related to the principles of pharmacology.

In recent years, the direct effects of foods and nutrition have been examined in a variety of aspects of pharmacology. The direct effect of food components on drug absorption and utilization has been reviewed, Roe, 1979; Smith and Bidlack, 1984). In addition, the impact of malnutrition on drug therapy and its effect on toxicity has been described (Buchanan, 1984; Krishnaswamy, 1987). These relationships have not been examined experimentally using physiological concentrations of toxicants.

A combined knowledge of both nutrition and toxicology can contribute to a better understanding of individual risk and may provide insight for selective protection against certain toxic agents. The impact of dietary status should be determined for all phases of toxicant handling, including absorption, disposition, metabolism, elimination, and mechanism of toxicity. These interactions are complex and are not completely understood, but should be examined under low dose exposures. Normally, high dose exposure scenerios are used in an effort to observe and study toxicity. Indeed, this model has proven useful to understand the sequel of toxic events that occur in accidental or industrial exposures.

However, a more thorough understanding of just how the body deals with low dose exposures may change the perception of low risk. This knowledge may also provide insight into the dose at which each agent exceeds the efficient handling and clearing mechanisms and initiates toxicity.

Many of these processes have been studied in the clinical situation involving drug therapy. However, the observations made would hold for both therapeutic as well as toxic xenobiotic agents. This chapter will examine many of the factors affecting these processes.

PHYSIOLOGICAL PARAMETERS

Following exposure to a toxicant, the xenobiotic (drug or toxicant) proceeds through one of several absorptive processes. The compound enters the general circulation and becomes bound in part to plasma proteins (Fig. 12.1). The free form of the xenobiotic remains available for further transport into tissues for metabolism and or excretion (Wilkinson, 1984). The accumulation of the agent or its metabolite within the tissues produces the resultant cellular damage identified as toxicity.

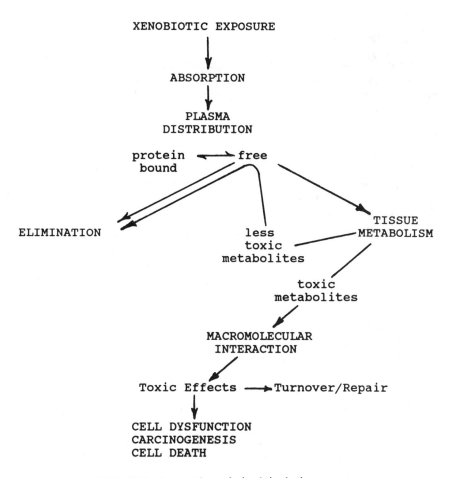

FIG. 12.1 Interaction of physiological parameters.

The intestine, liver, and kidney are the major organs controlling the movement of xenobiotic agents. Transport affects the accumulation of xenobiotics by determining intestinal absorption, liver metabolism, or liver and kidney elimination processes. The majority of drugs and toxicants are lipophilic or amphipathic in their chemical characteristics. As such, several transport mechanisms regulate their entry into the body and into the specific target tissues (Schwenk, 1987). Similar processes regulate the elimination of these agents and their metabolites.

Xenobiotic transport consists of movement across an initial barrier of epithelial cells. In each instance, xenobiotics can move either from the blood into the cells or vice versa. Although transport may vary for each organ, it occurs primarily by simple diffusion.

Xenobiotic Absorption

Routes of penetration. Drugs and toxicants are capable of entering the body by several routes, depending on the mode of the exposure. The physical form of the xenobiotics (volatiles or aerosols, liquids, or solids) can affect the degree of penetration into the body and the resultant toxicity.

Gastrointestinal. Related to the general consumer, the most common route of exposure occurs by oral ingestion. Therapeutic agents administered by this route, as well as the ingestion of a variety of toxicants, can potentially be absorbed at any location along the gastrointestinal tract. However, the actual site of absorption is dependent upon the chemical nature of the drug or toxicant. If the xenobiotic agent is a weak organic acid with some degree of lipid solubility, absorption will take place in the stomach. The high acid content of the stomach favors formation of the unionized (protonated) form of the xenobiotic agent. Under these conditions, passive diffusion across the gastric mucosal membrane will occur. Importantly, the neutral pH of the cell and the circulating plasma allows the unionized form to dissociate and reform the ionized species. This change results in the maintenance of the concentration gradient necessary for continued diffusion.

For those xenobiotics which are weak organic bases, the major site of absorption is the small intestine. In the small intestine, the pH of the lumen is close to neutrality (pH 7.0). Under these conditions, equilibrium between the protonated (charged) base and the uncharged base is shifted towards the base (unionized) form. Again, given sufficient lipid solubility, the uncharged form of the xenobiotic can readily pass across the epithelial cell membrane of the small intestine by passive diffusion.

Inhalation. The lungs are potentially an important site for xenobiotic agent absorption into the body. Particulate material is at least partially filtered by passage through the nasal cavity, while volatiles and fine aerosols can reach the lung surface.

Inhalation of toxicant substances, as aerosols, is a major route by which such substances enter the body. This route of exposure is of particular concern for industrial and chemical safety. Many substances are capable of forming aerosols. During large-scale industrial and chemical manufacturing operations, many highly toxic substances are inadvertently converted to aerosols. Workers exposed to such environments carry a high risk of toxic contamination due to inhalation of these aerosols. Under these conditions, worker safety must be carefully monitored.

Cigarette smoking represents a prime example of self-imposed toxicant exposure by this mechanism (Fielding, 1985; Remmer, 1987). Unfortunately, much of the tars accumulate on the lung surface because of their hydrophobicity and insolubility, but they leach into cells either by diffusion or following phagocytosis. The nicotine component crosses the epithelial cell membrane and enters the general circulation.

In medicine, many general anesthetics are gases which are administered via the inhalation route. These substances possess a relatively large oil in water partition coefficient and thus can be readily absorbed across the alveolar membranes. In addition, drugs can be administered as aerosols, providing extremely small particles of the drug which are suspended in air. The small particle size prevents the drug from sedimenting out of suspension due to gravitional forces. When these aerosols are inhaled, the solid particles are deposited on the surface of the bronchioles and the alveolar sacs of the lung. Once on the surface of the airways, absorption across the epithelial membrane cells can occur readily. In addition to passive and aqueous diffusion across the epithelial cells of the lung, solid particles can be absorbed by phagocytosis. The extensive supply of capillary blood flow to the lungs leads to a rapid rise in circulating levels of both administered drugs and inhaled toxicants. This procedure of drug administration is extremely useful in treating acute asthmatic attacks. A variety of drugs which act directly upon the smooth muscle of the bronchioles can rapidly relax bronchial constriction and thus relieve the asthmatic condition when administered by this route.

Percutaneous. The absorption of xenobiotics through the skin is another route of absorption. The outermost layer of the skin is composed of cells which are densely packed in a matrix of keratin. The combination of actively dividing cells along with structural elements provides a very tight surface which is resistant to water penetration. However, the skin is highly permeable to lipid-soluble substances (Bronaugh, 1982b). Drugs which are highly lipid-soluble such as antiinflammatory agents and steroids can be absorbed by topical application, and maintenance doses of certain agents can be provided by dermal patches, e.g., digoxin.

Many toxic substances are highly lipid-soluble (Kulkarni and Hodgson, 1980; Shah et al., 1981). When these substances come in contact with the skin, appreciable absorption can occur (Sato and Nakajima, 1979). This fact is often not considered with enough care. Individuals working with industrial chemicals, pesticides and herbicides, and many cleaning agents can unknowingly become contaminated with these agents. Thus, it is important to consider the potential for contamination and to use the appropriate protective clothing to minimize skin contact with these substances.

Injection. Drugs are frequently given by injection to bypass the absorptive restrictions of the skin or epithelial lining of the gastrointestinal tract. Depending on the rate of availability and the need to maintain a given plasma concentration, the drugs can be given plasma concentration, the drugs can be given intravenously, intramuscularly, or subcutaneously. The intravenous route of injection is most important when rapid response to the drug is required. This is often the case in intensive care units where rapid drug intervention is essential to the preservation of life. Intravenous injection bypasses the need for absorptive processes. Intravenous drips can be used to maintain therapeutic blood levels of a drug for prolonged periods.

Drugs may be injected intramuscularly. This route of administration can be used to administer relatively large volumes. Absorption can be rapid due to the high degree of vascular supply to muscles. The rate of absorption from the intramuscular site of injection is largely dependent upon the nature of the drug. Aqueous suspensions are rapidly absorbed if the molecular size of the drug is relatively small and the degree of lipid solubility and unionized form of the drug are relatively high. Under these conditions the drug readily enters the circulation via passive diffusion through the endothelial cells of the capillary vessels.

Drugs administered in oily vehicles are absorbed very slowly into the general circulation. In an oil suspension, the drug can be given intramuscularly and can provide slow, steady-state absorption for longer periods of time.

The subcutaneous injection of drugs limits the rate of availability. Since the vascular supply to this area is poor and contains a high amount of connective tissue, the degree to which the injected suspension can freely diffuse is restricted. The amount of drug available is dependent on the area occupied by the injected suspension.

Abrasion. Abrasive damage to the dermal layer allows for faster penetration by compounds that may otherwise be excluded. Since most toxic agents would not be injected, abrasion serves as a primary means of increased skin penetration.

Membrane permeation. Over 85 years ago, Overton (1902) demonstrated that a number of organic compounds penetrated cells at rates roughly related to their lipid:water partition coefficient, and he concluded that the cell membrane was similar to a lipid layer. Although it has since been demonstrated that other factors also govern passage of molecules through the membrane, the lipid bilayer membrane still plays a primary role in regulating rates of absorption of many substances. However, Hober and Hober (1937) specifically demonstrated that very water-soluble compounds could also readily enter cells as well. He termed the process physiological permeability, referring to the cell's need to acquire polar materials for cellular function. This observation served to stimulate characterization of additional transport processes.

Passive diffusion. The movement of substances, including xenobiotics, across the cell membrane by passive diffusion has the following characteristics: (a) only the unionized form of the substance can diffuse through the cell membrane; (b) the unionized form must be relatively lipid-soluble; (c) the size of the molecule also influences the rate of passive diffusion. With other properties being equal, smaller molecules tend to diffuse faster than molecules of greater molecular size.

Passive diffusion does not require energy input by the cell. The energy needed to drive passive transport is derived from the flow of the unionized substance through the membrane and down the concentration gradient. Ionized compounds do not move efficiently by diffusion, due to the ionic interactions between the compound and the proteins and polar phospholipids of the membrane.

Most of xenobiotic agents are either weak organic acids or weak organic bases. These compounds exist in aqueous solution as a mixture of both the ionized and the unionized form of the compound. The degree to which the xenobiotic exists as the unionized form is dependent on both the dissociation constant for that compound as well as the pH of the aqueous environment in which the drug is located. The relationship between pH, the dissociation constant for the drug (K_a), and the degree of dissociation is given by the Henderson-Hasselback equation (1):

$$pH = pK_a + \log[A^-]/[HA]$$

From equation (1), it can be seen that the degree of ionization of a weak acid $[A^-]/[HA]$ is a function of both the dissociation constant for the acid (K_a) and the pH of the environment which contains the acid.

From the Henderson-Hasselbach equation, it is apparent that weak organic acids are unionized (HA) at pH values lower than their respective pK_a value, whereas weak organic bases are unionized (BH) at pH values greater than their respective pK_a value.

In addition to a xenobiotic agent being unionized, passive diffusion is dependent upon the lipid solubility of the unionized form of the compound. The lipid solubility of unionized weak organic acids and bases can conveniently be represented by their oil in water partition coefficient (K_p), equation (2).

$$K_p = C_{org}/C_{aq}$$

where C_{org} represents the concentration of the compound in an organic solvent, such as olive oil, benzene, chloroform, or octanol, and C_{aq} represents the concentration of the compound in the water phase of the mixture. Unfortunately, use of different lipophilic compounds for the organic phase frequently results in different K_p values.

Substances having relatively large partition coefficients are readily soluble in the lipid matrix of membranes, whereas a relatively low partition coefficient indicates a high degree of water solubility, and those compounds would have difficulty entering the lipid matrix. Thus, it is the unionized, lipid-soluble form of a xenobiotic that can easily pass through cellular membranes by the process of passive diffusion.

Although lipid solubility is essential for initial uptake, other factors affect diffusion. Actual penetration may vary with the membrane characteristics and may be affected by some polar character on the molecule, as well as the size of the moelcule. However, if the molecule has high water solubility, its penetration by diffusion is usually very low.

Facilitated diffusion. The second process whereby substances can pass through cellular membranes is described as facilitated diffusion. Facilitated diffusion is one of two processes by which polar, water-soluble substances, which may be in their ionized or charged form, can be transported across cellular membranes. Facilitated diffusion requires the presence of a membrane carrier, usually a membrane associated protein molecule, to which the substance becomes associated through hydrogen bonding, weak ionic charges, and Van de Walls forces. The carrier complex is then translocated across the cell membrane. At least at lower concentrations of xenobiotic, the rate of transport by this mechanism exceeds the rate of simple diffusion. Once on the inside surface of the membrane, the substance then dissociates from the membrane carrier, thus being delivered to the inside of the cell. Facilitated diffusion also requires the presence of a concentration gradient across the cell membrane to produce transport.

A second facilitative carrier is required in the epithelial cells to assure movement down the concentration gradient. The second carrier assures transport of the substance out of the cell into the circulation.

Active membrane transport. The final process by which substances can enter cells is by active membrane transport. This process is similar to facilitated diffusion in that water-soluble, ionic substances pass through cellular membranes by means of specific membrane carriers. However, this process differs from facilitated diffusion in that substances can be transported against a concentration gradient. Such processes require the expenditure of cellular energy derived from the hydrolysis of ATP. Thus, active transport processes involve membrane ATPase activities which are associated with the translocation of the membrane carrier from one side of the cell membrane to the other side. Conversely, the carrier utilizes the transmembrane Na^+-gradient (provided in part by the Na^+-K^+ATPase) and/or the electrical potential as the energy source for uphill transport of the substance into the cell. The substance may then leave the cell at the opposite pole by facilitative diffusion (carrier), which assists active transport by keeping the gradient low. Sugars, amino acids, nucleotides, and many water-soluble vitamins are absorbed in this way. Although xenobiotic agents structurally similar to nutrients may share active transport pathways, there would not have been an evolutionary need to evolve specific transport sytems for the large number of xenobiotics available today. However, active transport of certain xenobiotic agents has been reported.

Gastrointestinal absorption.

Physiological absorptive processes. The gastrointestinal (GI) tract can be described as a tube-like structure through which dietary substances enter the body. Although continuously linked, various segments (the mouth, esophagus, stomach, small intestine, and colon) carry out specific physiological functions. In reality, the surface of the gastrointestinal tract is external to the body compartment.

In addition to the structural elements, several related structures are responsible for the synthesis, storage, and secretion of digestive substances into the GI tract. These include the salivary glands, oxyntic or gastric glands, the pancreas, the liver, and the gallbladder. As the ingested material passes through the GI tract, it is acted upon by a variety of GI tract secretions which lead to the emulsification, digestion, and absorption of the components present in the ingested material. Nondigestible and/or nonabsorbable substances pass completely through the GI tract and are excreted.

The intestinal structure provides a unique barrier to regulate the absorption of nutrients or xenobiotic materials. The lining of the GI tract is composed of epithelial cells and characterized by a lipid bilayer membrane which forms the luminal surface of the GI tract. The opposite membrane surface, the basement membrane, forms the barrier between the intercellular space, the capillary vessels, and the cells of each specific organ.

The spaces between adjacent epithelial cells of the GI lining form relatively tight junctions, which prevent the passage of most materials from the lumen to intercellular spaces. On the other hand, the junctions between the endothelial cells composing the capillary vessels are relatively large and thus allow many relatively small molecules to easily diffuse into the circulatory system. Thus, the epithelial lining probably constitutes the main barrier to the passage of solutes from the lumen to the blood stream.

Paracellular transport occurs through the tight junctions between cells. These junctions form a molecular sieve, permeable to water and small molecular weight substances. The major force for paracellular uptake is solvent drag (most of the water contained in the digestive juices (6 liter/day) is reabsorbed via the paracellular pathway). Solutes in this juice may be pulled through the tight junctions with the water. This process is called persorption, and particles pass through the loose junctions formed between dying enterocytes of the villus tips.

Due to the overall length of the GI tract, the large surface area, and the time it takes for materials to be excreted, the absorption of most compounds is quite efficient. The membrane surface of the epithelial cells contain protrusions (brush border), which contain certain digestive enzymes and the transport proteins.

In general, most xenobiotic agents are capable of being absorbed from the lumen of the gastrointestinal tract by passive diffusion. Transcellular (passive) diffusion processes allow small neutrally charged lipophilic substances to diffuse through the luminal membrane into the epithelial cell. These substances then diffuse through the basement membrane of the epithelial cell into the intercellular space and then continue to diffuse into the capillary vessels. Ionized substances which are poorly lipid-soluble, on the other hand, can only be absorbed through the epithelial lining of the GI tract by means of either facilitated diffusion or by active transport mechanisms.

Small, lipophilic molecules, such as ethanol, presumably diffuse rapidly through the brush border membrane, travel through the aqueous phase of the cell cytosol, and leave the cell at the basal membrane. Highly lipophilic compounds like Benzo(a)pyrene or DDT may be absorbed by the transcellular route as well, or, conversely, they may become integrated into the brush border membrane and move laterally along the plasma membrane (lipid matrix) toward the basal membrane.

The classic experiments that substantiated the role of pH and lipid solubility in xenobiotic diffusion are summarized here to support the above discussion:

Experimental results from human studies confirm the hypothesis that drug absorption from the stomach occurs by passive diffusion of the lipid-soluble unionized form of the drug (Hogben et al., 1957). Acidic drugs such as salicylic acid, thiopental, aspirin, secobarbital all having pK_a values less than 3.0, as well as the weak basic drug antipyrine with pK_a of 1.4 were all readily absorbed from the stomach. Conversely, basic drugs with pK_a values greater than 5 such as aminopyrine, quinine, and ephedrine were not absorbed from the stomach.

Schanker et al. (1957) reached similar conclusions in experiments using rat stomachs. When they made the stomach contents more basic, the absorption of the acidic drugs decreased and those of the basic drugs increased. These authors also demonstrated that the rate of absorption of the unionized form of the drug was dependent upon its lipid solubility as characterized by its oil in water partition coefficient. Thus, drug absorption from the stomach was via passive diffusion of the unionized drug through the gastric mucosa.

In support of the pH partition, Shore et al. (1957) evaluated the transfer of drugs from the plasma into the stomach acid. In this case, weak acid and bases were transferred, but strong bases produced the highest transfer. Bases having pK_a values between 5.0 and 10.0 produced a 40-fold excess in the stomach acid. Thus, again the gastric mucosa acted simply as a lipid membrane barrier.

In a continuing series of studies, Schanker et al. (1958) measured drug (salicylate and aniline) absorption from the rat small intestine, using an intestinal perfusion technique. Drug absorption from the small intestine was concluded to be by passive diffusion, since the rate of absorption was (a) related to the percentage of the drug in the unionized form and its lipid solubility, (b) directly proportional to concentration, and (c) the presence of a second drug did not alter the rate of absorption of a given drug. There was no apparent difference in absorption rates for drugs throughout the length of the small intestine.

Schanker (1959) then examined drug absorption from the rat colon using perfusion techniques. The results indicated that the rate of drug absorption from the colonic lumen into the blood was dependent on both the level of the unionized form of the drug and the lipid solubility of the unionized form of the drug. Thus, drug absorption from the alimentary tract appears to be largely by passive diffusion of the unionized form of the drug from the lumen of the gastrointestinal tract, through the epithelial cell membranes, into the general circulation (Schanker, 1960).

Physical interactions.   Absorption or adsorption interactions between drug and food molecules may influence drug availability (Toothaker and Welling, 1980). Food may also act as a purely physical barrier, preventing drug access to the mucosal surface of the gastrointestinal tract. This would affect both actively and passively absorbed compounds.

Gastric emptying.   Factors influencing gastric emptying have been reviewed by Bates and Gibaldi (1970). The predominant effect of food ingestion is that of inhibition of stomach emptying due to feedback mechanisms from the osmoreceptors, acid receptors, and fat and fatty acid receptors situated in the proximal small intestine. Stomach emptying is delayed by hot meals, by solutions of high viscosity, by high fat and, to a lesser extent, protein and carbohydrate meals. Solid meals almost double the stomach emptying time compared to liquid meals. Thus, ingestion of food may inhibit gastric emptying by one or more mechanisms and may influence drug absorption to a variable extent.

Compounds absorbed at specific intestinal sites or by saturable active transport mechanisms may exhibit increased absorption with delayed stomach emptying due to a decrease in the rate at which the xenobiotic passes the site of absorption.

Fluid volume.   The predominant driving force for the passive absorption of xenobiotics is the concentration gradient across the epithelial and capillary membrane. It would appear axiomatic that drugs should be absorbed more efficiently from concentrated solutions than from dilute solutions.

Numerous animal and human studies indicate the reverse may be the case. In animals, the toxicity of a large number of organic acids and bases, and also inorganic ions, was increased with increasing compound dilution. Ferguson (1962) gave equal doses of organic acids but diluted them to different concentrations in water equal to 1.25%, 2.5%, and 5.0% of body weight. The toxicity of all compounds increased with increasing dilution. In man, the initial absorption rate of aspirin was doubled when the volume of water consumed with the xenobiotic was increased from 75 mL to 150 mL (Borowitz et al., 1971).

One explanation for the increased absorption might be that the greater volume enhances stomach emptying, producing a more rapid exposure to the greater suface area of the intestine. However, Ochsenfahrt and Winne (1974) suggested the contributiion of solvent drag may increase intestinal absorbtion from hypotonic solutions. They examined absorption of the acidic xenobiotics benzoic acid and salicylic acid from the jejunum of the rat. Absorption of both unionized and ionized acidic molecules was greater in hypotonic solutions compared to hypertonic solutions. The rate of drug absorption was clearly related to net water flux, which was negative from the blood to the perfusing solution with hypertonic solutions, and positive with hypotonic solutions.

Gastric secretion.   Ingestion of food increases the gastric secretion of hydrochloric acid and of many enzymes that may affect drug dissolution and degradation. If large, the blood may actually become alkaline and may thereby affect the passage of ionizable compounds across the luminal membrane. Increased secretion of bile after food intake may accelerate dissolution of more lipophilic compounds and enhance micellar formation.

Gastric motility.   Food reaching the small intestine stimulates intestinal motility, and this may increase drug dissolution and decrease the diffusional path to the intestinal epithelium. Increased gastric motility may also lower absorption efficiency as a result of the increased transit rate of drug through the intestine.

Splanchic blood flow.   Interestingly, high protein liquid meals have been shown to increase the rate of estimated splanchic blood flow, while high glucose liquid meals cause a small, transient decrease (Brandt et al., 1955). Xenobiotic absorption may be affected by an altered splanchic blood flow due to an increase or decrease in the transluminal concentration gradient. Compounds transported by passive or facilitative diffusion would be affected, while compounds limited by luminal membrane transfer processes should not be affected by changes in the splanchic blood flow.

Altered splanchic blood flow may also influence the absorption of xenobiotics which are extensively metabolized due to changes in clearance during the first pass through the hepatoportal system (McLean et al., 1978).

Enterohepatic circulation.   From the enterohepatic circulation, the bile duct empties into the gastrointestinal tract. The bile acts as a detergent stimulating lipase activity and forming micelles to enhance lipid absorption. Lipid-soluble xenobiotics are absorbed by this mechanism.

The antifungal agent griseofulvin has a very low bioavailability when given orally, due to the very low solubility of the drug in aqueous solutions. In this study, the plasma level of griseofulvin was significantly increased when the drug was taken with a high fat meal (Crounse, 1961). Similar mechanisms would be involved in the absorption of the highly lipophilic compounds used as pesticides and herbicides.

During elimination, secondary absorption of the drug or toxicant can also occur due to the enterohepatic circulation. Elimination of the xenobiotics and their metabolites in the bile places them back into the gastric system for reabsorption.

Physiological effects of food on drug absorption.   Physiological changes caused by food and fluid can influence xenobiotic absorption. It has often been taken for granted that food generally impairs the absorption of drugs. The rate, and in part the extent, of drug absorption depends mainly on the rate of gastric emptying. Since food decreases the rate of emptying, it would therefore be assumed to decrease the rate of absorption. The conclusion is based on the assumption that the majority of drugs and toxicants are absorbed by passive diffusion (Melander, 1978).

Recent publications would question these simple assumptions. Food intake has been shown to improve the availability of several drugs (Melander et al., 1977,1978; Beerman and Groschinsky-Grind, 1978). Food may influence the rate of drug absorption without affecting the total amount absorbed, and both the rate and extent may be increased due to a decrease in the rate of emptying.

Nutritional alteration.   The pathophysiological changes due to protein-energy malnutrition (PEM), infection, infestation, and mineral or vitamin deficiencies can impair absorption of drugs or toxicants (Schneider and Viteri, 1974; Suskind, 1975). The absorptive efficiencies for nutrients such as fats, amino acids, vitamins, and mineral are also decreased.

PEM and various vitamin deficiencies result in vomiting, diarrhea, and steatorrhea, further affecting nutritional status. Changes include gastric dilation, gastric mucosal atrophy, hypochlorhydria, and a reduction of the gastric bacterial barrier (Mata et al., 1972). Gastric emptying time and intestinal transit time are significantly prolonged. Pancreatic structure and function, especially the exocrine function, are deranged (Barbezat and Hansen, 1968), with reduced enzyme levels including lipase, trypsin and chymotrypsin, and amylase (Schneider and Viteri, 1974).

In PCM, the small intestine undergoes a variety of changes. The mucous membrane becomes thinner with villous atrophy and increased transit time (Mayoral et al., 1972). Intestinal function, as determined by sugar, fat, or vitamin B12 absorption, is lower. Intradoudenal capacity to form fat micelles is also impaired in PCM.

Doluisio et al. (1969a,b) clearly indicated that in the rat short-term fasting had no effect on the rate of drug (highly lipid-soluble, weak bases–haloperidol and chlorpromazine) absorption from the gastrointestinal tract up to 20 hours. However, when fasting was continued for more than 20 hours, the rate of drug absorption from the gastrointestinal tract was found to decrease significantly. These results would agree with the above discussion and indicate the time required to initiate the physiological and biochemical changes to the gastrointestinal tract observed during starvation.

Protein deficiency was found to decrease both the rate of absorption of butylated hydroxyanisole from the gastrointestinal tract and its rate of excretion in urine by the kidneys (Kangsadalampai et al., 1986). In addition these results were also consistent with previous reports which indicated a decrease in the rate of drug clearance by the kidney under conditions of protein deficiency.

A unique experiment was described by Fortaine et al. (1987). Alteration of the polar head groups on membrane phospholipids were shown to effect several transport processes. The transport of thymidine, 2-deoxy-D-glucose, and 5-flurouracil was altered by these modifications to membrane phospholipids. However, there was no effect on the transport of uridine, α−aminoisobutyric acid, or the antineoplastic drugs daunorubicin, doxorubicin, and methotrexate. The mechanism by which an alteration in polar head group composition was responsible for an alteration in membrane transport is unclear. Possible mechanisms include alteration in the charged microenvironment of membrane bound enzyme activities upon the modification of the polar head groups of phospholipids, alteration in the fluid microdomain due to changes in the phospholipids, and an alteration in the asymmetric nature of the lipid bilayer which may be required for normal functioning of transmembrane transport proteins.

Xenobiotic Distribution

Compartments. Body fluids are divided between three compartments: vascular fluid, interstitial fluid, and intracellular water. Following the absorption of a drug or toxicant into the general circulation, the xenobiotic redistributes into one or more of these compartments.

In a 70 kg man, the body is composed of approximately 58% water, which is equivalent to 41 L. The extracellular fluid includes the plasma, interstitial-lymph, connective tissue, bone, and transcellular water. About 12–14 L of the total body water is located in this fraction. The plasma portion amounts to 3 L of fluid and serves as one of the keys to evaluation of xenobiotic distribution. The intracellular water comprises approximately 29 L of the total body water.

Following absorption of a xenobiotic into the plasma, the agent may be distributed to the site of toxic action, transferred to a storage depot, transported to organs for detoxification or interaction, or carried to the site of elimination. Transport in the lymphatic system is much less important since the flow rate is much less.

The volume of distribution (V_d) of drugs and toxicants can be calculated from the following equation:

$$V_d = \frac{x}{c} \qquad (3)$$

where x is the amount of the compound that is injected intravascularly and c is the concentration of the compound in the blood after sufficient time for the even distribution of the compound throughout the blood but prior to any appreciable metabolism or excretion of the compound has occurred.

Several assumptions are made when estimating the volume of distribution of drugs and toxicants using Equation (3). These assumptions include (a) no metabolism of the xenobiotic, (b) no binding or sequestration of the xenobiotic by other substances present in the body, and (c) no appreciable elimination of the xenobiotic has occurred. In most cases these assumptions are not completely valid, and the result varies from compound to compound. Thus, the volume of distribution so determined is only an apparent volume of distribution.

Xenobiotics bind to plasma and tissue proteins to a variable extent (Rowland, 1984). The agents form reversible protein interactions, which ensure their transport in the circulation. Importantly, the complex cannot cross the cell membrane barrier. Only the unbound xenobiotics are available to diffuse across membranes. In addition, protein binding can vary widely with disease, concommitant drug therapy, age, and many other factors (Jusko and Gretch, 1976).

The volume of distribution depends on the combination of tissue and body fluids in which the agent equilibrates and is affected by the chemical nature, ionic and lipophilic, of the agent. Certain tissues of the body may have an unusually high affinity for a given drug or toxicant, which will result in the sequestering of this substance by these tissues. The redistribution of highly lipid-soluble drugs and toxicants into highly lipophilic areas of the body such as adipose tissue is a good example of the tissue sequestering of substances. For this reason, distribution of lipophilic drugs can be altered by obesity (Abernathy and Greenblatt, 1982).

In cases such as these, protein binding and tissue squestration may be so great that the calculated V_d may exceed the total body volume. Understanding the relationship between altered protein binding and both pharmacokinetics and pharmacodynamics is therefore important.

If the clearance of the unbound xenobiotic is low, relative to organ blood flow, then the extraction ratio (and clearance) will also be low and dependent on plasma binding. If the extraction ratio is high, then elimination of the agent becomes limited by the perfusion rate. In this case, clearance will then be relatively insensitive to changes in binding.

Factors affecting distribution.

Protein binding. Many drugs and toxicants have been shown to be highly bound to plasma proteins (Wilkinson, 1983). Binding of the xenobiotic occurs as a result of hydrogen, ionic, or electrostatic bonds or from Van de Waals forces. Very rarely are covalent bonds involved.

The plasma is a complex solution containing different proteins, of which albumin, α_1-acid glycoprotein, lipoproteins, and globulins transport endogenous compounds (hormones and fatty acids) and exogenous compounds (drugs, toxicants, and other xenobiotics). Many agents bind to plasma proteins, principally to albumin and globulins. The extent of binding varies with the chemical nature of the agent, its binding affinity for the protein, and the concentration of the protein. Albumin is most important, although basic xenobiotics bind more specifically to the α_1-acid glycoprotein.

Many conditions impair albumin synthesis and its plasma concentration, including liver disease, renal disorders, endocrine disorders, stress, and aging. Nutritionally, protein and energy balance will influence the plasma protein profile by altering the rate of tissue protein synthesis and turnover. Xenobiotic-protein binding may be altered at different stages of malnutrition or nutrient deficiencies.

Since endogenous factors, such as fatty acids, bilirubin, bile acids, tryptophan, uric acid, steroid hormones, and thyroxine also bind to albumin, alterations in their availability can affect xenobiotic binding and distribution (Wilkinson, 1983).

The binding of endogenous and exogenous compounds to macromolecules in the circulating blood has been investigated. The reversibility of the interaction serves as a carrier mechanism for the functionally active unbound moiety. Most binding studies are carried out using plasma. However, the assumption that there are no differences between plasma and serum may be invalid (Wiegand et al., 1979,1980).

Albumin is the most abundant protein in the plasma, amounting to 58% of the total protein. A major physiological role of plasma albumin is as a transport protein for fatty acids. Additionally, albumin binds various anions, cations, steroids, bilirubin, and a variety of drugs, especially those with acidic and neutral characteristics (Table 12.1). Although these agents have been considered to bind nonspecifically, there are a few high-affinity sites and a variable number of different low-affinity sites currently being characterized and classified (Brodersen et al., 1977; Kragh-Hansen, 1981).

TABLE 12.1 Classification of Human Serum Albumin Binding Sites

---

ACIDIC XENOBIOTIC
Type I. Two separate specific sites
  1. *Warfarin binding site:* binds warfarin, dicoumarol, furosemide, iodopamide, iophenoxic acid, oxyphenylbutazone, phenybutazone, tolbutamide, valproic acid.
      Note: Bilirubin competitive binding free fatty acids can enhance or inhibit anionic ligand binding.
  2. *Benzodiazepine binding site:* binds diazepam, benzodiazepines, clofibric acid, dicoumarol, ethacrynic acid, glibenclamide, ibuprofen, iopanoic acid, naproxen.
      Note: Free fatty acids decrease binding.
  Note: Allosteric interactions between sites 1 and 2 results in noncompetitive inhibition of drug binding
Type II. First binding is saturable, but not the second: indomethacin, clometacin, and diclofenac
  Note: This site may be related to the type I site for high-affinity binding.
Type III. Nonsaturable binding
      Phenytoin binding site: phenobarbital, thiopental, pentobarbital, doxcyline, and tetracycline
Type IV. Nonsaturable binding of nonionizable xenobiotics *Digitalis glycosides binding:*
  Note: Binding is not modified by other drugs, but is decreased by free fatty acids.
BASIC XENOBIOTIC
Type V. Nonsaturable binding; α_1-Acid glycoprotein

Sources: Sjoholm et al., 1976, 1979; Sjodin, 1977; Soltys and Hsia, 1977; Lecompte et al., 1979; Piafsky, 1980; Tillement et al., 1980; Urien et al., 1980; Fehske et al., 1981.

The primary binding site is also the major binding region for bilirubin and serves as an important site of interaction for many other drugs such as sulfonamides, penicillin derivatives, and certain analgesics. Distinct from this region, another site binds D- and L-tryptophan. This site also binds benzodiazepine, certain antihypoglycemic agents, antibiotics, and analgesics (Jusko and Gretch, 1976; Wiegand et al., 1979; Fehske et al., 1979).

The binding of long-chain fatty acids involves two high-affinity sites, neither of which are directly involved in the binding of various drugs. A separate region, possibly the same as that involved in benzodiazepine binding, is responsible for interacting with medium-chain fatty acids.

The coumarin anticoagulants like warfarin, phenprocoumarin, and dicoumerol are strongly bound to human serum albumin (Fehske et al., 1979). The monomeric forms apparently interact with one high-affinity site on the albumin and at several sites of lower affinity. The dimeric form, dicoumerol, interacts with three sites of high affinity, one of which is the monomeric high-affinity site.

While compounds possessing basic characteristics do bind to albumin, the α_1-acid glycoprotein (α_1-AGP) plays a significant role in plasma binding (Piafsky, 1980). The α_1-AGP contains a high carbohydrate content and a large number of sialyl residues which contribute to its acidic nature. Although little is known about its physiological function, extensive binding of quinidine, dipyrimadole, lidocaine, other anesthetics, tricyclic antidepressants, chlorpromazine, and β-adrenergic blocking agents to a_1-acid glycoprotein was reported (Korngruth et al., 1981).

The major role of circulating lipoproteins is the transport of triglycerides, phospholipids, and cholesterol. Increasing evidence exists that lipoproteins may be important in the binding and distribution of very lipophilic and/or basic compounds (Bickel, 1975; Kates et al., 1978; Danon and Chen, 1979). For example, quinidine, chlorpromazine, imipramine, reserpine, propanolol, tetracycline, and various insecticides seem to simply dissolve into the lipids. The uptake and transport of carcinogens by the lipoproteins was described by Shu and Nichols (1981). However, binding of chlorpromazine and quinidine appeared to be saturable, which may suggest the binding is related to sites on the proteins covering the surface of the lipoprotein particles.

Upon evaluation of the relative distribution of insecticides in the plasma protein fractions, several interesting differences were observed. Seventy-five percent of nicotine was determined to be unbound. Of the 25% that was bound, 94% was associated with albumin, and very little was distributed into the lipoprotein (LDL or HDL) fractions. Carbaryl was almost entirely bound to the albumin, providing only 2.5% to be circulated in the unbound form. Parathion, dieldrin, and DDT were highly bound to the lipoprotein fractions. Two-thirds of the parathion was bound to albumin, but 21% was bound to the LDL and 12% was bound to the HDL fractions. DDT was distributed evenly between the three proteins, while dieldrin was found in higher concentrations in the LDL and HDL fractions.

Very specific proteins are responsible for the plasma binding and transport of certain hormones and other physiologically/biochemically important compounds: thyroxine binding and prealbumin globulins, transferrin, hemopexin, ceruloplasmin, and retinol-binding protein (Tillement et al., 1984). In addition, the membranes of red and white blood cells, as well as platelets, can bind drugs, especially basic drugs. Such binding is minor compared to the extensive interactions with the plasma proteins (Bickel, 1975).

The amount of the xenobiotic transferred to each tissue depends on the tissue ability to bind the agent. The specific binding to intracellular tissue constituents remains relatively uninvestigated (Jusko and Gretch, 1976; Kurz and Fichtl, 1983). Even though nucleic acids, polypeptides, and polysaccharides all have high binding capacity, difficulty arises in studying the binding under physiological conditions in vitro. These sites may be important serving as sites of damage as well as binding of the xenobiotic or its metabolites.

Effect of protein concentration.   The extent of xenobiotic binding is determined to a considerable extent by the concentration of the proteins and the number of binding sites on the macromolecules (Boobis and Chignell, 1979). Plasma binding may exhibit considerable intra- and intersubject variability because of this factor. For example, the normal concentration of albumin in men is 42 g/L (0.75 mM), while women have concentrations about 9% lower. Gender differences in drug binding have also been reported. In addition, disease states can lead to decreases in plasma albumin, as well as altered distribution of albumin between the intra- and extravascular spaces (Jusko and Gretch, 1976). Conversely, the plasma concentration of a_1-acid glycoprotein rises by four- to fivefold in inflammatory and other diseases, but is reduced by pregnancy and oral contraceptives.

The fluctuations of lipoprotein composition and concentration could also be expected to affect the interaction of these ligands. Although not extensively documented, effects have been reported when pronounced abnormalities occur (Kates et al., 1978; Korngruth et al., 1981).

Effect of xenobiotic concentration.   The concentration of xenobiotic may be an important determinant of binding. However, the relationship between the unbound fraction and total ligand concentration depends specifically on the affinity of the binding site. The dissociation constant serves as an inverse measure of affinity (Equations (4) and (5)). The binding affinity equals the unbound concentration at which 50% of the binding sites are saturated.

$$K_d = \frac{1}{K_a} \tag{4}$$

$$K_a = \frac{(\text{protein-bound drug})}{(\text{free drug})(\text{free protein})} \tag{5}$$

At low levels of xenobiotic relative to the dissociation constant, the change in binding is modest, but as the binding sites become increasingly occupied, an increase in the unbound fraction occurs. The higher the binding affinity, the sharper the change.

A significant concentration-dependent binding is present at these levels only if the dissociation constant is between 10^{-5} and 10^{-4} M_l. These concentrations only occur with compounds administered in large amounts and/or those not widely distributed outside the vascular system, e.g., salicylate and sulfonamide.

The plasma concentration of α_1-acid glycoproteins, 10–30 μM, could allow saturation to occur quite readily. The compounds that bind to the a_1-acid glycoproteins usually occur in small doses, either when given as a therapeutic agent or due to a toxicant exposure. However, salicylic acid when used in high doses for the treatment of arthritis exhibits concentration-dependent binding (Furst et al., 1979), and diisopyramide used in therapeutic doses may saturate the binding sites on the α_1-acid glycoprotein (Meffin et al., 1976). Thus, saturation of the α_1-AGP can occur, but probably does not occur under normal physiological conditions.

The relative contribution of each plasma protein to the overall binding of a xenobiotic may change as the concentration increases. Thyroxine and certain corticosteroids are normally transported in the plasma bound with high affinity to specific globulins. The capacity of such sites is limited. Thus, when the ligands are present in high concentrations, the binding shifts to secondary low-affinity sites on albumin (Bowmer and Lindup, 1980).

The unbound fraction increases with lower affinity and increasing concentration. In addition, the binding affinity for one agent may be reduced if the binding sites are already occupied by other ligands that are concomitantly present either by direct displacement or allosteric mechanisms (Gayte-Sorbier and Airaudo, 1984).

Influence of nutritional status. Hypoalbuminemia occurs in the majority of malnourished individuals, the degree depending on the duration and severity of undernutrition. The consequences of altered protein binding are quite different for drugs or toxicants that are extensively bound to tissues than for drugs that are highly bound to plasma proteins. Within the therapeutic plasma concentrations 96–99% of most drugs are protein bound. Thus, when more of the drug (xenobiotic) is not protein-bound, more is available to the tissues, increasing the potential for toxicity, but also enhancing elimination.

Malnutrition has been found to alter tissue uptake and tissue binding of a variety of drugs, e.g., tetracycline (Raghuram and Krishnaswamy, 1981) and phenylbutazone (Adithan et al., 1978). Adithan et al. (1978) and Krishnaswamy et al. (1981) reported the half-life of phenylbutazone was shortened and drug clearance was increased in malnourished patients.

The rate of albumin synthesis is directly related to the level of protein intake and amino acid supply (Waterlow, 1975). A decrease in the turnover rate of albumin occurs with a reduction in both synthesis and catabolism. The globulin proteins rise in malnutrition, perhaps as a result of infection (Coehn and Hansen, 1962). In addition, lipoproteins are reduced in malnutrition (Coward and Whitehead, 1972), but little has been reported on a_1-acid glycoproteins.

The binding of drugs in the serum was reduced by about 10% in undernourished subjects (Krishnaswamy et al., 1981). Buchanan (1977) evaluated drug binding in vitro, and noted a similar reduction in drug binding to serum.

As noted above, fatty acids bind to albumin by nonpolar interactions. The free fatty acid:albumin ratio of one is maintained (normal range 0.46–1.75). The binding affinity for free fatty acids is 5×10^5 times greater than that reported for drugs ($K_a = 5 \times 10^2 - 10^5/M$). Thus, competition occurs as a function of affinity and concentration, and perhaps conformational change in the albumin altering the binding.

A fatty meal can double the plasma free fatty acid levels within 12 hours, while fasting for 39 hours can triple the level (fasting free fatty acid:albumin ratio of 1.67–2.83). When greater than 2, the free fatty acids begin to bind to other proteins, red blood cell membranes, and lipoproteins.

Thus, in addition to lower albumin levels, a 5–15% change in drug binding may be produced by variations in free fatty. acid concentrations (Lichtenwalner et al., 1983).

Uremic patients produce substances that bind to albumin and displace drugs and endogenous ligands. Recently, 2-hydroxybenzoylglycine has been identified as one of the major inhibitors formed, although the synthetic steps have not been characterized.

Blood flow. A final physiological factor which may impact the volume of distribution of drugs and toxicants is the blood flow throughout the body. The distribution of drugs and toxicants is dependent on the rate of perfusion of the various tissues and organs of the body. There is considerable variation in the rates at which various tissues and organs of the body are perfused. As the perfusion rate is increased, the amount of drug available to tissues and organs for redistribution is increased. Depending upon the physical and chemical characteristics of a particular drug or toxicant, tissue perfusion rate can influence the volume of distribution of that substance.

Tissue solubility. Toxicants are often distributed and stored in specific tissues, either at sites of storage, in liver or kidney, or at the site of action. These agents can be squestered by binding to cellular proteins or solubilized into lipid stores of the adipose. Large amounts stored in these depots decrease immediate exposure, but increase potential hazard, if suddenly mobilized.

Xenobiotic Elimination

Kinetics. Following exposure, absorption of the xenobiotic would first enter the plasma compartment (Fig. 12.2). If the agent is tightly bound to the plasma proteins, very little of the xenobiotic can enter other tissues, nor can it undego metabolism or clearance. This would be an example of distribution to a single compartment (curve A). If, however, a second compartment is involved in the distribution, but the clearance remains low, then redistribution would appear more complex. Curve B might reflect the expected change in the plasma concentration.

If the xenobiotic undergoes rapid redistribution into multiple compartments and/or undergoes metabolism, the kinetic pattern of the xenobiotic in the plasma would appear as curve C. In this case the concentration would decrease in a nonlinear fashion, decreasing the rate of clearance as the concentration decreases. Finally, if redistribution, metabolism, and clearance are all ongoing processes, the plasma concentration of the xenobiotic would reflect curve D. The concentration would rise but would then fall rapidly as the xenobiotic was eliminated.

Biotransformation. The gastrointestinal tract serves as the main route of entry of compounds found in food and beverages and from administered

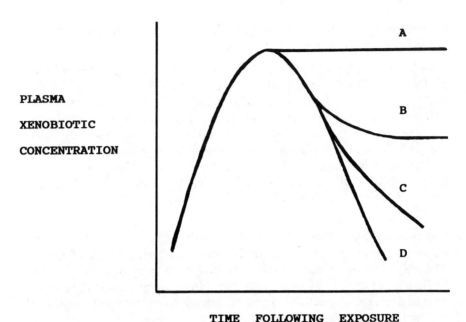

PLASMA

XENOBIOTIC

CONCENTRATION

TIME   FOLLOWING   EXPOSURE

FIG. 12.2 Effect of compartment distribution on elimination kinetics. See text for definitions of A–D.

therapeutic agents. This first line of defense against toxicity is provided by the mucosal lining. The mixed function oxidase activity is relatively low in the mucosa, as compared to the liver, but glucuronide and glutathione conjugation proceeds efficiently (Dawson and Bridges, 1981; Schwenk and Locher, 1985; Hanninen et al., 1987). The brush border region of the enterocyte is devoid of biotransformation enzymes. Thus, the metabolites formed in the enterocyte are simply released back into the lumen or passed on into the circulation.

The liver serves as the primary clearing site for the large variety of xenobiotics presented to it each day. The liver not only is the focus of the efficient portal delivery of the xenobiotics following absorption, but it is also very efficient at removing the majority of these agents by first pass elimination. In addition, the liver has the most abundant enzyme system available to metabolize, conjugate, and detoxify a large variety of chemically different xenobiotics.

The kidney contributes to a lesser degree but enhances clearance of detoxified agents. Compounds transported into renal cells may also be metabolized to more water-soluble forms. Metabolites thus formed may be handled differently than the parent compound. For example, catechol is a weak acid which enters the tubular cell by passive diffusion in its non-ionized form. Inside the cell it is conjugated to its sulfated and glucuronide form. These anions are actively excreted as organic ions in the tubular lumen (Rennick and Quebbemann, 1970; Rennick, 1972).

The respiratory tract is the major port of entry for airborne environmental chemicals. Different segments of the organ system, the nasal mucosa, trachea, and lung represent different levels of metabolism and express different sensitivities to chemically induced toxicities (Minchin and Boyd, 1983; Baron et al., 1988). High concentrations of enzymes occur in the nasal mucosa and the lung, including monooxygenase, epoxide hydatase, and the conjugating enzymes (Dahl, 1986; Dahl et al., 1988).

Hepatic toxicant-drug metabolism. The metabolism of xenobiotic agents has been reviewed previously: drug metabolism (Bidlack et al., 1986), toxic agents (Parke and Ioannides, 1981), carcinogens (Campbell, 1979), and chlorinated hydrocarbon insecticides (Varela et al., 1978).

Most of the foodborne chemicals that need to be cleared are presented at relatively low concentrations. In this situation, the body's defense mechanisms work very efficiently.

Hepatic mixed function oxidase. The hepatic enzyme system includes the mixed function oxidases (MFO) or monooxygenases and several conjugation enzymes, including sulfotransferase, glucuronyl transferase, and glutathione-S-transferase (Aitio, 1978; Schenkman and Kupfer, 1982). The MFO system first alters the existing functional groups, e.g., N- and O-dealkylation, to make the xenobiotic substrate more water-soluble (Table 12.2). A second group of enzymes specifically conjugates these polar groups, or inserts a polar group on those already present on the substrate, with endogenous cofactors including sulfate, glucuronic acid, and glutathione. The metabolism of a wide variety of compounds, including drugs, environmental chemicals, natural food toxicants, carcinogens, and even endogenous substrates like steroids have been studies in this system.

The MFO is composed of two enzymes coupled together in the endoplasmic reticulum—the flavoprotein, NADPH cytochrome P-450 reductase, and the terminal oxidase, cytochrome P-450 (Fig. 12.3). Two reducing equivalents from NADPH are transferred via the flavin moiety to the heme center of cytochrome P-450, which in the presence of molecular oxygen produces an oxygenated product and water. The flavoprotein is NADPH-specific and contains FAD and FMN (Iyanagi and Mason, 1973; Iyanagi et al., 1974). In addition, cytochrome P-450 has been determined to exist in multiple forms, including cytochrome P-448 (Lu

TABLE 12.2 Mixed Function Oxidase (Monooxygenase)
Reactions

Type of reaction	Example substrates
Aliphatic hydroxylation	DDT, hexobarbital, prostaglandins
Aromatic hydroxylation	Aniline, zoxazolamine
N-Dealkylation	Carbaryl, aminopyrine, morphine
O-Dealkylation	p-Nitroanisole, phenacetin
Epoxidation	Aldrin, safrole, bromobenzene
Dehalogenation	Carbontetrachloride, halothane
N-Oxidation	N-Acetyl-2-aminofluorene
Deamination	Amphetamines
S-Dealkylation	Methylmercaptans
S-Oxidation	Chlorpromazine
Desulfuration	Parathion, diazonin

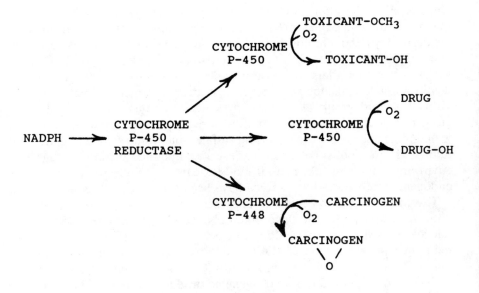

FIG. 12.3

and West, 1980). Each isozyme has different biochemical parameters as well as different substrate specificities (Guengerich, 1982). The isozymes can metabolize drugs, toxicants, and carcinogens. The system works so well that multiple substrates can be metabolized at the same time, e.g., aniline p-hydroxylation and p-nitroanisole O-demethylation (Lowery and Bidlack, 1978; Bidlack and Lowery, 1982).

Conjugation enzymes. The conjugating enzymes are located primarily in the cytosol and the endoplasmic reticulum (Table 12.3). Sulfotransferase (ST) conjugates phenols, as well as alcohols, amines, and thiols, with sulfate. The high-energy cofactor, PAPS (3'-phosphoadenosine-5'-phosphosulfate), is used to form the sulfate esters. Several forms of these enzymes, differing in substrate specificity, have been identified in the cytosol (Dodson, 1977; Singer, 1985). Another group of ST enzymes does exist in the endoplasmic reticulum/golgi membranes, but these enzymes form sulfate esters with mucopolysaccharide and do not appear to participate in xenobiotic metabolism. Unfortunately, sulfation can also increase the toxicity and carcinogenicity of certain agents, e.g., N-acetyl-2-aminofluorene, by increasing their electrophilic character.

Glucuronyl transferase (GT) is the most versatile of the conjugation reactions, transferring glucuronic acid from UDPGA (uridine diphosphate glucuronic acid) to the xenobiotic (Dutton, 1976; Zakim et al., 1985). Glucuronyl transferase is located in the endoplasmic reticulum and exists in multiple forms. Substrates for GT include plant and drug phenolic

TABLE 12.3 Conjugation Reactions: Cofactors and Substrates

Enzymes	Cofactor	Substrate reactive groups
Glucuronyl transferase	Uridine diphosphate glucuronic acid	Phenols, alcohols, primary amines
Sulfotransferase	3'-Phosphoadenosine-5'-phosphosulfate	Phenols, alcohols, aromatic amines
Glutathione transferase	Glutathione	Epoxides, arene oxides, halides, nitro-groups
Epoxide hydrolase	Water	Epoxides, arene oxides
Acetyl transferase	Acetyl CoA	Primary amines
Methyl transferase	S-Adenosyl methionine	Catechols
	5-Methyltetrahydrofolic acid	Catecholamines
Glycine transferase	CoA derivatives carboxylic acids	Aromatic, heterocyclic, arylacetic acids

compounds, as well as endogenous substrates such as steroids and bilirubin.

Sulfotransferase and glucuronyl transferase can compete for similar substrates. However, at lower substrate concentrations more sulfation occurs than glucuronidation, but as the concentration of the substrate increases the amount of glucuronidation then exceeds sulfation (Moldeus, 1976). The simultaneous metabolism of aniline and p-nitroanisole by the MFO produces both p-aminophenol and p-nitrophenol, respectively; yet, even at lower concentrations the p-nitrophenol was preferentially conjugated. In fact, Caldwell (1980) reported an increase in drug toxicity when multiple drugs were given to patients, resulting from competition between drugs for similar conjugation reactions.

Glutathione-S-transferases (GSH-T) are a family of enzymes located primarily in the cytosol, but they may also occur in the endoplasmic reticulum (Morgenstern et al., 1979). Cellular glutathione (GSH) is used to conjugate a variety of substrates, including halogen- or nitrobenzenes, or aromatic epoxides (Habig et al., 1974; Chasseud, 1979; Boyer and Kenney, 1985). To increase the detoxification of the epoxide metabolites produced from metabolism of aryl hydrocarbons, GSH transferase competes with epoxide hydratase to inactivate the carcinogenic products (Oesch, 1980). In addition, under normal physiological conditions, GSH can catalyze many detoxification reactions nonenzymatically.

Metabolic cofactors.   The major determinant of the detoxification reactions is the availability of the required enzymatic cofactors—NADPH, PAPS, UDPGA, and GSH. Each of these cofactors are closely regulated and affected by nutritional status.

NADPH is generated from three enzymatic processes (Thurman and Kauffman, 1980). Using glucose-6-phosphate, generated from plasma glucose, glucogen stores, or gluconeogenesis, the pentose phosphate shunt produces two NADPHs from the enzymes glucose-6-phosphate dehydrogenase and 6-phosphogluconate dehydrogenase. In the absence of glucose or glycogen, cytosolic NADPH is generated from mitochondrial oxidations. Isocitrate diffuses through the mitochondrial membrane and is oxidized to α-ketoglutarate into the mitochondria, isocitrate is regenerated at the expense of intramitochondrial NADPH. The second substrate to leave the mitochondria is malate. It is converted to pyruvate and NADPH by malic enzyme. Again the product, pyruvate, reenters the mitochondria, and additional malate is regenerated at the expense of ATP and NADH. Thus, both of these enzyme systems utilize mitochondrial-reducing equivalents to generate cytosolic NADPH.

PAPS is synthesized from inorganic sulfate by two enzyme reactions (DeMeio, 1975). The first, ATP sulfuryltransferase, forms an ester between ATP and sulfate releasing pyrophosphate and adenosine-5′-phosphosulfate (APS). The second enzyme, APS-phosphokinase, also uses an ATP to phosphorylate APS, generating PAPS. Formation of PAPS is primarily regulated by the availability of sulfate and energy (ATP).

Dietary inorganic sulfate only provides for a small portion of the intracellular sulfate pool. The majority of cellular sulfate is obtained from the desulfuration and oxidation of the amino acid cysteine.

The synthesis of UDPGA occurs as a normal metabolic pathway branching from glucose-1-phosphate, used for glycogen synthesis, to the uronic acid pathway (Dutton and Burchell, 1975; Dutton, 1976). At the expense of UTP, UDP-glucose is formed by UDPG-phosphorylase. Then UDP-glucose dehydrogenase uses two NAD+ to oxidize UDP-glucose to UDPGA, also forming two NADHs. Thus, UDPGA availability is regulated by the presence of glucose, energy (UTP) and NAD+.

Glutathione is synthesized from three amino acids (glutamate, cysteine, and glycine) by two enzymatic reactions. Each reaction utilizes one ATP for energy. First, the dipeptide glutamylcysteine is formed by g-glutamylcysteine synthetase. Then, glycine is added by GSH synthetase to complete the tripeptide (Meister and Anderson, 1983). Thus, it is apparent that the maintenance of cellular GSH is dependent on the availability of cellular amino acids.

Dietary factors.   In man and animals, dietary factors are important to the regulation of xenobiotic metabolism and clearance. Nutrient availability is most important for the maintenance of these reactions, but nonnutrient components also affect the MFO and conjugation reactions.

Induction of enzyme activities.   Chemicals endogenous to our foods, such as indoles, safrole, and flavones, as well as manmade chemicals such as BHA (2(3)-tert-butyl-4-hydroxyanisole), chlorinated hydrocarbon pesticides and herbicides, as well as drugs and ethanol can selectively increase the enzyme activities (Snyder and Remmer, 1982). The major mechanism by which these compounds increase enzyme activities is induction, which produces an actual increase in the amount of the enzymes affected, rather than a simple activation of existing enzyme activities.

Naturally occurring plant constituents have been determined to induce the components of the MFO system. In both animal and human experiments, the inclusion of the cruciferous vegetables, cabbage and cauliflower, in the diets of animals and men produced an increase in the rate of MFO metabolism for many drugs (Pantuck et al., 1976;1979). When indoles found in these vegetables were added to purified diets, similar responses were noted, suggesting their role as inducers of drug metabolism. (Evarts and Mostafa, 1981).

Safrole (4-allyl-1,2-methlenedioxybenzene), another natural plant constituent which was used as a flavoring agent, was determined to induce cytochrome P-450, ethylmorphine-N-demethylase, nitroreductase, arylhydrocarbon hydroxylase, and biphenyl hydroxylase (Ioannides et al., 1981).

In addition, charcoal broiled beef has also been demonstrated to increase the metabolism of phenacetin (Conney et al., 1976). In this case aryl hydrocarbons are formed by pyrolysis of the fat drippings. In various animal species, these compounds increase the isozyme, cytochrome P-448, and the associated MFO activity, aryl hydrocarbon hydroxylase, which is related to the metabolism of carcinogens.

DDT and dieldrin enhance their own metabolism by induction of MFO components (Snyder and Remmer, 1982). In addition, certain pharmacological agents, e.g., phenobarbital, and even ethanol, may also induce certain isozymes of the MFO.

Less well studied are the effects of these agents on the conjugation enzymes. However, BHA, 7,8-benzoflavone, aryl hydrocarbons, aldrin, and DDT each produce increases in GT activity, apparently increasing different isozyme forms of the transferase (Lilienbaum et al., 1982). In addition, indoles, benzylisothiocyanate, and BHA induce GSH-transferases (Benson et al., 1979).

Since each of the experiments presented were idealistically evaluated in animals and humans, a perspective must be maintained on the actual daily exposure of such materials from our diet. The MFO and conjugation enzymes in individuals consuming a balanced diet are most likely under combined regulation. That is, multiple agents maintain the intestinal and perhaps the liver MFO at a relatively constant level. Only dietary extremes, such as avoidance or focused consumption of individual foods, would result in major changes in activity.

Starvation.   The state of nutrition can influence a variety of the reactions involved in xenobiotic detoxification. During starvation, cellular metabolism shifts toward catabolism. To provide energy, glycogen stores are quickly depleted, then as fatty acids are oxidized for energy, amino acids are degraded to provide glucose via gluconeogenesis. Eventually cellular enzymes, including the MFO and conjugation enzymes, would be expected to be lost. In addition, the availability of the intracellular cofactors (NADPH, PAPS, UDPGA, and GSH) would become limited.

However, many conflicting reports exist concerning human drug metabolism during starvation. For example, overweight patients who fasted for 7–10 days did not alter their clearance of either tolbutamide or antipyrine (Reidenberg and Vesell, 1975), while protein-calorie malnutrition in children caused a decreased clearance of tolbutamide, antipyrine, or chloramphenicol (Mehta et al., 1975). Decreased metabolism was indicated by increased plasma peak levels and decreased conjugated drug in the urine. Other factors, such as plasma binding proteins, may be decreased and thereby increase the availability of the drug for metabolism and clearance. Thus, interpretation of results must be made with caution.

Patients admitted for peptic ulcer were determined to be undernourished (mean albumin was 18% less and a 15% smaller body mass). From liver biopsy samples, no differences was observed for cytochrome P-450 or GSH-S-transferase, while UDPGT activity was reduced about 20% for both p-nitrophenol and chloramphenicol. Uniquely, arylhydrocarbon hydroxylase activity was increased about 20% (Rajpurohit et al., 1985).

In animal studies, the protein:carbohydrate ratio in calorically adequate diets has been shown to have an effect. Primarily, high protein diets increased drug metabolism and the MFO components while low protein and high carbohydrate diets decreased these activities. Only a few experiments have evaluated these dietary factors in man.

Although conflicts exist, authors have reported increased N- and O-dealkylation in 72-hour fasted male rats (Marcelos and Laitinen, 1975). Even following one day of food deprivation, increased metabolism and enhanced liver damage was reported for a variety of chlorinated hydrocarbons, including CCl_4 and 1,1-dichloroethylene (Nakajima and Sato, 1979). Fasting has also been found to induce a specific form of cytochrome P-450 (P-450j) (Hong et al., 1987).

Sachan and Su (1986) noted that food restriction (50% of the control) for 7 weeks resulted in a twofold increase in activity of the NADPH-generating enzymes (malic enzyme, glucose-6-phosphate dehydrogenase, and 6-phosphogluconate dehydrogenase). A slight increase in GT activity was also noted.

Interestingly, UDPGA levels decreased only 10–20% over 3 days of starvation. However, in the presence of alcohol, UDPGA levels fell more than 30% initially and by more than 60% over 72 hours (Minnigh and Zemaitis, 1982). Glucuronidation of acetaminophen was decreased in the presence of alcohol. Most likely, metabolism of alcohol by alcohol dehydrogenase increased the intracellular NADH/NAD ratio, which decreased the conversion of UDP-glucose to UDP-glucuronic acid and diminished UDPGA levels needed for glucuronidation.

Dietary protein.   Alterations of dietary protein, decreasing both quality and quantity, affects the MFO activities and the resulting xenobiotic toxicity. Both cytochrome P-450 and the reductase were reduced, as were the related metabolism of ethylmorphine, aniline, heptachlor, and aryl hydrocarbons. Certain activities were increased such as epoxide hydratase and glucuronyl transferase (Campbell and Hayes, 1976; Hietanen, 1980).

Mgbodile and Campbell (1972) showed a decrease in MFO activity in weanling rats fed a 5% casein semipurified diet for 2 weeks, compared to control animals fed a 20% casein diet. The V_{max} for ethylmorphine and aniline was decreased 66%, with equal decreases in the activity of cytochrome P-450 and the reductase. The authors noted that during this interval of time the cells had increased in size by 50%, including a threefold increase in lipid and glycogen content; yet, the microsomal protein content was depressed.

Clinton et al. (1979) reported that feeding rats a low protein diet fed from weaning decreased hepatic cytochrome P-450 content. In addition, Magdalou et al. (1979) showed that protein depletion decreased cytochrome P-450 content, total protein, and total phospholipid. Previously, Hayes et al. (1973) reported altered substrate interaction with cytochrome P-450 during protein deficiency, as well as altered induction of the MFO components by 3-methylchloanthrene (Hayes and Campbell, 1974).

When studied over a 2-month period, protein deficiency was determined to produce a biphasic decrease in microsomal cytochromes (Kuwano and Hiraga, 1980). The most rapid change occurred within the first 4 days. Aminopyrine demethylase, p-nitroanisole O-demethylase, and aniline hydroxylase also decreased in a parallel manner.

Short-term dietary deficiency has no significant effect (Hietanen, 1980). Some of the differences reported in the literature may simply result from the initial age of the animals used and the variable duration of the experimental feeding period.

The relative toxicity of a variety of insecticides, herbicides, and fungicides (captan, carbaryl, diazinon, DDT, endosulfan, lindane, and malathion) are increased from 2- to 2100-fold in protein-deficient diets (Boyd et al., 1970). In addition, increased drug toxicity has been reported for pentobarbital, phenacetin, and zoxazolamine (Kato et al., 1968). In each of these examples, the increase in toxicity results primarily from a loss of detoxification reactions. Each agent is toxic in its parent form and was not cleared.

Decreased conjugation also contributed to the increased toxicity of these compounds. As might be expected, restricted dietary protein should limit the availability of cysteine needed for synthesis of both PAPS and

GSH (Krijgsheld et al., 1981). Indeed, glutathione levels were determined to be reduced during protein deficiency (Glazenburg et al., 1983).

Protein depletion also produced changes in liver UDP-glucuronyl-transferase activity. Hietanen (1980) noted a decrease in activity, while others have reported the GT activity was increased (Wood and Woodcock, 1970; Woodcock and Wood, 1971). These differences may result from differences in methodology and substrate selection, as well as differences in dietary composition.

The main determinant of toxicity is the requirement for metabolism. If the xenobiotic is toxic to begin with, then a lower MFO activity would result in increased toxicity, whereas, if the xenobiotic agent must be activated to become toxic, then lower MFO activities would decrease the toxicity of that compound. Interestingly, protein deficiency has been associated with a decreased, but never a total, absence of the MFO activity. Alterations in the specific isozymes and their turnover may well determine the noted changes in MFO and conjugation activities.

Protein-energy malnutrition. Buchanan et al. (1980) noted an increase in the $t_{1/2}$ of acetanilide in children suffering from kwashiorkor, which decreased following increased dietary protein. Similar responses were noted for both theophylline and antipyrine in humans (Anderson et al., 1982).

Individual isozyme changes were reported by Kato et al. (1981, 1982). Soy protein diets supplemented with methionine depressed aniline hydroxylase activity but slightly elevated the aminopyrine N-demethylase activity. NADPH cytochrome c reductase and the level of cytochrome P-450 were both increased. The relative biological values of proteins were positively correlated with the aniline hydroxylase, cytochrome P-450, and reductase.

In addition, rats fed 48% of their dietary requirement of sulfur amino acids, methionine and cysteine, have reduced levels of cytochrome P-450 and an increased UDP-glucuronyl transferase activity (Magdalou et al., 1979). Mainigi and Campbell (1981) found that a low protein diet also reduced hepatic glutathione levels within a few hours, and these low levels remained low for 6 weeks. No further evaluation of this unique effect has been reported.

The hepatic glutathione concentration increased with addition of aflatoxin B_1 to the animals' diet, regardless of the dietary protein level. The acute lesions that developed in the liver were more pronounced in the rats fed a high protein diet. The latter effect reflects an increase in metabolism to the active toxicant, exceeding the detoxification pathway involving glutathione.

Methionine deficiency also reduced the glutathione levels in the liver of mice and increased the hepatotoxicity of acetaminophen (Reicks and Hathcock, 1984).

These observations are important, but more sophisticated evaluations are needed in which individual isozymes are evaluated. Again, the major changes are observed in experiments using extreme swings in protein or amino acid composition.

Dietary carbohydrates. Diets high in sucrose, glucose, or fructose produced decreased metabolism of several drugs and increased the sleeping times of animals given several different barbiturates (Strother et al., 1971). In partial explanation of these effects, Dickerson et al. (1971) reported that when diets high in sugar were fed to rats, the MFO enzyme activities and cytochrome P-450 were decreased. The mechanism of this effect remains unresolved.

Using a liquid diet in which calories were held constant, the amounts of carbohydrates, protein, and fat were varied (Nakajima et al., 1982; Sato et al., 1983). For a series of aromatic and chlorinated hydrocarbons, the rate of metabolism was inversely related to the carbohydrate content. Hepatotoxicity was also greater for animals fed the low carbohydrate diets. Uniquely, the concentration of cytochrome P-450 was determined not to be altered.

The relative quantity of carbohydrate and fat in the diet was more important than the type of carbohydrate. In most studies evaluating the effect of dietary fat and protein on drug and toxicant metabolism, substitution of carbohydrate for fat or protein nutriture has been employed to balance calories with little regard for resulting effects of carbohydrate modification. There is no specific role for carbohydrate in the MFO reaction system.

In human subjects, high carbohydrate diets have been reported to not affect drug metabolism of antipyrine and theophylline when compared to normal diets (Alvares et al., 1976; Kappas et al., 1976; Anderson et al., 1982).

The effect of diabetes on drug metabolism has been examined as well. Watkins et al. (1988) used long-term experimental insulin-dependent diabetes in adult male Sprague-Dawley rats. The development of diabetes following injection of streptozotocin was rapid and persisted over the 90-day experimental period. They evaluated benzphetamine demethylase, styrene oxide hydrolase, and UDP GT activity toward several substrates, including 1-naphthol, diethystibesterol, estrone and testosterone, and

GSH S-transferase, evaluating 1-chloro-2,4-dinitrobenzene, ethacrynic acid, and sulfobromopthalein.

Elevation of glucose was apparent (123 vs 557 mg/dL) in the diabetic animals, but no differences were noted in the circulating aminotransferase or in hepatic protein levels. Interestingly, cytochrome P-450 was reduced by 25%, epoxide hydratase was decreased slightly, and glutathione transferase activities were decreased 30–40% by the diabetes treatment. Diabetes had little effect on the N-demethylase activity or the GT activity for 1-naphthol or estrone GT activity, while the diabetic animals increased the DES GT activity and decreased testosterone GT activity. Following acute challenge by bromobenzene or carbon tetrachloride the hepatotoxicity of these agents was greater in the diabetic animals than in the controls. Similar observations have been reported by Hanasono et al. (1977a,b), who characterized the potentiation of carbon tetrachloride hepatotoxicity in alloxan- or streptozotocin-treated diabetic rats.

Skett and Joels (1985) compared differences between acute and chronic diabetes mellitus on hepatic drug metabolism. The mechanism by which sugar, or diabetes, affects changes in the components of the MFO and conjugation enzymes remains undefined. However, the changes identified above indicate that specific isozymes were affected, suggesting a higher level of regulation and specificity than previously recognized.

Dietary lipids. The integrity of the microsomal membrane is essential for maintaining interaction between the reductase and cytochrome P-450. In reconstituted enzyme systems, inclusion of phosphatidylcholine was determined to be essential for maximum activity (Strobel et al., 1970). Since the B-position fatty acid of this phospholipid is highly unsaturated, it might be expected that dietary lipids could affect MFO activity.

The role of dietary lipids in regulating the fatty acid content of the endoplasmic reticulum has been well established (Hammer and Wills, 1978). Indeed, without the essential fatty acids in the diet, the membrane lipids become more saturated. Although the reductase was unaffected, cytochrome P-450 and several MFO activities were decreased (Marshall and McLean, 1971; Norred and Wade, 1972; Wade et al., 1978). In addition, the inclusion of unsaturated lipids in the diet provided higher MFO activities and allowed a greater induction of cytochrome P-450 and the MFO activities.

Species differences may affect these membrane changes as well. Unsaturated dietary fat enhanced drug metabolism in cebus monkeys but not in squirrel monkeys (Meyandi et al., 1985). Only a few studies have examined these effects in man, and no changes have been noted (Anderson et al., 1979). The lack of an effect may be due to the short duration of the dietary changes or due to the limited number of drug substrates evaluated or another species difference.

Alcohol. Ethanol inhibits drug metabolism in vivo and in vitro. However, the in vitro concentrations require much higher levels to produce similar effects than those seen in cells. For example, in perfused liver, drug metabolism was inhibited 50% by 2–5 mM ethanol, while in microsomes 130 mM ethanol was required to provide the same inhibition. If 4-methylpyrazole was included to inhibit alcohol dehydrogenase, pNA metabolism was greatly reduced. Thus, either the metabolite, acetaldehyde, or the resultant NADH formed, or both, contributed to the decreased metabolism (Reinke et al., 1980a).

Using phenobarbital-treated animals, Reinke et al. (1980b) reported that inclusion of xylitol and sorbitol stimulated pNA metabolism in perfused livers from fasted but not fed animals. NADH generated by the metabolism of the sugar alcohols enhanced pNA metabolism. In vitro addition of NADH increased pNA metabolism by the MFO but was unaffected by ethanol or sorbitol directly, whereas acetaldehyde addition inhibited pNA metabolism in both microsomes (Ki = 5 mM) and perfused livers (Ki = 0.5 mM). Thus, the acetaldehyde by-product may be responsible for MFO inhibition.

Another possible interpretation of these results could be based on the availability of NADPH. If the rate of the MFO activity in the intact cells is limited by the generation of cytosolic NADPH, then during metabolism of alcohol NADH is produced. Accumulation of reducing equivalents by the mitochondria inhibits the TCA cycle and limits the availability of malate and α-ketoglutarate necessary for the generation of cytosolic NADPH via the mitochondrial shuttle. This interpretation would also provide an explanation for the greater impact of ethanol on drug metabolism in the livers from the fasted animals. Thus, the MFO activity may well be inhibited indirectly by the limitation of NADPH.

Reinke et al. (1986) observed that the rates of glucuronidation and sulfation were diminished in perfused rat livers after chronic alcohol administration. Since both processes were inhibited, a decrease in cytosolic energy may be produced.

Glucuronidation in isolated hepatocytes is inhibited by ethanol, but not by acetaldehyde. The change in the intracellular NADH/NAD ratio may reduce the formation of UDPGA from UDPG. This interpretation has been supported using sorbitol and lactate, both of which also inhibited glucuronidation (Moldeus et al., 1978). Long-term exposure to alcohol may result in the induction of glucuronyl transferase similar to the induction of a specific isozyme of cytochrome P-450 (Lieber, 1984).

Vitamins.   Both the water-soluble and fat-soluble vitamins have an effect on the MFO system in experimental animals. Deficiencies of individual or multiple B vitamins have decreased specific isozymes of the cytochrome P-450 system, as well as GT (Miltenberger and Oltersdorf, 1978). Considering the critical roles played by vitamins in cellular energy metabolism as well as their interaction in metabolizing each other into their active coenzymes, these results are not surprising.

Deficiency of thiamin increased hepatochlor and aniline metabolism in liver microsomes, while supplementation with thiamin decreased the same activities (Wade et al., 1969). The supplemented animals were found to have lowered cytochrome P-450 and b5 content (Grosse and Wade, 1971). The reductase was reduced as well. However, Wade et al. (1975) concluded that the decrease was due to the type of carbohydrate rather than to the vitamin itself. Rats fed high thiamin diets containing sucrose had decreased cytochrome P-450 content, while rats fed similar diets containing starch did not have the depressed cytochrome levels. Uniquely, the metabolism was reduced in both carbohydrate diets.

The direct effect of riboflavin deficiency is of major interest since the NADPH cytochrome P-450 reductase is a flavoprotein, containing one mole each of FMN and FAD. During dietary depletion, the FMN moiety is lost while the FAD moiety is retained (Hara and Taniguchi, 1982). This is not unexpected, since FMN is more loosely bound to the protein. In addition, the level of FMN in the liver was below the concentration necessary to saturate the reductase, and when an excess of FAD was available it became bound to the FMN site. The loss of the reductase activity was paralleled by a decrease in the metabolism of aniline, acetanilide, aminopyrine, and ethylmorphine. Similar decreases in drug metabolism were reported by Patel and Pawar, (1974). Catz et al. (1970) and Yang (1974) reported a decrease in the content of cytochrome P-450 and aryl hydrocarbon hydroxylase activity.

Iyanagi et al. (1974) indicated separate roles for the two species of flavins in the reductase. FAD served as an electron receptor for NADPH, and FMN served as the electron donor for the cytochrome P-450 system (Vermilion and Coon, 1978; Vermilion et al., 1981).

In vitro addition of flavins has also been shown to stimulate reduction of nitro and azo compounds (Williams et al., 1970; Shargel and Mazel, 1973). Thus, the azo-reductase appears to be a flavoprotein sensitive to the availability of flavin as well.

Numerous experiments have been reported evaluating the effect of vitamin C deficiency on drug metabolism (Holloway and Petersen, 1984). Ascorbic acid–deficient guinea pigs had longer sleep times than did the control animals following pentobarbital administration. In addition,

Conney et al. (1961) reported an increased paralysis time in ascorbic acid–deficient guinea pig treated with zoxazolamine, related to reduced metabolism of the drugs by the MFO system.

Using guinea pigs, the deficiency of vitamin C produced a progressive change in the microsomal components of the MFO. During the first 10–12 days, no changes in the reductase or in cytochrome P-450 were noted, but hydroxylation reactions were decreased. By 21 days, which is necessary to produce vitamin C deficiency, both N- and O-dealkylation reactions were also decreased (Zannoni et al., 1977; Sikic et al., 1977). GSH-transferase was also decreased. Upon resupplementation with vitamin C, the hepatic vitamin C levels returned to normal within 3 days, while recovery of the MFO activities required 6 days. These results might suggest an effect of the vitamin deficiency on protein synthesis, but induction of the MFO components by phenobarbital was not impaired. Thus, further clarification is needed.

Depletion of vitamin A stores, produced a decrease in cytochrome P-450 and a variety of MFO activities, suggesting a generalized effect of retinol deficiency on xenobiotic metabolism (Colby et al., 1975; Miranda et al., 1979). These effects occurred prior to the appearance of other symptomologies of vitamin A deficiency.

It should also be noted that the MFO is involved in metabolism and clearance of retinol and retinoic acid. Induction of the MFO by phenobarbital led to an increased rate of vitamin A depletion and initiating the onset of vitamin A deficiency. After treatment with ethanol, a specific isozyme of Cytochrome P-450 is induced that not only metabolizes ethanol, but also increases the metabolism of retinoic acid (Sato and Lieber, 1982; Leo et al., 1984). Retinoic acid is also cleared in part by UDPGA conjugation via GT to retinoyl glucuronide (DeLuca et al., 1981). Although the glucuronide is a well established pathway, little work has focused on characterization of the specific glucuronyl transferase isozyme involved.

Vitamin E deficiency also produced decreases in MFO activities, specifically N-dealkylation reactions for codeine and aminopyrine (Carpenter, 1972; Horn et al., 1976). Uniquely, neither the reductase nor the cytochrome P-450 were altered, and the MFO activities were still induced by both phenobarbital and 3-methylcholanthrene. In addition, dietary repletion of vitamin E returned the MFO activity to normal within 48 hours. This effect may suggest that vitamin E participates as an integral part of the lipid matrix, coupling the reductase to cytochrome P-450 for electron transfer.

Chen et al (1982) found no change in the reductase or cytochrome b5. However, cytochrome P-450 was decreased, as was ethyl morphine N-demethylase and benzo(a)pyrene hydroxylation (Chen et al., 1982). Aminolevulinic acid dehydrogenase was also decreased (Carpenter, 1972; Horn et al., 1976), but this would not explain the discrepancy between a loss in cytochrome P-450 and no loss in cytochrome b5 concentration. Since vitamin E scavenges free radicals, it may protect the membrane integrity and thereby preserve MFO activity. The loss was predicted to be secondary to increased oxidative damage, either as a loss of membrane integrity or simply the loss of the vitamin E stabilizing factor.

Minerals. Due to the complex alterations that occur in cellular metabolism during mineral depletion, very little information has been reported concerning their effects on xenobiotic metabolism and clearance.

Iron has a central role in the synthesis of heme and hemoproteins, including cytochrome P-450. Iron deficiency is normally characterized by anemia and is most prevalent among children and young women.

Related to the essential role played by iron in heme synthesis, it would be expected that iron deficiency might alter metabolism of xenobiotics in the body. In adult mice, iron deficiency (hematocrits reduced to 35% of controls) produced no change in either nitroreductase or arylhydrocarbon hydroxylase activities, while metabolism of aminopyrine and hexobarbital was increased (Catz et al., 1970).

In iron depletion studies in rats, Becking (1972,1976) did not find changes in cytochrome P-450 or cytochrome b5 concentrations. In one case, iron depletion for 40 days increased aniline metabolism in vitro and in vivo by 30%. No change in cytochrome P-450 was noted, but an apparent increase in the reductase was noted after 25–35 days. Becking (1976) also noted that upon refeeding of the deficient animals, the enzyme activities returned to normal within 7 days.

Peters and Fouts (1970a,b) noted that the NADPH oxidase and NADPH cytochrome C reductase activities were increased when magnesium was added to the in vitro rat hepatic microsomal preparation. Magnesium appeared to enhance electron flow to the substrate bound to the cytochrome. With elevated magnesium concentrations, the oxidase was decreased while the reductase activity was increased.

Dietary magnesium alters in vivo and in vitro MFO systems in rats. After 12 days on a magnesium-deficient diet, decreased reductase, cytochrome P-450, and metabolism of aminopyrine and aniline was determined (Becking, 1976). In vivo and in vitro metabolism of pentobarbital was affected. Since magnesium is required for optimum drug metabolism in vitro, it seems important to separate the results obtained from the changes that would be produced by diminished availability of cellular energy, such as starvation or altered protein synthesis.

Magnesium depletion (10 days) was compared to 18 days of magnesium deficiency (Brown and Bidlack, 1988). At 10 days, the growth rate was not yet affected, there were no overt signs of deficiency, nor was there a change in hepatic concentration of magnesium. Metabolism of p-nitroanisole and aniline were reduced 16% and 30%, respectively, in the depleted animals compared to pair-fed controls. Importantly no alterations in the total cytochrome P-450 or reductase levels occurred. Thus, the possibility exists that specific isozymes may have been affected.

However, by 18 days cytochrome P-450 was reduced 30% and p-nitroanisole O-demethylation was reduced 60%. These animals had symptoms of deficiency and were growing at a diminished rate.

Uniquely at 10 days, the glucuronyl transferase activity was decreased by 50% in the magnesium-depleted animals. When the microsomal membranes were washed with EDTA to remove residual cations, it was noted that the magnesium-depleted animals had either lost a specific isozyme or the cation regulation site had been altered (Brown et al., 1988). This observation is especially intriguing since multiple isozymes of GT have been characterized, and various inducing agents affect different izozyme activities (Lilienblum et al., 1982).

In isolated hepatocytes, p-nitroanisole metabolism and p-nitrophenol glucuronidation were diminished. The evaluation of glucuronidation suggested the Km was shifted to a higher concentration of p-nitrophenol (Brown and Bidlack, unpublished). Again the data would suggest a specific regulation of certain isozyme activities in magnesium depletion. Additional examination of these observations continue, extending to the potential molecular regulation of certain isozymes by magnesium.

An improved understanding of the integral roles played by dietary factors in the regulation of hepatic drug and toxicant metabolism can only be examined by animal studies. The results obtained may eventually provide us with the ability to diminish xenobiotic initiated hepatotoxicity, but extrapolation to the human situation must be handled with care.

Kidney filtration.   Urinary excretion is the primary route for elimination of water-soluble drugs and their metabolites. They are handled by filtration, selective resorption, and secretion (Hewitt and Hook, 1983).

The kidney has a filtration apparatus, which extracts unbound drugs into the tubules. After filtration, weak acids like barbituates or weak bases such as amphetamines may be reabsorbed in a pH-dependent manner. Primarily, transport occurs by diffusion.

Strong acids and bases act differently. They are handled in the proximal tubule cells by specific transport processes. These processes appear to be bidirectional. For example, penicillin is almost exclusively secreted, while bile acids are almost exclusively reabsorbed.

Drugs are transported from the blood by a sodium-dependent or sodium-independent process. The former occurs in conjunction with a facilitative diffusion process. The xenobiotics are then eliminated at the brush border site by diffusion. The overall process leads to a 30-fold tubule/blood concentration difference.

Transport can be produced by the chemical nature of the compounds as well. Cations are taken up from the blood by facilitated diffusion, driven by the elctrical membrane potential. In this case, their secretion into the lumen is coupled with protons to an antiport.

Glomerular filtration. Glomerular filtration is a passive process whereby a nearly protein-free filtrate of plasma enters the tubular lumen by ultrafiltration through the glomerular capillaries. The glomerular membrane selectively permits the passage of small molecules and ions such as water, urea, sodium, chloride, and glucose, but not large molecules such as most proteins or cells. However, albumin and hemoglobin will pass through the membrane in small amounts, but in general they are resorbed.

The forces which determine fluid exchange across extrarenal capillary endothelia are also those producing glomerular ultrafiltration. Glomerular capillary hydrostatic pressure, the main driving force, is generated by the arterial blood pressure. The drop in hydrostatic pressure, which occurs in capillaries as the fluid passes from the arterial end of the capillary to the venous end, diminishes net ultrafiltration across the capillaries. Conversely, in the glomerular capillary the hydrostatic pressure is maintained by the presence of an arteriole at the distal end of the capillary. The constant hydrostatic pressure is associated with increasing oncotic pressure along the glomerular capillary owing to the extrusion of water, resulting in a fall in ultrafiltration pressure along the length of the glomerular capillary. Although the net ultrafiltration pressures are similar in systemic and glomerular capillaries, the rate of fluid flow is greater in the glomerular capillaries. Thus, surface area and permeability must be greater in the glomerular capillaries, allowing for rapid filtration of materials across the glomerulus.

The urinary excretion of a drug or toxicant or their metabolites will depend on the rate of delivery of the substance to the kidney. The rate will depend on plasma flow to the kidney and the volume of distribution of the drug. On the other hand, the rate of elimination will be determined by the percentage of unbound drug. If a drug is not protein bound and is neither secreted nor reabsorbed, the rate of clearance will approach the

372 Bidlack and Riebow

glomerular filtration rate, e.g., gentamicin and inulin (Pastoriza-Munoz et al., 1979). Any factor that affects protein binding alters the pharmacokinetics and the rate of excretion.

Reabsorption.   Reabsorption is the transport, either passive or active, of substances out of the tubular fluid. The kidney has a primary function to reabsorb the bulk of glomerular filtrate, allowing for the excretion of water and the retention of essential elements. From 98 to 99% of the salt and water, and essentially all of the filtered bicarbonate, glucose, and amino acids, are reabsorbed.

The active reabsorption of salt and reabsorption of water in the proximal tubule causes drugs and other substances in the urine to become highly concentrated, providing then the driving force for passive reabsorption. The rate of reabsorption is dependent on concentration and urine flow. Diffusion across the tubular cell will be affected by the solubility of the compound in urine versus the plasma and by the ability of the compound to penetrate the lipid cell membrane.

Urinary pH can also impact diffusion. If the compound is an acid, and the urine is made alkaline with bicarbonate, more acid will be charged and therefore retained in the urine. The principles for transport are the same as those discussed earlier for absorption from the stomach.

Active processes in the proximal tubule enhance the reabsorption of certain organic compounds. Most of these compounds are endogenous compounds, such as sugars, amino acids, vitamin C, urate, etc. Few drugs are actively transported; however, lithium, fluoride, bromide, and 1-methyldopa are examples of those agents actively reabsorbed (Young and Edwards, 1966; Reidenberg, 1971).

Secretion.   Tubular secretion is the movement of compounds from plasma into the tubular lumen. The clearance of a substance that is secreted and not reabsorbed will be greater than the clearance of inulin (not secreted). Consequently, secreted substances will be rapidly eliminated from plasma and will be found in relatively high concentrations in the urine. Tubular secretion occurs by active transport. The efficiency of (secretion) transport is not limited by plasma protein binding (Keen, 1971). Organic anions and cations are secreted into the proximal tubule by separate transport processes (Rennick, 1981; Hewitt and Hook, 1983).

The binding of xenobiotics to plasma proteins has been shown to alter the rate at which the agents are filtered at the glomerulus but does not alter the rate of tubular secretion of most compounds. The rapid removal of phenol red, penicillins, and PAH, all 80–90% bound, by the tubular secretory mechanism serve as classic examples which support this theory.

There are exceptions; Bowman (1975) demonstrated that the extensive binding of furosemide to albumin retarded the secretory process. the rate of secretion was determined to be dependent in part on the concentration of unbound drug. Hook et al. (1976) also observed the influence of plasma protein binding on the secretory process in the studies of 2,4,5-trichlorophenoxyacetic acid, an herbicide.

Protein intake influences glomerular filtration and endogenous creatinine clearance (Bosch et al., 1983). Dietary-induced changes in urine pH and ionization of drugs also alter drug reabsorption.

Pullman et al. (1954) reported that feeding of a low protein diet to healthy young subjects lowered their glomerular filtration rate, effective renal plasma flow, and the tubular excretion of p-aminohippurate, while a high protein diet raised each of the test parameters.

Normal dietary subjects had significantly higher creatinine clearance than normal vegetarians. An increased protein intake in normal volunteers produced a significant increase in creatinine clearance. The capacity of the kidney to increase its level of function with protein intake suggests a renal function reserve.

However, if the number of nephrons is reduced, i.e., by disease or age, the renal function reserve may be diminished (Brenner et al., 1982). Alleyne (1967) noted specifically that malnourished children had several functional renal lesions. A reduction in glomerular filtration rate and renal plasma flow and evidence of impaired tubular function was shown by the existence of aminoaciduria, renal phosphaturia, impaired urinary concentration, and ability to excrete an acid load. With recovery there was steady improvement in renal function. The etiology of the lesions may have been related to the deficiencies of magnesium and potassium which occur in malnourished children.

Severe malnutrition decreases the elimination of several antibiotics, including tetracycline, cefoxitin, gentamycin, penicillin, and tobramycin (Buchanan, 1984). Mild or moderate undernutrition without kidney damage causes more rapid drug elimination.

Many food additives and environmental toxicants are excreted through the kidney. When BHA was given as an oral dose, Hirose et al. (1987) determined that 87–96% was excreted in the urine within 48 hours. Following an oral dose of 2-amino-3-methylimidazo[4,5-f] quinoline, metabolites were excreted in the urine (Peleran et al., 1987). The metabolites included N-acetylated imidazole quinoline and 3-N-dimethyl imidazole quinoline. Similar compounds have been identified as metabolites produced from pyrolysates of meat and sardines (Yamazoe et al., 1984; Shinohara et al., 1984).

Enterohepatic circulation.   After intestinal absorption, xenobiotics are carried with the portal blood to the liver, where they move from the periportal region of the lobules to the pericentral region. The fenestrated endothelium of the hepatic sinusoids brings the xenobiotic in close contact with the hepatocytes. These cells form a barrier between the blood and the bile, sealed by tight junctions.

The daily formation of bile acids accounts for a major portion of cholesterol turnover (Klassen and Watkins, 1984). The initial oxidation products of cholesterol are chenodeoxycholic and cholic acid. Cholate is further oxidized to deoxycholic acid or conjugated with taurine or glycine to form taurocholate and glycocholate, respectively. Lipophilic substances that pass into the bile are readily solubilized. Upon entry into the gastrointestinal tract, the bile acids serve to form lipid micelles to assure absorption of fats and fat-soluble vitamins. In addition, certain xenobiotics may also reenter the body as part of those micelles.

Xenobiotics are taken up by hepatocytes by a a variety of mechanisms. Uncharged agents, such as nitrosdimethyamine, 1-naphthol, and PCBs, appear to be transported by diffusion. Drugs associated with lipoproteins may be taken up by receptor-mediated endocytosis. Inulin is taken up by fluid-phase endocytosis. Some heavy metals are taken up by cation channels, but a wide variety of drugs are transported by highly efficient drug-specific carrier systems in the sinusoidal membrane.

These carriers are probably specific for endogenous compounds but have been characterized using xenobiotic agents of interest or having special characteristics (Schwenk, 1987). Three groups of carriers exist: those which actively transport drugs into liver cells, those which release newly formed conjugates from the liver cell into the blood, and those which transport drugs and conjugates into the bile. None of these systems has been unequivocally characterized, and thus the mechanism of their function remains a mystery.

Sinusoidal transport.   The liver sinusoidal membrane is a highly dynamic structure. About 20 xenobiotics are among the compounds studied in isolated hepatocytes. Many of these compounds compete for transport with each other. Kinetic analysis allows distinction between four different types of carrier systems with overlapping specificities (Schwenk, 1987):

Carrier 1.   The first carrier is identical to the active bile acid carrier, but also transports a variety of drugs. In this carrier, active transport system transport is promoted by an active sodium gradient (Ziegler et al., 1984; Wieland et al., 1984.)

Carrier 2.   The second carrier transports a variety of organic anions, which contain strong or weak acid groups. These anions are accumulated in the hepatocyte, probably by binding to intracellular macromolecules. A specific carrier protein associated with carrier 2 has been isolated, which binds bilirubin and bromosulphophthalein (Reichen and Berk, 1979; Inagaki et al., 1985).

Carrier 3. The third carrier transports a variety of organic cations by active transport produced by the sodium gradient.

Carrier 4. The fourth carrier transports ouabain by an ATP-dependent active transport system (Schwenk et al., 1981).

Canicular transport. Canicular membrane vesicles suggest bile acid secretion is an active, carrier-mediated process and is not dependent on a sodium gradient. The driving force appears to be provided by the membrane potential which pushes the anions out of the cell (Meier et al., 1984).

The high bile/plasma concentration gradient (sometimes more than 1000) of many drugs is the result of various cellular-biological events (active hepatocellular uptake, transcellular transport, active biliary secretion, ductular water reabsorption) and physiochemical interactions (integration of drugs into pericanalicular membranes and mixed biliary micelles).

Intestinal secretion. Excretion of absorbed xenobiotics into the feces has been considered to occur primarily through biliary excretion. However, recent studies have indicated that for some xenobiotics, intestinal excretion may be a major route of elimination. To be transported from the serosa to the lumen of the intestine, a xenobiotic has to diffuse (or be transported) across the capillary endothelium, the longitudinal, circular and submucosal muscles, and the mucosa (Bohlen, 1984).

The mechanisms involved in the transport of xenobiotics from the blood to the lumen are similar to those already discussed for absorption (Binder, 1979). For most lipophilic compounds, passive diffusion is the major process contributing to the transport across the gut wall. The nature of the translumenal transport may vary along the length of the gastrointestinal tract with respect to physiological membrane changes, pH of the lumen, contents of the lumen, fluid content, etc. Hydrophilic substances may be secreted via the cellular and paracellular routes.

The turnover of fluids includes 3 L secreted into the intestines each day. However, depending on the point of entry, resorption may conserve the agent rather than providing for its excretion.

Schanker (1959) first suggested that intestinal excretion occurred based on quinine secretion into the intestine of a rat preparation. More recently, Mu et al. (1975) reported that prior to bile diversion 77% of an injected dose of quinoline methanol appeared in the feces, while after bile diversion 14% was still excreted into the intestinal contents.

Endogenous urate is secreted into the gastrointestinal tract, accounting for 25-30% of the daily output. In the rat, urate is transported across the proximal and distal segments of small intestine by a nonsaturable process (Dukes et al., 1983). Although chemically similar, hydroxanthine and xanthine are actively secreted in the GI tract (Kolassa et al., 1980).

During absorption, many agents are metabolized in the mucosal lining of the gastrointestinal tract. During excretion, a chemical may also be metabolized in the mucosa before reaching the intestinal lumen. In the lumen the compound or its metabolite may be reabsorbed, metabolized enzymatically or nonenzymatically by gut microflora, or become adsorbed to the fecal mass and thereafter excreted.

In an experiment related to a clinical therapeutic situation, elimination of digoxin was examined (Lauterbach, 1975). The digoxin, administered intravascularly, was eliminated extensively in jejunal perfusates in guinea pigs with both kidney and bile duct cannulations in place. These experiments also supported the role of intestinal excretion. The process was further characterized to be an active excretion process (Holland and Quay, 1976).

Many organochlorine compounds such a chlordecone, mirex, and dieldrin appear in feces after parenteral administration. However, in these experiments the amounts recovered closely match those calculated for biliary excretion alone (Health and Vandekar, 1964; Pittman et al., 1976; Boyan et al., 1979; Bungay et al., 1981).

Finally, these processes have been determined to occur in man as well. A man, having a cholecystostemy, was exposed to chlordecone and the agent was isolated from the gastrointestinal tract (Guzelian, 1982).

CONCLUSIONS

From the detailed discussion presented in this chapter, it should now be apparent that the body is under tight physiological regulation. Each of the biochemical and physiological processes described interact efficiently to handle nutrient absorption, distribution, and utilization to assure the health of the whole animal. In addition, many of the components of this intricate system have evolved to handle endogenously generated products in a manner necessary to prevent potential toxicity.

During evolution, these same transport and metabolism processes also became our major defense network, protecting the body from exogenous toxicants. This system is so efficient that in order to study toxicity or carcinogenesis, extremely high levels of the xenobiotic agent must be given to override the defense mechanisms. Unfortunately, these results are constantly being extrapolated back linearly to suggest a direct dose risk at low levels. In most cases these correlations do not stand up under careful scrutiny.

First, the body handles hundreds to thousands of individual chemicals every day without any sign of toxicity or cellular damage. These compounds are natural constituents of our food supply and our environment, and yet our life expectancy continues to rise with each generation.

Second, daily exposure to a multitude of environmental agents occurring as a by-product of urbanization and industrialization has not produced illness or disease in large population groups so exposed. The greatest self-exposure has been the use of cigarettes and alcohol. It is quite certain that the incidence of cancer rises for this population group, but it should be noted that the majority of individuals using these toxicants do not become ill. Those who do contract lung disease or cancer have continually exposed themselves to these agents over a lifetime.

Third, animal experiments are necessary to gain insight into the mechanism of toxicity of individual xenobiotics. With such data, decisions can be made on risk vs benefit. Unfortunately, the evaluation of how well the animals handled low dose exposures usually goes unmentioned. If extrapolations are to be made for toxicity, then consideration should also be expressed for the efficiency of handling physiological exposure levels. In addition, most toxicology studies make little effort to standardize the diets used, not just for nutrient content but for other components which may alter enzyme rates and physiological response.

Lastly, a large number of studies have now been completed examining the role of food and food components in xenobiotic absorption from the gastrointestinal tract, the role of nutritional status in altering transport and metabolism of xenobiotics, and the elimination reactions which clear these agents from the body. Much of the knowledge gained in this area has developed with the evaluation of therapeutic efficacy in patients having less than ideal nutritional status (Arcy and Merkus, 1980; Berchtold et al., 1984; Meydani, 1987). Very little practical knowledge has been generated evaluating direct interactions between toxicants and dietary components.

Hopefully, this chapter has provided a sufficient overview of these interactions to provide the reader with new insight. At the same time we hope the material stimulated the young and older researcher alike to consider examining some of these areas further.

ACKNOWLEDGMENT

This work was supported in part by a grant provided by Calreco, Inc.

REFERENCES

Abernathy, D. R. and Greenblatt, D. J. 1982. Pharmacokinetics of drugs in obesity. *Clin. Pharmacokinet.* 7: 108–124.

Adithan, C., Gandhi, I. S., and Chandrasekar, S. 1978. Pharmacokinetics of phenylbutazone in undernutrition. *Indian J. Pharmacol.* 10: 301–308.

Aitio, A. (Ed.). 1978. *Conjugation Reactions in Drug Biotransformation.* Elsevier/North Holland Biomedical Press, New York.

Alleyne, G. A. O. 1967. The effect of severe protein calorie malnutrition on the renal function of Jamaican children. *Pediatrics* 39: 400–411.

Alvares, A. P. 1976. Interactions between environmental chemicals and drug biotransformation in man. *Clin. Pharmacokinetic* 3: 452–477.

Alvares, A. P., Anderson, K. E., Conney, A. H., and Kappas, A. 1976. Interaction between nutritional factors and drug biotransformations in man. Proc. *Natl. Acad. Sci.* 73: 2501–2504.

Anderson, K. E., Conney, A. H., and Kappas, A. 1982. Nutritional influences on chemical biotransformations in humans. *Nutr. Rev.* 40: 161–171.

Anderson, K. E., Conney, A. H., and Kappas, A. 1979. Nutrition and oxidative drug metabolism in man: Relative influence of dietary lipids, carbohydrates, and protein. *Clin. Pharmacol. Ther.* 26: 493–501.

Anderson, K. E., Conney, A. H., and Kappas, A. 1982. Nutritional Influences on chemical biotransformation in humans. *Nutr. Rep. Int.* 40: 161–171.

Arcy, P. F. D. and Merkus, F. W. H. M. 1980. Food and drug interactions: influence of food on drug bioavailability and toxicity. *Pharmacy International* Dec.: 238–244.

Barbezat, G. O. and Habsen, J. D. L. 1968. The exocrine pancreas and protein calorie malnutrition. *Pediatrics* 42: 77–92.

Baron, J., Burke, J. P., Guergerich, P., Jakoby, W. B., and Voigt, J. M. 1988. Sites for xenobiotic activation and detoxification within the respiratory tract: Implications for chemically induced toxicity. *Toxicol. Appld. Pharm.* 93: 493–505.

Bates, T. R. and Gibaldi, M. 1970. *Current Concepts in the Pharmaceutical Sciences: Biopharmaceutics,* (Ed.) Swarbrick, J., pp. 57–99. Lea and Febiger, Philadelphia, PA.

Becking, G. C. 1972. Influence of dietary iron levels on hepatic drug metabolism in vivo and in vitro in the rat. *Biochem. Pharmacol.* 21: 1585–1593.

Becking, G. C. 1976. Hepatic drug metabolism in iron, magnesium, and potassium deficient rats. *Fed. Proc.* 35: 2480–2486.

Beermann, B. and Groschinsky-Grind, M. 1978. Enhancement of the gastrointestinal absorption of hydrochlorothiazide by propantheline. *Europ. J. Clin. Pharmacol.* 13: 385–387.

Benson, A. M., Cha, Y. N., Bueding, E., Heine, H. S., and Talalay, P. 1979. Elevation of extrahepatic glutathione S-transferase and epoxide hydratase activities by 2(3)-tert-butyl-4-hydroxyanisole. *Cancer Res.* 39: 2971–2977.

Berchtold, P., Weihrauch, T. R., and Berger, M. 1984. Food and drug interactions on digestive absorption. *Wld. Rev. Nutr. Diet.* 43: 10–33.

Bickel, M. H. 1975. Binding of chlorpromazine and imipramine to red cells, albumin, lipoproteins and other blood components. *J. Pharm. Pharmacol.* 27: 733–738.

Bidlack, W. R. 1982. Toxicant metabolism and the role of nutrients. *Food Technol.* 36: 106–113.

Bidlack, W. R. and Lowery, G. L. 1982. Multiple drug metabolism: p-nitoanisole reversal of acetone enhanced aniline hydroxylation. *Biochem. Pharmac.* 31: 311–318.

Bidlack, W. R. and Smith, C. H. 1984. Effect of nutritional factors on hepatic drug and toxicant metabolism. *J. Amer. Dietetic Assoc.* 84: 892–898.

Bidlack, W. R., Brown, R. D., and Mohan, C. 1986. Nutritional parameters that alter hepatic drug metabolism, conjugation and clearance. *Fed. Proc.* 45: 142–148.

Binder, H. J. 1979, *Mechanisms of Intestinal Secretion.* A. R. Liss, New York.

Bohlen, H. G. 1984. Regional vascular behavior in the gastrointestinal wall. *Fed. Proc.* 43: 7–15.

Boobis, S. W. and Chignell, C. F. 1979. Effect of protein concentration on the binding of drugs to human serum albumin. I. sulfadiazine, salicylate and indomethacin. *Biochem. Pharmacol.* 29: 752–755.

Borowitz, J. L., Moore, P. F., Yim, G. K. M., and Miya, T. S. 1971.

Mechanism of enhanced drug effects produced by dilution of the oral dose. *Toxicol. Appl. Pharmacol.* 19: 164–168.

Bosch, J., Saccaggi, A., Lauer, A., and Ronco, C. 1983. Renal function reserve in humans: Effect of protein intake on glomerular filtration rate. *Am. J. Med.* 75: 943–949.

Bowman, R. H. 1975. Renal secretion of [^{35}S]flurosemide and its depression by albumin binding. *Amer. J. Physiol.* 220: 93–98.

Bowmer, C. J. and Lindup, W. E. 1980. Inverse dependence of binding constants upon albumin concentration: results for L-tryptophan and three anionic dyes. *Biochim. Biophys. Acta* 624: 260–270.

Boyd, E. M., Dobos, I., and Krijnen, C. J. 1970. Endosulfan toxicity and dietary protein. *Arch. Envir. Health.* 21: 15–21.

Boyer, T. D. and Kenney, W. C. 1985. Preparation, characterization and properties of glutathione-S-transferases. In *Methodological Aspects of Drug Metabolizing Enzymes, Biochemical Pharmacology and Toxicology,* Vol. 1, (Ed.). Zakim, D. and Vessey, D. A., p. 297. John Wiley and Sons, New York.

Boylan, J. J., Cohn, W. J., Egle, J. L., Blanke, R. V. and Guzelian, P. S. 1979. *Clin. Pharmacol. Ther.* 25: 579–585.

Brandt, J. L., Castleman, L., Ruskin, H. D., Greenwald, J., Kelly, J. J., and Jones, A. 1955. The effect of oral protein and glucose feeding on splanchic blood flow and oxygen utilization in normal and cirrhotic subjects. *J. Clin. Invest.* 34: 1017–1025.

Brenner, M. B., Meyer, T. W., and Hostetter, T. H. 1982. Dietary protein intake and the progressive nature of kidney disease: the role of hemodynamically mediated glomerular sclerosis in aging, renal ablation and intrinsic renal disease. *N. Engl. J. Med.* 307: 652–659.

Brodersen, R., Sjodin, T., and Sjoholm, I. 1977. Independent binding of ligands to human serum albumin. *J. Biol. Chem.* 252: 5067–5072.

Brodie, M. J., Boobis, A. R., Toverud, E. L., Ellis, W., Murray, S., Dollery, C. T., Webster, S., and Harrison, R. 1980. Drug metabolism in vegetarians. *Br. J. Clin. Pharmacol.* 9: 523–525.

Bronaugh, R. L., Stewart, R. F., and Congdon, E. R. 1982a. Methods for in vitro percutaneous absorption studies. I. Comparison with in vivo results. *Toxicol. Appl. Pharmacol.* 62: 474–480.

Bronaugh, R. L., Stewart, R. F., and Congdon, E. R. 1982b. Methods for in vitro percutaneous absorption studies. II. Animal models for human skin. *Toxicol. Appl. Pharmacol.* 62: 481–488.

Brown, R. C., Meskin, and Bidlack, W. R. 1988.

Brown, R. C. and Bidlack, W. R. 1988. Altered glucuronyl transferase activity in magnesium depleted rats. *TEMA-6* in press.

Buchanan, N. 1977. Drug protein binding and protein energy malnutrition. *S. Afr. Med. J.* 52: 733–737.

Buchanan, N. 1984. Effect of protein energy malnutrition on drug metabolism in man. *World Rev. Nutr. Diet.* 43: 129–139.

Buchanan, N., Davis, M. D., Henderson, D. B., Mucklow, J. C., and Rawlins, M. D. 1980. Acetanilide pharmacokinetics in kwashiorkor. *Br. J. Clin. Pharmacol.* 9: 525–526.

Bungay, P. M., Dedrick, R. L., and Matthews, H. B. 1981. Enteric transport of chlordecone (kepone) in the rat. *J. Pharmacokinet. Biopharm.* 9: 309–341.

Caldwell, J. 1980. Conjugation reactions. In *Concepts in Drug Metabolism.* (Ed.) Jenner, P. and Testa, B., New York, Ch. 4, pp. 211–250. Marcel Dekker, New York.

Campbell, T. C. and Hayes, J. R. 1976. The effect of quantity and quality of dietary protein on drug metabolism. *Fed. Proc.* 35: 2470–2474.

Campbell, T. C. 1979. Influence of nutrition on metabolism of carcinogens. *Adv. Nutr. Res.* 2: 29–55.

Carpenter, M. P. 1972. Vitamin E and microsomal drug hydroxylations. *Ann. N.Y. Acad. Sci.* 203: 81–92.

Catz, C. S., Juchau, M. R., and Yaffe, S. J. 1970 Effects of iron, riboflavin, and iodine deficiencies on hepatic drug metabolizing enzyme systems. *J. Pharmacol. Exp. Ther.* 174: 197–205.

Chasseud, L. F. 1979. The role of glutathione and glutathione S-transferases in the metabolism of chemical carcinogens and other electrophilic agents. *Adv. Cancer Res.* 29: 175–274.

Chen, J., Goetchius, M. P., Combs, G. F. Jr., and Campbell, T. C. 1982. Effects of dietary selenium and vitamin E on covalent binding of aflatoxin to chick liver cell macromolecules. *J. Nutr.* 122: 350–355.

Clinton, S. K., Truex, C. R., and Visek, W. J. 1979. Dietary protein, aryl hydrocarbon hydroxylase and chemical carcinogenesis in rats. *J. Nutr.* 109: 55–62.

Cohen, S. and Hansen, J. D. L. 1962. Metabolism of albumin and g-globulin in kwashiorkor. *Clin. Sci.* 23: 351–359.

Colby, H. D., Kramer, R. E., Greiner, J. W., Robinson, D. A., Krausse, R. F., and Canady, W. J. 1975. Hepatic drug metabolism in retinol-deficient rats. *Biochem. Pharmacol.* 24: 1644–1646.

Conney, A. H., Bray, G. A., Evans, C., and Burns, J. J. 1961. Metabolic interactions between L-ascorbic acid and drugs. *Ann. N.Y. Acad. Sci.* 92: 115–127.

Conney, A. H., Pantuck, E. J., Hsiao, K-C., Garland, W. A., Anderson, K. E., Alvares, A. P., and Kappas, A. 1976. Enhanced phenacetin metabolism in human subjects fed charcoal broiled beef. *Clin. Pharmacol. Ther.* 20: 633–642.

Coward, W. H. and Whitehead, R. G. 1972. Changes in serum lipoprotein concentration during development of kwashiorkor and recovery. *British J. Nutr.* 27: 383–394.

Crounse, R. G. 1961. Human pharmacology of griseofulvin: the effect of fat intake on gastrointestinal absorption. *J. Invest. Dematol.* 37: 529–533.

Dahl, A. R. 1986. The role of nasal xenobiotic metabolism in toxicology. In *Respiratory Toxicology,* (Ed.) Hollinger, M. A., pp. 143–184. Elsevier, New York.

Dahl, A. R., Bond, J. A., Petridou-Fischer, J., Sabourin, P. J., and Whaley, S. J. 1988. Effects of the respiratory tract on inhaled materials. *Toxicol. Appld. Pharmac.* 93: 484–492.

Danon, A. and Chen, Z. 1979. Binding of imipramine to plasma proteins: effect of hyperlipoproteinemia. *Clin. Pharmacol. Ther.* 25: 316–325.

Dawson, J. R. and Bridges, J. W. 1981. Intestinal microsomal drug metabolism. A comparison of rat and guinea pig enzymes and of rat crypt and villous tip cell enzymes. *Biochem. Pharmacol.* 30: 2415–2420.

DeLuca, H. F., Zile, M., and Sietzema, W. K. 1981. The metabolism of retinoic acid to 5,6-epoxyretinoic acid, retinoyl-β-glucuronide, and other polar metabolites. *Ann. N.Y. Acad. Sci.* 359: 25–36.

DeMeio, R. H. 1975. Sulfate activation and transfer. In *Metabolic Pathways,* (Ed.) Greenberg, D. M.: Vol. 7, 3rd ed., Ch. 8, pp. 287–358.

Dickerson, J. W. T., Basu, T. K., and Parke, D. V. 1971. Activity of drug metabolizing enzymes in the liver of growing rats fed on diets high in sucrose, glucose, fructose or an equimolar mixture of glucose and fructose. *Proc. Nutr. Soc.* 30: 27A.

Dodson, K. S. 1977. Conjugation with sulfate. In *Drug Metabolism from Microbe to Man.* (Ed.) Parke, D. V. and Smith, R. L. Taylor and Francis, London.

Doluisio, J. T., Billups, N. F., Dittert, L. W., Sugita, E. T., and Swintosky, J. V. 1969a. Drug Absorption. I. An in situ rat gut technique yielding realistic absorption rates. *J. Pharmaceut. Sci.* 58: 1196–1200.

Doluisio, J. R., Tan, G. H., Billups, N. F., and Diamond, B. L. 1969b. Drug Absorption II. Effect of fasting on intestinal drug absorption. *J. Pharmaceut. Sci.* 58: 1200–1204.

Dukes, C. E., Steplock, D. A., Kahn, A. M., and Weinman, E. J. 1983. The transport of urate in the small intestine of the rat (41471). *Proc. Soc. Exp. Biol. Med.* 171: 19–23.

Dutton, G. J. and Burchell, B. 1975. Newer aspects of glucuronidation. In *Progress in Drug Metabolism,* (Ed.) Bridges, J. W. and Chasseaud, L. F., Vol. 2, Ch. 1, pp. 1–70. Wiley, London.

Dutton, G. J. (Ed.) 1976. *Glucuronic Acid, Free and Combined.* Academic Press, New York.

Evarts, R. P. and Mostafa, M. H. 1981. Effects of indole and tryptophan on cytochrome P-450, dimethylnitrosamine demethylase, and aryl hydrocarbon hydroxylase. *Biochem. Pharmacol.* 30: 517–522.

Fehske, K. J., Muller, W. E., and Wollert, U. 1981. The location of drug binding sites in human serum albumin. *Biochem. Pharmacol.* 30: 687–692.

Fehske, K. J., Muller, W. E., Wollert, U. and Velden, U. 1979. The lone tryptophan residue of human serum albumin as part of the specific warfarin binding site: Binding of dicoumerol to the warfarin, indole and benzodiazepine binding sites. *Mol. Pharmacol.* 16: 778–789.

Ferguson, H. C. 1962. Dilution of dose and oral toxicity. *Toxicol. Appl. Pharmacol.* 4: 759–762.

Fielding, J. E. 1985. Smoking: Health effects and control. *N. Engl. J. Med.* 313: 491–480, 555–561.

Fortaine, R. N., Doi, O., and Schroeder, F. 1987. Membrane phospholipids alter nutrient transport and drug toxicity in tumorigenic fibroblasts. *Drug. Nutr. Interact.* 5: 49–60.

Furst, D. E., Tozer, T. N., and Melmon, K. L. 1979. Salicylate clearance, the resultant protein binding and metabolism. *Clin. Pharmacol. Ther.* 26: 380–389.

Gayte-Sorbier, A. and Airaudo, C. B. 1984. Nutrition and drug protein binding. *Wld. Rev. Nutr. Diet.* 43: 95–116.

Glazenburg, E. J., Jekel-Halsema, I. M. C., Scholtens, E., Baars, A. J., and Mulder, G. J. 1983. Effects of variation in the dietary supply of cysteine and methionine on liver concentrations of glutathione and "active sulfate" (PAPS) and serum levels of sulfate, cystine, methionine and taurine: Relation to the metabolism of acetaminophen.*J. Nutr.* 113: 1363–1373.

Grosse, W. and Wade, A. E. 1971. The effect of thiamine consumption on liver microsomal drug metabolizing pathways. *J. Pharmacol. Exp. Ther.* 176: 758–785.

Guengerich, F. P. 1982. Isolation and purification of cytochrome P-450 and the existence of multiple forms. In *Hepatic Cytochrome P-450 Monooxygenase System.* (Ed.) Schenkam, J. B. and Kupfer, D., Ch. 19, pp. 497–521. Pergamon Press, New York.

Guzelian, P. S. 1982. Chlordecone poisoning: A case study in approaches for detoxification of humans exposed to environmental chemicals. *Drug Metab. Rev.* 13: 663–679.

Habig, W. H., Pabst, M. J., and Jakoby, W. B. 1974. Glutathione-S-transferases—The first enzymatic step in mercapturic acid formation. *J. Biol. Chem.* 249: 7130–7139.

Hammer, C. T. and Wills, E. D. 1978. The role of lipid components of the diet in the regulation of the fatty acid composition of rat liver endoplasmic reticulum and lipid peroxidation. *Biochem. J.* 174: 585–593.

Hanasono, G. K., Cote, M. G., and Plaa, G. L. 1975a. Potentiation of carbon tetrachloride induced hepatotoxicity in alloxan-or streptozotocin-diabetic rats. *J. Pharmacol. Exp. Ther.* 192: 592–604.

Hanasono, G. K., Witschi, H., and Plaa, G. L. 1975b. Potentiation of the hepatotoxic responses to chemicals in alloxan-diabetic rats. *Proc. Soc. Exp. Biol. Med.* 149: 903–907.

Hanninen, O., Lindstrom-Seppa, P., and Pelkonen, K. 1987. Role of gut in xenobiotic metabolism. *Arch. Toxicol.* 60: 34–36.

Hara, T. and Taniguchi, M. 1982. Abnormal NADPH cytochrome P-450 reductase in the liver microsomes of riboflavin deficient rats. *Biochem. Biophys. Res. Commun.* 104: 394–401.

Hayes, J. R., Mgbodile, M. U. K., and Campbell, T. C. 1973. Effect of protein deficiency on the inducibility of the hepatic microsomal drug-metabolizing enzyme system. I. Effect of substrate interaction with cytochrome P-450. *Biochem. Pharmacol.* 22: 1005–1014.

Hayes, J. R. and Campbell, T. C. 1974. Effects of protein deficiency on the inducibility of the hepatic microsomal drug metabolizing enzyme system, III. Effect of 3-methylcholanthrene induction on activity and binding kinetics. *Biochem. Pharmacol.* 23: 1721–1731.

Heath, and Vandekar, 1964.

Hewitt, W. R. and Hook, J. B. 1983. The renal excretion of drugs. *Prog. Drug. Metabo.* 7: 11–56.

Hietanen, E. 1980. Modification of hepatic drug metabolizing enzyme activities and their induction by dietary protein. *Gen. Pharmacol.* 11: 443–450.

Hirose, M., Hagiwara, A., Inoue, K., Sakata, T., Ito, N., Kaneko, H., Yoshitake, A., and Miyamoto, J. 1987. Metabolism of 2- and 3-tert-butyl-4-hydroxyanisole (2-and 3-BHA) in the rat I: Excretion of BHA in urine, feces and expired air and distribution of BHA in the main organs. *Toxicology* 43: 139–147.

Hober, and Hober, 1937.

Hogben, C. A. M., Schanker, L. S., Tocco, D. J., and Brodie, B. B. 1957. Absorption of drugs from the stomach. II. The human. *J. Pharmacol. Exp. Therm.* 120: 540–545.

Holland, D. R. and Quay, J. F. 1976. Intestinal secretion of erythromycin base, *J. Pharm. Sci.* 65: 417–419.

Holloway, D. E. and Peterson, F. J. 1984. Ascorbic acid in drug metabolism. In *Drugs and Nutrients* (Ed.) Roe, D. A. and Campbell, T. C., Marcel Dekker, New York.

Hong, J., Pan, J., Gonzalez, F. J., Gelboin, H. V., and Yang, C. S. 1987. The induction of a specific form of cytochrome P-450 (P-450j) by fasting. *Biochem. Biophys. Res. Commun.* 142: 1077–1083.

Hook, J. B., Cardona, B., Osborn, J. L., and Bailie, M. D. 1976. The renal handling of 2,4,5-trichlorophenoxyacetic acid (2,4,5-T) in the dog. *Food Cosmet. Toxicol.* 14: 19–23.

Horn, L. R., Machlin, L. J., Barker, M. O., and Brin, M. 1976. Drug metabolism and hepatic heme proteins in the vitamin E deficient rat. *Arch. Biochem. Biophys.* 172: 270–277.

Inagaki, T., Stockert, R. J., Novikoff, P. M., Novikoff, A. B., and Wolkoff, A. W. 1985. Immunocytochemical localization of OABP in liver and heart. *Hepatology* 5: 1018–1024.

Ioannides, C., Delaforge, M., and Parks, D. V. 1981. Safrole: Its metabolism, carcinogenicity and interactions with cytochrome P-450. *Food Cosmet. Toxicol.* 19: 657–666.

Israili, Z. H. and Dayton, P. G. 1984. Enhancement of xenobiotic elimination: Role of intestinal excretion. *Drug Metabolism Rev.* 15: 1123–1159.

Iyanagi, T. and Mason, H. S. 1973. Some properties of hepatic reduced nicotinamide adenine dinucleotide phosphate-cytochrome C reductase. *Biochemistry.* 12: 2297–2308.

Iyanagi, T., Makino, N., and Mason, H. S. 1974. Redox properties of the reduced nicotinamide adenine dinucleotide phosphate-cytochrome P-450 and reduced nicotinamide adenine dinucleotide-cytochrome b5 reductases. *Biochemistry* 13: 1701-1710.

Jusko, W. J. and Gretch, M. 1976. Plasma and tissue protein binding of drugs in pharmacokinetics *Drug. Metab. Rev.* 5: 43-140.

Kangsadalampai, K. R. P., Sharma, M. J., Taylor, M. J., and Salunkhe, D. K. 1986. Effect of protein deficiency and Tween 60 on the pharmacokinetics of butylated hydroxyanisole and metabolites in male Sprague-Dawley rats. *Drug-Nutrient Interactions* 4: 289-297.

Kappas, A., Anderson, K. E., Conney, A. H., and Alvares, A. P. 1976. Influence of dietary protein and carbohydrate on antipyrine and theophylline metabolism in man. *Clin. Pharmacol. Ther.* 20: 643-653.

Kates, R. E., Sokoloski, T. D., and Comstock, T. J. 1978. Binding of quinidine to plasma proteins in normal subjects and in hyperproteinemias. *Clin. Pharmacol. Ther.* 23: 30-35.

Kato, R. and Gillette, J. R. 1965. Effect of starvation on the NADPH-dependent enzymes in liver microsomes of male and female rats. *J. Pharmacol. Exp. Therap.* 150: 279-284.

Kato, N., Mochizuki, S., Kawai, K., and Yoshida, A. 1982. Effect of dietary level of sulfur amino acids on liver drug-metabolizing enzymes, serum cholesterol and urinary ascorbic acid in rats fed PCB. *J. Nutr.* 112: 848-854.

Kato, R., Oshima, T., and Tomizawa, W. 1968. Toxicity and metabolism of drugs in relation to dietary protein. *Jap. J. Pharmacol.* 18: 356- 366.

Kato, N., Tani, T., and Yoshida, A. 1981. Effect of dietary quality of protein on liver microsomal mixed function oxidase system, plasma cholesterol and urinary ascorbic acid in rats fed PCB. *J. Nutr.* 111: 123-133.

Keen, P. 1971. Effect of binding to plasma proteins on the distribution, activity and elimination of drugs. *Handbook Exp. Pharmacol.* 28: 213-233.

Klassen, C. D. and Watkins, J. B., III. 1984. Mechanisms of bile formation, hepatic uptake, and biliary excretion. *Pharmacol. Rev.* 36: 1-67.

Kolassa, N., Schutzenberger, W. G., Weiner, H., and Turnheim, K. 1980. Active secretion of hypoxanthine and xanthine by guinea pig jejunum in vitro. *Am. J. Physiol.* 238: G141-G149.

Kornguth, M. L., Hutchins, L. G., and Eichelman, B. S. 1981. Binding of psychotropic drugs related to isolated a1-acid glycoprotein. *Biochem. Pharmacol.* 30: 2435-2441.

Koster, A. S. and Noordshock, J. 1983. Glucuronidation in isolated perfused rat intestinal segments after second administration of 1-naphthol. *J. Pharma. Exp. Ther.* 226: 533–538.

Kragh-Hansen, U. 1981. Molecular aspects of ligand binding to serum albumin. *Pharmacol. Rev.* 33: 17–53.

Krijgsheld, K. R., Scholtens, E., and Mulder, G. J. 1981. An evaluation of methods to decrease the availability of inorganic sulfate for sulfate conjugation in the rat in vivo. *Biochem. Pharmacol.* 30: 1973–1979.

Krishnaswamy, K. 1987. Effects of malnutrition on drug metabolism and toxicity in humans. In *Nutritional Toxicology,* II, (Ed.) Hathcock, J. pp. 105–128. Academic Press, New York.

Krishnaswamy, K., Ushasri, V., and Naidu, A. N. 1981. The effect of malnutrition on the pharmacokinetics of phenylbutazone. *Clin. Pharmacokin.* 6: 152–159.

Kulkarni, A. P. and Hodgson, E. 1980. Metabolism of insecticides by mixed function oxidase systems. *Pharmac. Ther.* 8: 379– 475.

Kurtz, H. and Fichtl, B. 1983. Binding of drugs to tissues. *Drug Metab. Rev.* 14: 467–510.

Kuwano, S. and Hiraga, K. 1980. Effect of dietary protein deficiency on the rat hepatic drug metabolizing system. *Jpn. J. Pharmacol.* 30: 75–83.

Lauterbach, F. 1975. Resorption and Sekretion von arzneistoffen durch die Mukosaepithelien des Gastrointestinaltraktes. *Arzneim. Forsch.* 25: 479–488.

Lecomte, M., Zini, R., D'Athis, P., and Tillement, J. P. 1979. Phenytoin binding to human albumin. *Eur. J. Drug Metab. Pharmacokinet.* 4: 23–28.

Leo, M. A., Iida, S., and Lieber, C. S. 1984. Retinoic acid metabolism by a system reconstituted with cytochrome P-450. *Arch. Biochem. Biophys.* 234: 305–312.

Lichtenwalner, D. M., Suh, B., and Lichtenwalner, M. R. 1983. Isolation and chemical characterization of 2-hydroxybenzoyl-glycine as a drug binding inhibitor in uremia. *J. Clin. Invest.* 71: 1289–1296.

Lieber, C. S. 1984. Alcohol and the liver: 1984 update. *Hepatology* 4: 1243–1260.

Lilienblum, W., Walli, A. K., and Bock, K. W. 1982. Differential induction of rat liver microsomal UDP glucuronyl transferase activities by various inducing agents. *Biochem. Pharmacol.* 31: 907–913.

Lowery, G. L. and Bidlack, W. R. 1978. Multiple drug metabolism in isolated hepatocytes: Enhancement of aniline metabolism. *Biochem. Biophys. Res. Commun.* 83: 747–753.

Lu, A. Y. H. and West, S. B. 1980. Multiplicity of mammalian microsomal cytochrome P-450. *Pharmacol. Rev.* 31: 227–295.

Magdalou, J., Steimetz, D., Balt, A. -M., Poullin, B., Siest, G., and Debry, G. 1979. The effect of dietary sulfur-amino acids on the activity of drug metabolizing enzymes in rat liver microsomes. *J. Nutr.* 109: 864–871.

Mainigi, K. D. and Campbell, T. C. 1981. Effects of low dietary protein and dietary aflatoxin on hepatic glutathione levels in F-344 rats. *Toxicol. Appl. Pharmacol.* 59: 196–203.

Marcelos, M. and Laitinen, M. 1975. Starvation and phenobarbital treatment effects on drug hydroxylation and glucuronidation in the rat liver and small intestine mucosa. *Biochem. Pharmacol.* 24: 1529–1535.

Marshall, W. J. and McLean, A. E. M. 1971. A requirement for dietary lipids for induction of cytochrome P-450 by phenobarbitone in rat liver microsome fraction. *Bioch. J.* 122: 569–573.

Mata, L. J., Jimenez, F., Cordon, M., Rosales, R., Prera, E., Schneider, R. E., and Viteri, F. 1972. Gastrointestinal flora of children with PCM. *Amer. J. Clin. Nutr.* 25: 1118–1126.

Mayoral, L. G., Tripathy, K., Bolanas, O., Lotero, H., Doque, E., Garcia, F. T., and Ghitis, J. 1972. Intestinal, functional and morphological abnormalities in severely protein malnourished adults. *Amer. J. Clin. Nutr.* 25: 1084–1091.

McLean, A. J., McNamara, P. J., duSouich, P., Gibaldi, M., and Lalka, D. 1978. Food, splanchic blood flow and bioavailability of drugs subject to first pass metabolism. *Clin. Pharmacol. Ther.* 24: 5–10.

Meffin, P. J., Robert, E. W., Winkle, R. A., Harapat, S., Peters, F. A., and Harrison, D. C. 1979. Role of concentration dependent plasma protein binding of disopyramide disposition. *J. Pharmacokin. Biopharm.* 7: 29–46.

Mehta, S., Kalsi, H. K., Jayaraman, S., and Mathur, V. S. 1975. Chloramphenicol metabolism in children with protein calorie malnutrition. *Am. J. Clin. Nutr.* 28: 977–986.

Meier, P. J., Meier-Abt, A. S., Barrett, C., and Boyer, J. L. 1984. Mechanisms of taurocholate transport in canalicular and   basolateral rat liver plasma membrane vesicles. *J. Biol. Chem.* 259: 10614–10622.

Meister, A. and Anderson, M. E. 1983. Glutathione. *Ann. Rev. Biochem.* 52: 711–760.

Melander, A. 1978. Influences of food on the bioavailability of drugs. *Clin. Pharmacokinet.* 3: 337–351.

Melander, A., Danielson, K., Scherstein, B., and Wahlin, E. 1977. Enhancement of the bioavailability of propanolol and metroprolol by food. *Clin. Pharmacol. Ther.* 22: 108–112.

Melander, A., Brante, G., Johansson, O., Lindberg, T., and Wahlin, E. 1978. Influence of food intake on the absorption of phenytoin in man. *Eur. J. Clin. Invest.*

Meydani, M. 1987. Dietary effects on detoxification processes. In *Nutritional Toxicology*, II., (Ed.) Hathcock, J. pp. 1–39. Academic Press, Inc, New York.

Meydani, M., Blumberg, J. B., and Hayes, K. C. 1985. Dietary fat unsaturation enhances drug metabolism in cebus but not in squirrel monkeys. *J. Nutr.* 115: 573–578.

Mgbodile, M. U. K. and Campbell, T. C. 1972. Effect of protein deprivation in male weanling rats on the kinetics of hepatic microsomal enzyme activity. *J. Nutr.* 102: 53–60.

Miltenberger, R., and Oltersdorf, U. 1978. The B-vitamin group and the activity of hepatic microsomal mixed function oxidases of the growing Wistar rat. *Brit. J. Nutr.* 39: 127–137.

Minchin, R. F. and Boyd, M. R. 1983. Localization of metabolic activation and deactivation systems in the lung: Significance to the pulmonary toxicity of xenobiotics. *Ann. Rev. Pharmacol. Toxicol.* 23: 217–238.

Minnigh, E. B. and Zemaitis, M. A. 1982. Altered acetaminophen disposition in fed and food-deprived rats after acute ethanol administration. *Drug Metab. Dispos.* 10: 183–188.

Miranda, C. L., Mukhtar, H., Bend, J. R., and Chhabra, R. S. 1979. Effects of vitamin A deficiency on hepatic and extrahepatic mixed function oxidase and epoxide metabolizing enzymes in guinea pig and rabbit. *Biochem. Pharmacol.* 28: 2713– 2716.

Moldeus, P., Anderson, B., and Norling, A. 1978. Interaction of ethanol oxidation with glucuronidation in isolated hepatocytes. *Biochem. Pharmacol.* 27: 2583–2588.

Moldeus, P., Vadi, H., and Berggren, M. 1976. Oxidative and conjugative metabolism of p-nitroanisole and p-nitrophenol in isolated rat liver cells. *Acta Pharmacol. et Toxicol.* 39: 17–32.

Morgenstern, R., DePierre, J. W., and Ernster, L. 1979. Activation of microsomal glutathione S-transferase activity by sulfhydryl reagents. *Biochem. Biophys. Res. Commun.* 87: 657–663.

Mu, J. Y., Israili, Z. H., and Dayton, P. G. 1975. Studies of the disposition and metabolism of mefloquine HCl (WR 142,490), a quinolinemethanol antmalarial, in the rat. *Drug Metab. Dispos.* 3: 198–210.

Nakajima, T. and Sato, A. 1979. Enhanced activity of liver drug-metabolizing enzymes for aromatic and chlorinated hydrocarbons following food deprivation. *Tox. Appl. Pharmac.* 50: 549–556.

Nakajima, T., Koyama, Y., and Sato, A. 1982. Dietary modification of metabolism and toxicity of chemical substances—with special reference to carbohydrate. *Biochem. Pharmacol.* 31: 1005–1011.

Norred, W. P. and Wade, A. E. 1972. Dietary fatty acid induced alterations of hepatic microsomal metabolism. *Biochem. Pharmacol.* 21: 2887–2897.

Ochsenfahrt, H. and Winne, D. 1988. The contribution of solvent drag to the intestinal absorption of the acidic drugs benzoic acid and salicylic acid from the jejunum of the rat. *Naunyn Schmiedeberg's Arch. Pharmacol.* 281: 197–217.

Oesch, F. 1980. Influence of foreign compounds on formation and disposition of reactive metabolites. In *Environmental Chemicals, Enzyme Function and Human Disease,* CIBA Foundation 76, pp. 169–183. Excerpta Medica, New York.

Oie, S. and Tozer, T. N. 1979. Effects of altered plasma protein binding on apparent volume of distribution. *J. Pharm. Sci.* 68: 1203–1205.

Overton, 1902.

Pantuck, E. J., Hsiao, K. -C., Loub, W. D., Wattenberg, L. W., Kuntzman, R., and Conney, A. H. 1976. Stimulatory effect of vegetables on intestinal drug metabolism in the rat. *J. Pharmac. Exp. Ther.* 198: 278–283.

Pantuck, E. J., Pantuck, C. B., Garland, W. A., Min, B. H., Wattenberg, L. W., Anderson, K. E., Kappas, A., and Conney, A. H. 1979. Stimulatory effect of Brussels sprouts and cabbage on human drug metabolism. *Clin. Pharmacol. Ther.* 25: 88–95.

Parke, D. V. and Ioannides, C. 1981. The role of nutrition in toxicology. *Ann. Rev. Nutr.* 1: 207–234.

Pastoriza-Munoz, E., Bowman, R. L., and Kaloyanides, G. J. 1979. Renal tubular transport of gentamicin in the rat. *Kidney Int.* 16: 440–450.

Patel, J. M. and Pawar, S. S. 1974. Riboflavin and drug metabolism in adult male and female rats. *Biochem. Pharmacol.* 23: 1467–1477.

Peleran, J. C., Rao, D., and Bories, G. F. 1987. Identification of the cooked food mutagen 2-amino-3-methylimidazo [4,5-f] quinoline (IQ) and its N-acetylated and 3-N-demethylated metabolites in rat urine. *Toxicology* 43: 193–199.

Peters, M. A. and Fouts, J. R. 1970a. A study of some possible mechanisms by which magnesium activates hepatic microsomal drug metabolism in vitro. *J. Pharmacol. Exptl. Ther.* 173: 233–241.

Peters, M. A. and Fouts, J. R. 1970b. The influence of magnesium and some other divalent cations on hepatic microsomal drug metabolism in vitro. *Biochem. Pharmacol.*. 19: 533-544.

Piafsky, K. M. 1980. Disease induced changes in the plasma binding of basic drugs. *Clin. Pharmacokinet.* 5: 246-262.

Pittman, K., Wiener, M., and Treble, J. H. 1976. Mirex kinetics in the Rhesus monkey. *Drug Metab. Dispos.* 4: 288-295.

Pullman, T. N., Alving, A. S., Dern, R. J., and Landowne, M. 1954. The influence of dietary protein intake on specifric renal functions in normal man. *J. Lab. & Clin. Med.* 44: 320-332.

Raghuram, T. C. and Krishnaswamy, K. 1981. Tetracycline absorption in malnutrition. *Drug-Nutr. Interact.* 1: 23-25.

Raypurohit, R., Kalamegham, R., Chary, A. K., and Krishnaswamy, K. 1985. Hepatic drug metabolising enzymes in undernourished men. *Toxicology* 37: 259-266.

Reichen, J. and Berk, P. D. 1979. Isolation of an organic anion binding protein from rat liver plasma membrane fractions by affinity chromatography. *Biochim. Biophys. Res. Commun.* 91: 484-489.

Reicks, M. M. and Hathcock, J. N. 1984. Effects of dietary methionine and ethanol on acetaminophen hepatotoxicity in mice. *Drug-Nutr. Interact.* 3: 43-52.

Reidenberg, M. M. 1971. Mechanisms of excretion of drugs. In *Renal Function and Drug Action.* Ch. 2, pp. 5-7. W.B. Saunders Company, Philadelphia, PA.

Reidenberg, M. M. and Vesell, E. S. 1975. Unaltered metabolism of antipyrine and tolbutamine in fasting man. *Clin. Pharmacol. Ther.* 17: 650-656.

Reinke, L. A., Kauffman, F. C., Belinsky, S. A., and Thurman, R. G. 1980a. Interactions between ethanol metabolism and mixed function oxidation in perfused rat liver: Inhibition of p-nitroanisole O-demethylation. *J. Pharmacol. Exp. Ther.* 213: 70-78.

Reinke, L. A., Moyer, M. J., and Notley, K. A. 1986. Diminished rates of glucuronidation and sulfation in perfused rat liver after chronic ethanol administration. *Biochem Pharmacol* 35: 439-447.

Reinke, L. A. Moyer, M. J., and Notley, K. A. 1986. Diminished rates of glucuronidation and sulfation in perfused rat liver after chronic ethanol administration. *Biochem Pharmacol* 35: 439-447.

Remmer, H. 1987. Review. Passively inhaled tobacco smoke: A challenge to toxicology and preventive medicine. *Arch. Toxicol.* 61: 89-104.

Rennick, B. R. 1972. Renal excretion of drugs: Tubular transport and metabolism. *Ann. Rev. Pharmacol.* 12: 141–156.

Rennick, B. R. 1981. Renal tubule transport of organic cations. *Amer. J. Physiol.* 240: F-83–F89.

Rennick, B. R. and Quebbemann 1970.

Roe, Daphne A. 1979. Interactions between drugs and nutrients. *Medical Clinics of North America* 63: 985–1007.

Rowland, M. 1984. Protein binding and drug clearance. *Clin. Pharmacokinet.* 9. Supp.: 10–17.

Sachan, D. S. and Su, P. K. 1986. Effects of level of food restriction on in vivo and in vitro alterations in drug metabolism and associated enzymes. *Drug-Ntr. Interact.* 4: 363–370.

Sato, M. and Nakajima, T. 1979.

Sato, M. and Lieber, C. S. 1982. Increased metabolism of retinoic acid after chronic ethanol consumption in rat liver microsomes. *Arch. Biochem. Biophys.* 213: 557–564.

Sato, A.,Nakajima, T., and Koyama, Y. 1983. Interaction between ethanol and carbohydrate on the metabolism in rat liver of aromatic and chlorinated hydrocarbons. *Tox. Appl. Pharmacol.* 68: 242–249.

Schanker, L. S. 1959. Absorption of drugs from the rat colon. *J. Pharmacol. Exp. Ther.* 126: 283–290.

Schanker, L. S. 1960. On the mechanism of absorption of drugs from the gastrointestinal tract. *J. Med. Pharm. Chem.* 2: 343–359.

Schanker, L. S., Shore, P. A., Brodie, B. B., and Hogben, C. A. M. 1957. Absorption of drugs from the stomach I. The rat. *J.Pharmacol. Exp. Ther.* 120: 528–539.

Schanker, L. S., Tacco, D. J., Brodie, B. B., and Hogben, C. A. M. 1958. Absorption of drugs from the rat small intestine. *J. Pharmacol. Exp. Ther.* 123: 81–88.

Schenkman, J. B. and Kupfer, D. eds. 1982. *Hepatic Cytochrome P-450 Monooxygenase System.* Pergamon Press, New York.

Schneider, R. E. and Viteri, F. E. 1974. Studies on the luminal events of lipid absorption in PCM children: Its relation with nutritional recovery and diarrhea. I. Capacity of the doudenal contents to achieve micellar solubilization of lipids. *Amer. J. Clin. Nutr.* 27: 777–787.

Schwenk, M. 1987. Drug transport in intestine, liver and kidney. *Arch. Toxicol.* 60: 37–42.

Schwenk, M. and Locher, M. 1985. 1-Naphthol conjugation in isolated cells from liver, jejunum, ileum, colon and kidney of the guinea pig. *Biochem. Pharmacol.* 34: 679–701.

Schwenk, M., Wiedmann, T., and Remmer, H. 1981. Uptake accumulation and release of ouabain by isolated rat hepatocytes. *Naunyn-Schmiedeberg's Arch. Pharmacol.* 316: 340–344.

Shah, P. V., Monroe, R. J., and Guthrie, F. E. 1981. Comparative rates of dermal penetration of insecticides in mice. *Toxicol. Appl. Pharmacol.* 59: 414–423.

Shargel, L. and Mazel, P. 1973. Effect of riboflavin deficiency on phenobarbital and 3-methylcholanthrene induction of microsomal drug metabolizing enzymes of the rat. *Biochem. Pharmacol.* 22: 2365–2373.

Shinohara, A., Yamazoe, Y., Saito, K., Kamataki, T., and Kato, R. 1984. Specific differences in the N-acetylation by liver cytosol of mutagenic hetercyclic aromatic amines in protein pyrolysates. *Carcinogenesis* 5: 683–686.

Shore, P. A., Brodie, B. B., and Hogben, C. A. M. 1957. The gastric secretion of drugs: a pH partition hypothesis. *J. Pharmacol. Exp. Ther.* 119: 361–369.

Shu, H. P. and Nichols, A. V. 1981. Uptake of lipophilic carcinogens by plasma lipoproteins. Structure-activity studies. *Biochim, Biophys. Acta* 665: 376–384.

Sikic, B. I., Mimnaugh, E. G., Litterest, C. L., and Gram, T. E. 1977. The effects of ascorbic acid deficiency and repletion on pulmonary, renal and hepatic drug metabolism in the guinea pig. *Arch. Biochem. Biophys.* 179: 663–671.

Singer, S. S. 1985. Preparation and characterization of the different kinds of sulfotransferases. In *Methodological Aspects of Drug Metabolizing Enzymes, Biochemical Pharmacology and Toxicology,* Vol. 1, (Ed.) Zakim, D. and Vessey, D. A., p. 95. John Wiley and Sons, New York.

Sjodin, T. 1977. Circular dichroism studies on the inhibiting effect of oleic acid on the binding of diazepam to human serum albumin. *Biochem. Pharmac.* 26: 2157–2161.

Sjoholm, I., Ekman, B., Kober, A., Lungstedt-Pahlman, I., Seiving, B., and Sjodin, T. 1979. Binding of drugs to human serum albumin: XI. The specificity of three binding sites as studied with albumin immobilized in microparticles. *Molec. Pharmac.* 16: 767–777.

Sjoholm, I., Kober, A., Odar-Cederlof, I., and Borge, O. 1976. Protein binding of drugs in uremic and normal serum: the role of endogenous binding inhibitors. *Biochem. Pharmacol.* 25: 1205–1213.

Skett, P. and Joels, L. A. 1985. Different effects of acute and chronic diabetes mellitus on hepatic drug metabolism in the rat. *Biochem. Pharmacol.* 34: 287–289.

Smith, C. H. and Bidlack, W. R. 1984. Dietary concerns associated with the use of medications. *J. Am. Dietet.* 84: 901–914.

Snyder, R. and Remmer, H. 1982. Classes of hepatic microsomal mixed function oxidase inducers. In *Hepatic Cytochrome P-450 Monooxygenase System.* (Ed.) Schenkman, J. B. and Kupfer, D. Ch. 8, pp. 227–268. Pergammon Press, New York.

Soltys and Hsia, 1977.

Strobel, H. W., Lu, A. Y. H., Hedema, J., and Coon, M. J. 1970. Phosphatidylcholine requirement in the enzymatic reduction of hemoprotein P-450, and in fatty acid, hydrocarbon and drug hydroxylation. *J. Biol. Chem.* 245: 4851–4854.

Strother, A., Throckmorton, J. K., and Herzer, C. 1971. The influence of high sugar consumption by mice on the duration of action of barbiturates and in vitro metabolism of barbiturates, aniline and p-nitoanisole. *J. Pharmacol. Exp. Ther.* 179: 490–498.

Suskind, R. M. 1975. Gastrointestinal changes in the malnourished child. *Pediatric Clinics of North America* 22: 873–883.

Thurman, R. G. and Kauffman, F. C. 1980. Factors regulating drug metabolism in intact hepatocytes. *Pharm. Reviews* 31: 229–251.

Tillement, J. P., Houin, G., Zini, R., Urien, S., Albengres, E., Barre, J., Lecomte, M., D'Athis, P., and Sebille, B. 1984. The binding of drugs to blood plasma macromolecules: Recent advances and therapeutic significance. *Adv. Drug. Res.* 13: 60–94.

Tillement, J. P., Zini, R., Lecomte, M., and D'Athis, P. 1980. Binding of digitoxin, digoxin and gitoxin to human serum albumin. *Eur. J. Drug. Metab. Pharmacokinet.* 5: 129–134.

Toothaker, R. D. and Welling, P. G. 1980. The effect of food and drug bioavailability. *Annual Rev. Pharmacol. Toxicol.* 20: 173–199.

Urien, S., Albengres, E., and Tillement, J. P. 1981. *Int. J. Clin. Pharmac. Ther. Toxicol.* 19: 319–325.

Urien, S., Albengres, E., Zini, R., D'Athis, P. and Tillement, J. P. 1980. Serum binding and interactions of chlorophenoxyisobutyric acid, itanoxone and fenofibric acid according to their different HSA binding sites. In *Drugs Affecting Lipid Metabolism,* pp. 201–209. Elsevier, Amsterdam.

Varela, G., Andujar, M. A. M., and Navarro, M. A. P. 1978. Chlorinated hydrocarbon insecticides and nutrition. *Wld. Rev. Nutr. Diet.* 30: 148–188.

Vermillion, J. L., Ballou, D. P., Massey, V., and Coon, M. J. 1981. Separate role for FMN and FAD in catalysis by liver microsomal NADPH cytochrome P-450 reductase. *J. Biol. Chem.* 256: 266–277.

Vermillion, J. L. and Coon, M. J. 1978. Identification of the high and low potential flavins of liver microsomal NADPH cytochrome P-450 reductase. *J. Biol. Chem.* 253: 8812–8819.

Vessell, E. S. 1977. Genetic and environmental factors affecting drug disposition in man. *Clin. Pharmacol. Ther.* 22: 659–679.

Wade. A. E., Greene, F. E., Ciordia, R. M., Meadows, J. S., and Caster, C. O. 1969. Effects of dietary thiamine intake on hepatic drug metabolism in the male rate. *Biochem. Pharmacol.* 18: 2288–2291.

Wade, A. E. and Norred, W. P. 1976. Effect of dietary lipid on drug metabolizing enzymes. *Fed. Proc.* 35: 2475–2479.

Wade, A. E. et al. 1975.

Wade, A. E., Norred, W. P., and Evans, J. S. 1978. Lipids in drug detoxication. In *Nutrition and Drug Interactions,* (Ed.) Hathcock, J. N. and Coon, J., pp. 475–503. Academic Press, New York.

Waterlow, J. K. 1975. Adaption of low protein intake. In *Protein Calorie Malnutrition,* (Ed.) Olson, R. E. pp. 23–24. Academic Press, New York.

Watkins, J. B. III, Sanders, R. A., and Beck, L. V. 1988. The effect of long term streptozotocin induced diabetes on the hepatotoxicity of bromobenzene and carbon tetrachloride and hepatic biotransformation in rats. *Toxicol. & Applied Pharmacol.* 93: 329–338.

Welling, P. G. 1977. Influence of food and diet on gastrointestinal drug absorption: A review. *J. Pharmacokin. Biopharm.* 5: 291–334.

Welling, P. G., Huang, H., Koch, P. A., Craig, W. A., and Madsen, P. O. 1977. Bioavailability of Ampicillin and Amoxicillin in fasted and non-fasted subjects. *J. Pharm. Sci.* 66: 549–552.

Welling, P. G. and Tse, F. L. S. 1982. The influence of food on the absorption of antimicrobial agents. *J. Antimicrob. Chemother.* 9: 7–27.

Wiegand, U. W., Hintze, K. L., Slattery, J. T., and Levy, G. 1980. Protein binding of several drugs in serum and plasma of healthy subjects. *Clin. Pharmacol. Ther.* 27: 297–300.

Wiegand, U. W., Slattery, J. T., Hintze, K. L., and Levy, G. 1979. Differences in the protein binding of several drugs and bilirubin in serum and heparinized plasma of rats. *Life Sci.* 25: 471–477.

Wieland, T., Nassal, M., Kramer, W., Fricker, G., Bickel, U., and Kurz, G.

1984. Identity of hepatic membrane transport systems for bile salts, phalloidin and antamanide by photoaffinity labeling. *Proc. Natl. Acad. Sci.* 81: 5232–5236.

Wilkinson, G. R. 1983. Plasma and tissue binding considerations in drug disposition. *Drug Metabolism Rev.* 14: 427–465.

Wilkinson, G. R. 1984. Plasma binding, distribution and elimination. In *Drugs and Nutrients,* (Ed.) Roe, D. A. and Campbell, T. C., pp. 21–49. Marcell Dekker, New York.

Wilkinson, G. R. and Shand, D. G. 1975. A physiological approach to hepatic drug clearance. *Clin. Pharmacol. Ther.*. 18: 377–390.

Wilkinson, G. R., and Schenker, S. 1976. Effects of liver disease on drug disposition in man. *Biochem. Pharmacol.* 25: 2675–2681.

Williams et al. 1970.

Wood, G. C. and Woodcock, B. G. 1970. Effect of dietary protein on the conjugation of foreign compounds in rat liver. *J. Pharm. Pharmacol.* 22: Suppl. 605–635.

Woodcock, B. K. and Wood, G. C. 1971. Effect of protein free diet on UDP glucuronyl transferase and sulfotransferase activities in rat liver. *Biochem Pharmacol.* 20: 2703–2731.

Yamazoe, Y., Shimada, M., Kamataki, T., and Kato, R. 1983. Microsomal activation of 2-amino-3-methyl imidazo[4,5-f]quinoline, a pyrolysate of sardine and beef extracts, to a mutagenic intermediate. *Cancer Res.* 43: 5768–5774.

Yang, C. S. 1974. Alterations of the aryl hydrocarbon hydroxylase system during riboflavin depletion and repletion. *Arch. Biochem. Biophys.* 160: 623–630.

Young, J. A. and Edwards, K. D. G. 1966. Clearance and stop-flow studies on histidine and methyldopa transport by rat kidney. *Amer. J. Physiol.* 210: 667–675.

Zakim. D., Vessey, D. A., and Hochman, Y. 1985. Methods for the characterization of UDP-glucuronyltransferase. In *Methodological Aspects of Drug Metabolizing Enzymes, Biochemical Pharmacology and Toxicology,* Vol. 1, (Ed.) Zakim, D and Vessey, D. A. pp. 161–174. John Wiley and Sons, New York.

Zannoni, V. G., Flynn, E. J., and Lynch, M. 1977. Ascorbic acid and drug metabolism. *Biochem. Pharmacol.* 21: 1377–1392.

Ziegler, K., Frimmer, M. and Fasold, H. 1984. Further characterization of membrane proteins involved in the transport of organic anions in hepatocytes. *Biochem. Biophys. Acta* 769: 117–129.

13
Regulatory Distinctions Between Naturally Occurring and Added Substances in Food

Clausen Ely, Jr.

Covington & Burling
Washington, D.C.

The federal food safety regulatory scheme is a patchwork of separate statutory standards for different categories of food constituents. Virtually all state food safety laws mirror the federal design. Although federal food safety standards are complex, overlapping, and sometimes inconsistent, they incorporate a number of sound underlying principles. The safety standard applicable to a particular type of food constituent depends upon its origin, history of use, benefits, and avoidability.

Food and color additives are governed by rigorous safety standards. Environmental contaminants are subject to more flexible regulatory constraints. Naturally occurring substances are regulated under the most lenient safety test. The different standards applicable to these basic categories of food constituents reflect a balanced approach that accomodates the public's desire for safety with its need for a plentiful and inexpensive food supply.

The Federal Food and Drug Administration (FDA) has effectively regulated the United States food supply for many years, giving due consideration to different categories of food substances. This legacy is now threatened by California Proposition 65 and similar proposals in other states that portend a radical departure in regulatory approach. These laws blur the distinction between naturally occurring and added substances in food, elevate warnings to a preferred method of regulation, and put undue focus on trivial and insignificant risks.

REGULATION OF NATURALLY OCCURRING SUBSTANCES IN FOOD

The statutory safety standard for naturally occurring substances in food is contained in section 402(a)(1) of the Federal Food, Drug and Cosmetic Act (FD&C Act), which provides that:

> A food shall be deemed to be adulterated—if it bears or contains any poisonous or deleterious substance which may render it injurious to health; but in case the substance is not an added substance such food shall not be considered adulterated under this clause if the quantity of such substance in such food does not ordinarily render it injurious to health.[1]

The critical distinction under section 402(a)(1) is between "added" and "not added" poisonous or deleterious substances. Neither term is defined in the Act, but the "not added" category is generally regarded as embracing naturally occurring toxicants, while all other toxicants fall within the "added" classification.

The "ordinarily injurious" safety standard for naturally occurring toxicants is more lenient than that for all other types of food substances. The "ordinarily injurious" adulteration test was introduced in the 1938 Act. Congress's purpose in crafting this standard is not fully elucidated in the legislative history. However, there are a number of strong practical reasons to support a more lenient safety standard for naturally occurring food substances, and Congress evidently recognized those reasons. Naturally occurring poisonous or deletrious substances are ubiquitous in food, often pose only trivial or modest risks, and, in many cases, would be extremely expensive or impossible to eliminate.

Judicial interpretation of the "ordinarily injurious" safety standard has been rare. This is not surprising. It reflects the demanding standard of proof imposed on FDA and the fact, implicitly recognized by Congress, that the great majority of naturally occurring toxicants in food are generally regarded as posing acceptable risks. In the leading case interpreting the "ordinarily injurious" standard, involving FDA seizure of oysters containing shell fragments, the court stressed that shell fragments cannot be entirely eliminated from oysters and that there was no evidence that consumers had actually been injured from consumption of the oysters in question.[2] This is consistent with statements during the hearings prior to passage of the 1938 Act which indicate that Congress did not intend to ban commonly consumed naturally occurring toxicants, such as caffeine in coffee and oxalic acid in rhubarb, and only intended to prohibit natural food substances, such as poisonous mushrooms, that are highly toxic in small amounts.[3] Consistent with this approach, in the most recent decision involving a naturally occurring toxicant, the court held that amygdalin in apricot kernels is not ordinarily injurious despite the fact that it might be toxic to those who consome unusually large amounts.[4]

In order successfully to prosecute an adulteration action against a food product containing a naturally occurring toxicant, FDA must weigh the relative danger and importance of the food involved and must demonstrate a probability of harm to a significant number of consumers. The key distinction between this adulteration standard and that applicable to added substances is the greater probability of harm the government must show to restrict a natural constituent.

There is no distinction between carcinogens (either animal or human) and other types of toxicants under the safety standard for naturally occurring food constituents. FDA is free to ignore naturally occurring carcinogens in food that do not pose a significant probability of harm, and it has often done so. Given the mounting evidence that many foods contain low levels of natural carcinogens,[5] the absence of a categorical prohibition against naturally occurring carcinogens appears to reflect a sensible and realistic approach.

It is important to note, however, that the safety standard for naturally occurring food constituents has increasingly little practical importance. This is because FDA and the courts have adopted a very restricted definition of naturally occurring substances. As a result, virtually all food toxicants are classified by FDA as "added" substances and are thus subject to the more rigorous safety standard for those substances.

FDA has narrowly defined a naturally occurring poisonous or deleterious substance as one that is an "inherent natural constituent of a food and is not the result of environmental, agricultural, industrial, or other contamination."[6] Under the FDA definition, virtually any substance not produced by or essential for the life processes of a food organism would be regarded as "added," regardless of whether such substance is introduced into the environment by human activity or could be avoided by the best feasible handling and preservation techniques. In adopting this peculiar definition of naturally occurring, FDA's obvious unstated purpose was to avoid whenever possible the demanding standard of proof under the ordinarily injurious adulteration standard.

In the absence of definitive legislative history, FDA's interpretation of the Act is ordinarily given deference by the courts.[7] Accordingly, the courts have also adopted a narrow definition of naturally occurring or not added substances, and a correspondingly broad definition of added substances. The courts have held, for example, that salmonella in shrimp[8] and aflatoxin in corn[9] are "added poisonous or deleterious substances." The courts have reasoned that "added" substances include natural bacteria and fungi that can be avoided by optimal food handling and sanitary practices and that FDA has no duty to demonstrate human intervention with respect to the contamination of any particular article of food it wishes to regulate as an added substance.

In the leading decision in this area, *United States v. Anderson Seafoods Inc.,* the United States Court of Appeals for the Fifth Circuit upheld FDA's seizure of swordfish containing mercury on the ground that the mercury was an added substance.[10] Although the court acknowledged that the vast majority of mercury in swordfish is derived from natural geologic sources, it found that a small amount is contributed by human pollution and ruled that the entire mercury content must be judged under the stricter safety standard for added substances.

Because of the prevailing narrow interpretation of naturally occurring substances under the FD&C Act, the safety standard for "added" poisonous or deleterious substances takes on greater importance, especially as applied to unavoidable toxicants, such as environmental contaminants, that are not directly attributable to the activities of food growers or processors and that might be regarded as fitting a common perception of "natural."

REGULATION OF ADDED SUBSTANCES IN FOOD

All food substances that are not naturally occurring are regarded as "added" under the FD&C Act. Congress has created several different categories under the broad class of "added" food constituents, and has established different safety standards and procedures for each category. For simplicity, three broad groups of added food substances can be identified: (1)unintended added substances that are neither necessary nor unavoidable; (2) substances whose use is necessary in the production of food or unavoidable by good manufacturing practice; and (3) substances that become constituents of food through their intended use. The latter category includes food and color additives and pesticide residues.

Food and color additives, unlike other added substances, are regulated through an elaborate premarket review and approval process, must be proven safe by the intended user and are subject to the Delaney Clause, which prohibits any additive found to induce cancer when ingested by man or animal.[11] In addition, FDA is not permitted to take account of the benefits of a food or color additive in determining whether to approve its use. Pesticide residue tolerances are also subject to premarket approval. However, pesticide tolerances are not governed by the Delaney Clause, and the Environmental Protection Agency (EPA) has explicit authority to consider the economic benefits of pesticides in setting tolerances.[12]

Section 402(a)(1) of the Act provides that a food containing an added poisonous or deleterious substance will be regarded as adulterated where the added substance may render the food injurious to health. The "may render injurious" standard was authoritatively interpreted by the Supreme Court in the *Lexington Mill* case in 1914.[13] The Court held that the key issue is the quantity of the added substance in food. To meet the section 402(a)(1) adulteration test, there must be a sufficient amount of a poisonous or deleterious substance in food to creat a significant possibility that the food may be injurious. There is no requirement, however, that FDA prove conclusively that a particular food will cause injury, and consideration must be given to possible harm to the most vulnerable segments of the public (e.g., the old, the young, and the ill).

It is notable that, in contrast to the Delaney Clause, the adulteration standard for added substances embodies a risk threshold concept and clearly permits the approval of carcinogenic substances that pose a *de minimis* or insignificant risk. The recent court decision overturning FDA's approval of two carcinogenic color additives that were found to pose a *de minimis* risk was based exclusively on the extraordinary rigidity of the Delaney Clause and does not call into question the flexibility of the basic adulteration standard for added substances.[14]

In view of FDA's restrictive interpretation of naturally occurring substances, an increasingly important category of added food constituents is unavoidable environmental contaminants. FDA has authority under section 406 of the FD&C Act to establish tolerances for added poisonous or deleterious substances that are required in the production of food or cannot be avoided by good manufacturing practice.[15] As with the basic section 402(a)(1) adulteration standard, there is no special treatment of carcinogens under section 406. Moreover, under the unavoidability criterion in section 406, FDA may give implicit consideration to the benefits of added substances.[16]

Under authority of section 406, FDA has established tolerances for polychlorinated biphenyls (PCBs) in milk and fish[17] and has issued action levels for a number of environmental contaminants in food, including aflatoxin in corn and peanuts, lead in pottery, and mercury in fish.[18] The Supreme Court recently confirmed that FDA is not required to establish formal tolerances for unavoidable added poisonous or deleterious substances in food and that the Agency is free to employ action levels when it chooses.[19] This gives FDA the flexibility to initiate or revise action levels in light of new scientific developments without undertaking the prolonged rulemaking required under section 406.

Through use of its authority under section 406, FDA has regulated unavoidable environmental contaminants under a flexible safety standard comparable to that for naturally occurring toxicants. FDA has determined that environmental contaminants are not food additives, because they are not intended to be added to and serve no functional purpose in food,[20] and it has interpreted section 406 as permitting a rough balancing of the value of the food, the toxicity of the contaminant, and the feasibility of reducing or eliminating the contaminant.

The multiplicity of safety standards for different categories of food constituents is undeniably complex. Moreover, there is growing controversy over whether the Delaney Clause is justified in light of modern scientific advances.[21] Nevertheless, there is a rough underlying logic to the federal food safety scheme, and it has proven remarkably durable and effective. Although a simpler and more logical food safety system might be devised in the abstract, it is doubtful whether a proposed wholesale revision of the statutory scheme would survive the legislative process in any better form than current law.

There are sound practical reasons for the disparate safety standards for naturally occurring constituents and other food substances. The relatively lenient safety standard for naturally occurring food substances reflects a reasonable judgment that such substances have been historically acceptable to consumers, often provide significant benefits, and are disproportionately difficult to avoid. New food additives, on the other hand, logically should be subject to more rigorous safety controls prior to introduction into the food supply. The approach to regulation of environmental contaminants under the Act, including consideration of avoidability and benefits, has proven to be flexible and reasonably protective.

REGULATION UNDER CALIFORNIA PROPOSITION 65

Federal regulation of poisonous or deleterious food substances contrasts sharply with the regulatory scheme embodied in California Proposition 65 and similar laws recently proposed in other states. The growth in such laws thus poses a serious threat to the federal food safety system.

California Proposition 65, which was passed by voter initiative on November 4, 1986, includes a requirement to provide a clear and reasonable warning in connection with any business activity that causes a person to be exposed to a listed carcinogen or reproductive toxicant.[22] The warning requirement applies to food products, and the California governor has listed over 200 chemicals for which warnings will be required. The California law has fundamentally different premises than the federal food safety system.

First, unlike federal law, Proposition 65 does not differentiate between exposures to naturally occurring chemicals in food and exposures to chemicals added by man. Because low levels of naturally occurring carcinogens and reproductive toxicants are ubiquitous in food, strict interpretation of Proposition 65 would require warnings on virtually all food products. To avoid this absurd result, the California Health and Welfare Agency has issued emergency regulations exempting naturally occurring substances from the food warning requirement.[23]

The California Health and Welfare Agency recently published a proposal to convert the emergency exemption for naturally occurring toxicants to a final regulation. It explained the basis for the proposal as follows:

> This exemption is derived from the distinction in state and federal food adulteration laws between naturally occurring substances in food and those which are added substances.... The laws make it easier to prove adulteration where a deleterious substance was introduced into food by man, than where a substance was naturally occurring in the food.... The rationale for this special treatment of food is the historical desire to preserve naturally occurring foods in the American food supply, despite the presence in those foods of small amounts of potentially deleterious substances, as well as a recognition of the general safety of unprocessed foods as a matter of consumer experience.... For these same reasons, it is reasonable and appropriate to implement the Act so that warnings are not required for naturally occurring chemicals in food.[24]

In spite of the Health and Welfare Agency's cogent reasoning, it is important to bear in mind that there is no textual basis for the naturally occurring exemption in Propositioin 65; the exemption may be subject to legal challenge, and similar laws passed in other states may not be interpreted in the same manner.

There are two important differences between the Proposition 65 exemption and the FDA definition of naturally occurring poisonous or deleterious substances. First, the California regulation exempts from the warning requirement "toxins produced by the natural growth of fungi" (i.e., aflatoxin), whereas FDA has taken the position that fungi are not naturally occurring because they are not inherent constituents of food.

Second, the California regulation provides that where a chemical in food is in part naturally occurring and in part added as a result of human activity, the naturally occurring portion remains subject to the exemption. By contrast, in the Anderson Seafoods case, the court held under the federal Act that where any portion of a food contaminant is added the entire amount will be treated as such.

The California Health and Welfare Agency's naturally occurring exemption is more detailed than the FDA definition, but the precise parameters of the California exemption are unclear. The exemption provides that a chemical is naturally occurring only to the extent that the chemical did not result from any "known human activity," except that "human activity" does not include sowing, planting, plowing, or irrigation. An important unanswered question is whether the exemption applies to environmental contaminants in food that are not attributable to the grower or processor but that were introduced into the environment, at a remote time and location, by some form of human activity. For example, what is the status under the California regulation of lead in food that is derived from soil levels attributable to air pollution from remote manufacturing activities or automobile exhaust?

The California exemption further provides that a chemical is naturally occurring only to the extent that "it was not avoidable by good manufacturing practices or other intervening measures." It is not clear what types of "intervening measures" must be taken into account in determining whether a chemical is sufficiently avoidable to fall outside the exemption.

The second important difference between California Proposition 65 and federal law is the relative importance given to carcinogens and reproductive toxicants as compared to other food hazards. There is no special safety standard for reproductive toxicants under federal law. Although the Delaney Clause ostensibly imposes a blanket prohibition on food and color additives that are animal carcinogens, federal law does not otherwise differentiate between carcinogens and other poisonous or deleterious substances in food. By contrast, Proposition 65 imposes warning requirements *only* with respect to carcinogens and reproductive toxicants and ignores all other types of food hazards.

A third fundamental difference between Proposition 65 and federal food safety regulation is that Proposition 65 relies exclusively on a warning mechanism, whereas warnings are eschewed by FDA. Although FDA has statutory power to require warnings for toxicants in food, which it has occasionally exercised,[25] the Agency has expressed a strong policy preference for regulations that limit exposure to toxicants in food rather than warning consumers of their presence. FDA has reasoned that levels of toxicants which pose a significant risk ordinarily should not be permitted in food and that warnings for toxicants that pose an insignificant risk would merely confuse consumers.

For example, in 1977, FDA rejected a proposal that warnings be required for hazardous contaminants, for which tolerances or action levels were prescribed, finding that such warnings would be "unnecessary and inappropriate," and explaining that "if any food is found to be hazardous to health, FDA will not permit it to be distributed in interstate commerce."[26] Similarly, in 1979, FDA held that any requirement for warnings on foods containing carcinogens "would apply to many, perhaps most foods, in a supermarket, ...[that] such warnings would be so numerous they would confuse the public, would not promote informed consumer decision making, and would not advance the public health."[27]

CONCLUSION

Under Federal law, there are important regulatory distinctions between naturally occurring and added substances in food. Naturally occurring substances are subject to a more lenient and flexible safety standard than other categories of food constituents, and there are sound public policy reasons for this distinction. This long-standing regulatory framework is threatened by California Proposition 65 and similar proposals in other states, which do not distinguish between naturally occurring and added substances in food and which embody fundamentally different regulatory mechanisms than federal law.

NOTES

1. 21 U.S.C. § 342(a)(1).

2. *United States* v. *1232 Cases of American Beauty Brand Oysters,* 43 F. Supp. 749 (W.D. Mo. 1942).

3. Merrill, "Regulating Carcinogens in Food: A Legislator's Guide to the Food Safety Provisions of the Federal Food Drug and Cosmetic Act," 77 Mich. L. Rev. 171, 186, footnote 59 (1978).

4. *Millet, Pit and Seed Company, Inc.* v. *United States,* 436 F. Supp. 84 (E.D. Tenn. 1977).

5. Ames, "Dietary Carcinogens and Anticarcinogens," *Science,* Vol. 211, p. 1256 (September 1983).

6. 21 (C.F.R. § 109.3 (1987).

7. *Young* v. *Community Nutrition Institute,* 106 S. Ct. 2360 (1986).

8. *Continental Seafoods, Inc.* v. *Schweiker,* 674 F. 2d 38 (D.C. Cir. 1982).

9. *United States* v. *Boston Farm Center, Inc.,* 590 F.2d 149 (5th Cir. 1979).

10. *United States* v. *Anderson Seafoods, Inc.,* 622 F.2d 157 (5th Cir. 1980).

11. 21 U.S.C. § § 348 and 376.

12. 21 U.S.C. § 346a.

13. *United States* v. *Lexington Mill & Elevator Co.,* 232 U.S. 399 (1914).

14. *Public Citizen* v. *Young,* 831 F.2d 1108 (D.C. Cir. 1987).

15. 21 U.S.C. § 346.

16. Merrill, "Regulating Carcinogens," supra, p. 200.

17. 21 C.F.R. § 109.30 (1987).

18. 39 Fed. Reg. 42748 (1974).

19. *Young* v. *Community Nutrition Institute,* 106 S. Ct. 2360. (1986).

20. 39 Fed. Reg. 42743 (1974).

21. *See,* Merrill, "FDA's Implementation of the Delaney Clause: Repudiation of Congressional Choice, or Reasoned Adaptation to Scientific Progress?," 5 Yale J. on Reg. 1 (1988); Blank, "The Delaney Clause: Technical Naivete and Scientific Advocacy in the Formulation of Public Health Policies," 62 Calif. L. Rev. 1084 (1974).

22. California Health and Safety Code, Section 25249.6.

23. California Administrative Code, Title 22, Section 12501(b).

24. California Health and Welfare Agency, Notice of Proposed Rulemaking to Adopt New Title 22, Sections 12501 to 12503, page 1 (May 25, 1988).

25. See, e.g., 21 C.F.R. § 101.17 (1987).

26. 42 Fed. Reg. 52814 (1977).

27. 44 Fed. Reg. 59509, 5913 (1979).

14

Strengths and Limitations of Toxicological Testing Procedures

Andrew G. Ebert

The Robert H. Kellen Company
Atlanta, Georgia

INTRODUCTION

"Absolute safety is the ideal toward which many individuals concerned with food protective measures aspire. Establishing the absence of potential harm, however, entails proving a negative which is a practical impossibility." That quote, from Siu et al. (1977) in the paper published by the members of the SCOGS (Select Committee on GRAS Substances), illustrates that which is considered in this paper.

As the straight line to many shaggy dog stories goes, there is good news and bad news. The good news is that there exists the science and art of toxicology. Perhaps the greatest strength of toxicologic testing is that there is a series of sometimes simple, sometimes complex tests in which the potential for xenobiotics to engender harm in a biological system may be studied. Basically, it has served society well. As far as food safety is concerned, these tests have, by and large, been accepted by industry and academia, food industry regulators, and the regulated industry in protecting the health and safety of consumers while allowing our complex system of food production, processing, distribution, marketing, and sales to proceed on a relatively sound economic basis.

The bad news, and hence, at least in this writer's view, one of the great limitations of toxicologic testing is that, as Siu et al. (1977) accurately point out, we cannot provide absolute proof of safety to society and the general population cannot understand why not. Who among us has not been involved in dialogue of the following type? We can (an example is given) and you (fill in name of scientist-like toxicologist) cannot (fill in name of problem). For example, we can put a man on the moon, but you toxicologists cannot assure us that our food is safe.

SYSTEMS IN TOXICOLOGY TESTING—THE DECISION TREE

Let's review the situation in more detail. First, there *is* a system for toxicologic testing in place. It has evolved over the years and provided a basic, generally agreed upon system to study food components, direct and indirect food additives, pesticides, and the preclinical phase of new drug evaluation. The Safety Decision Tree (see Fig. 14.1), developed some years ago by the Food Safety Council, is an agreed-upon system for testing in toxicology. This concordance in toxicologic research protocols is one of the basic strengths in toxicologic testing.

First the test material is defined, an easy task in the case of a drug, or single component food additive, a difficult task in the case of a complex chemical mixture such as a food. Next some estimate of exposure is made,

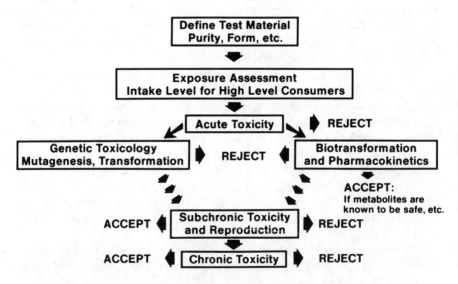

FIG. 14.1 Safety Decision Tree. (*Adapted from Hayes and Campbell, 1986.*)

often a difficult task in the case of new substances. I might add that the substances evaluated must represent the same materials to which humans will be or are exposed; highly purified samples do not necessarily represent the item of commerce.

There follows genetic toxicology as a predictor of carcinogenicity. Longer-term animal studies follow. They usually involve two species— one a nonrodent—utilizing several dose levels and periods of study from months to years.

Ideally, low doses given in a study should give little biological effect in the test system so that a NOEL (no observed effect level) may be calculated. High doses should also be given to induce toxic effects. Once toxicity has been induced, it is then possible to observe and measure the intensity of the effect noted. Estimates of safety factors may then be made or its reciprocal, risk ascertained. Risk is defined as the probability that a substance will inherently produce harm under specified conditions and, related to it, the probability that harm will occur under the conditions of use is called hazard.

Those of us who have bench experience in the metabolic fate of drugs and foods also emphasize the strength of absorption, distribution, metabolism, and excretion tests in toxicology. Measurement of the ADME of a test compound in experimental animals and man can provide data in two important areas. First, if a given laboratory animal metabolizes the test compound in a similar fashion to humans, a strong argument is provided that that laboratory animal is a good model for the effects of the compound in humans. Second, knowing where a xenobiotic agent goes within an organism and how that organism detoxifies it and excretes it provides valuable information to the toxicologist in potentially pinning down the toxicologic site, that is, knowing where to look and what to look for.

FDA's Redbook

Although committing to rigid protocols has been anathema to toxicologists for years, there has been sufficient agreement for the FDA to draft for comment a proposed text for testing food and color additives. Its existence should be known to all scientists. Its content will be known to all toxicologists. Its potential implementation represents another strength in toxicologic testing and had better be known to food technocologists. This so-called FDA "Redbook," officially titled *Toxicologic Principles for the Safety Assessment of Direct Food Additives and Color Additives Used in Food,* (FDA, 1982), essentially associates structure of the test compound and

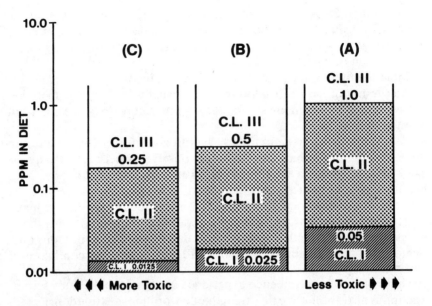

FIG. 14.2 FDA Redbook structure categories (*Adapted from Toxicologic Principles for the Safety Assessment of Direct Food Additives and Color Additives Used in Food, U.S. Food and Drug Administration, 1982.*)

potential population exposure and bases the testing requirements on the creation of "levels of concern."

The toxicologic tests in the Redbook are a tiered system of recommended studies—with more research required on food and color additives assigned a greater"concern level." Concern level is, in turn, based upon estimates of consumer exposure and assignment to one of three toxicity categories based on structural similarities to known toxicants. The basic Redbook algorithm for concern is illustrated in Fig. 14.2. Note that dietary exposure is on a log plot of dietary levels ranging from a low of 0.0125 ppm to 1.0 ppm across three structure levels. Parts per million in diet increases 20-fold for "C" compounds, 20-fold for "B" level compounds, and 20-fold for "A" level compounds.

Structure Category A contains compounds believed to be of a lower order of toxicity, such as many simple aliphatic noncyclic, saturated hydrocarbons,and monofunctional alcohols and ketones of chain length C2–C20.

The highest toxicity group is Structure Category C. It includes alpha and beta unsaturated aldehydes, ketones, aromatic amines, nitro and nitroso groups on compound safrole-like structures, and furans, among others. Category B is intermediate in toxicity estimation, based on structure. It contains many olefins, fatty acids, inorganic salts, peptides, and proteins.

The amount of toxicity testing required is then based on the derived "concern level." Figure 14.3 describes studies listed in the Redbook for Concern Level I. Only two short-term tests are called for—short-term rodent feeding and short-term carcinogenicity potential. Corresponding dietary levels for 1 are 0.0125 ppm to 0.05 ppm corresponding to 0.00031 to 0.0012 mg/kg/day, depending on structure. Figure 14.4 describes studies indicated for Concern Level II following STTs for carcinogenicity. These include a rodent reproduction and teratology study and 90-day feeding studies in rodents and nonrodents.

For the highest concern level, number III, the most research is required, as illustrated in Fig. 14.5. Here carcinogenicity evaluation in two rodent species is required. A chronic feeding of at least one year is called for in two species, one nonrodent and one rodent. The rat or mouse work is usually linked to the carcinogenicity study. In addition to the multigeneration study called for in Concern Level II compounds, a long-term study of at least one year's duration in nonrodents is required as is the short-term carcinogenicity evaluation required for Concern Level I and II compounds.

Our firm manages IFAC, the International Food Additives Council, and thus has considerable interest in the Redbook. As toxicologic testing is a common practice in the laboratories of IFAC members, like the

STUDIES REQUIRED
- ● Short-Term (28 Day) Rodent Feeding
- ● Short-Term Carcinogenicity Potential

EXPOSURE - STRUCTURE / LEVEL

STRUCTURE CATEGORY	INTAKE	
	PPM (DIET)	mg/kg/day
A	‹0.0500	0.00120
B	‹0.0250	0.00063
C	‹0.0125	0.00031

FIG. 14.3 Toxicology tests required for concern level I compounds. (*Modified from Toxicologic Principles for the Safety Assessment of Direct Food Additives and Color Additives Used in Food, U.S. Food and Drug Administration, 1982.*)

STUDIES REQUIRED

- Short-Term Carcinogenicity Potential
- Multi-Generation (NLT 2) Study
  Reproduction Plus Teratology - Rodent
- Subchronic (NLT 90 Days) Feeding in 2 Species
  1 Rodent, 1 Non-Rodent

EXPOSURE - STRUCTURE/LEVEL

STRUCTURE CATEGORY	PPM (DIET)	INTAKE mg/kg/day
A	0.0500	0.00120
B	0.0250	0.00063
C	0.0125	0.00031

FIG. 14.4   Toxicology tests required for concern level II compounds. (*Modified from Toxicologic Principles for the Safety Assessment of Direct Food Additives and Color Additives Used in Food, U.S. Food and Drug Administration, 1982.*)

STUDIES REQUIRED

- Short-Term Carcinogenicity
- Multi-Generational (NLT 2) Study
  Reproduction Plus Teratology - Rodent
- Carcinogenicity Studies - 2 Rodent Species
- Chronic (NLT 1 Year) Feeding Study in
  1 Rodent and 1 Non-Rodent Species

EXPOSURE - STRUCTURE/LEVEL

STRUCTURE CATEGORY	PPM (DIET)	INTAKE mg/kg/day
A	1.00	0.0250
B	0.50	0.0125
C	0.25	0.0063

FIG. 14.5   Toxicology tests required for concern level III compounds. (*Modified from Toxicologic Principles for the Safety Assessment of Direct Food Additives and Color Additives Used in Food, U.S. Food and Drug Administration, 1982.*)

assigned topic of this paper, our members have examined the strengths and limitations of the methods proposed in the Redbook. There is an obvious limitation in that the Redbook is inapplicable to complex mixtures, natural products, and other test substances where the structure of the potential toxicant is unknown. Also, in the case of new compounds, the anticipated use of a food additive, hence exposure to the population, may exist only in the fertile mind of the marketing executive who will be charged with the commercial success of the material once cleared.

If a new food component is commercially successful, its total level of exposure, hence its concern level, may have to be adjusted upward. Therefore, IFAC felt that the Redbook algorithm needed to be expanded beyond its existing bounds. Our suggestion is illustrated in Fig. 14.6. IFAC has proposed that the FDA algorithm be "exploded," because many direct food additives are ingested at dietary levels exceeding 1 ppm. IFAC proposed that a new category be added. We call it "AA." At Concern Level III, its break-off points are at 25.0 and 250.0 ppm, respectively. Concern level break-off points have also been expanded to 100-fold across each of the structure categories. IFAC believes that for "Double A" compounds, no

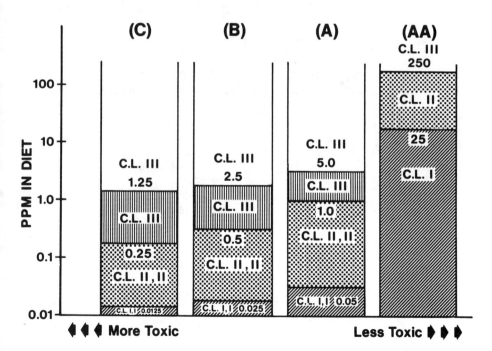

FIG. 14.6 Structure categories algorithm proposed by the International Food Additives Council for Extension of the FDA Redbook Algorithm.

toxicity studies are required. The category is to reflect those food additives of defined purity used at higher levels than Categories A, B, or C. We are optimistic that the FDA will adapt an "exploded" algorithm. To us it appears workable and realistic of food additive use.

Based on the data derived from the estimated population exposure and the lowest effect level derived from the toxicologic studies completed, it is then possible to calculate an "R value." This is the quotient obtained by dividing the human exposure in milligrams of additive per kilogram of body weight per day by the lowest effect level of the substance, also expressed in milligrams of additive per kilogram of body weight per day. R values relate toxicity and exposure, thus providing an estimation of relative concern. A relatively high intake on a daily basis of a substance that induced animal toxicity at a relatively low dose would yield a high R value and vice versa. It follows then that the reciprocal of R, 1/R, gives an es-

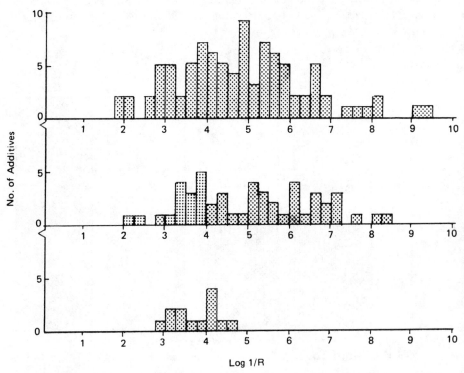

FIG. 14.7 Frequency distribution of 1/R values in various Redbook structure categories. (*Adapted from Rulis and Hattan, 1985.*)

timate of safety margins—at least against those substances similarly evaluated.

Using the algorithm described in Fig. 14.2, Rulis and Hattan have calculated frequency distributions for log 1/R across the three structure categories, as illustrated in Fig. 14.7, for 159 food additives for which the lowest effect level (LEL) was known and there were accurate poundage consumption data. There is great range—over eight units in log 1/R partly from the extreme variability in exposure values—even within a given structure group like "C." When Rulis and Hattan (1985) sum the number of additives in each column for values of log 1/R vs the number of additives, the 159 additives well fit a nonlinear least squares fit normal distribution curve (see Fig. 14.8). The most probable number—the peak— lies between log 1/R 4 and 5. If one calculates the lowest effect level that would result in a log 1/R value between 4 and 5, the corresponding amount to show a lowest effect level in animals would be enormous and 1/R safety factor in the thousands. Rules and Hattan point out that the histogram is vacant to the left of log 1/R = 2.

A value of log 1/R = 1 could correspond to, for example, an additive whose lowest effect level in animals is 1 mg/kg/day and whose use by 10% of the U.S. population is 10^6 lb/yr. As Fig. 14.8 shows, only a few additives are used in that high amount, and in animal studies few were shown to have a low effect level as low as 1 mg/kg/day.

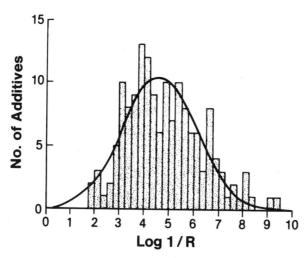

FIG. 14.8 Frequency distribution of R values. Accumulated across the three Red-book structure categories. (*Adapted from Rulis and Hattan, 1985.*)

My point is this: The construction of the Redbook algorithm followed by specific evaluations of numerous food additives indicates that it is a toxicologic method, a system, that works.

Whether Decision Tree, Redbook, or custom-designed by the toxicologist, there is general greement that toxicologic tests represent powerful, biological research activities that can illustrate the harm of a substance to an organism. However, these tests are largely done retrospectively. The reciprocal, predicting harm, that is, risk assessment, has spawned an entire new science encompassing biology, medicine, epidemiology, and most certainly statistics. Food technologists interested in risks and food safety are referred to the Scientific Status Summary on this subject published by IFT's Office of Scientific Public Affairs (Newsome, 1988).

LIMITATIONS IN TOXICOLOGICAL TESTING

Now that we have examined some systems used in toxicologic testing, some consideration of the limitations is in order—a quality audit of the power of these tests, if you will. As one could observe from both the Decision Tree and/or Redbook approach, long-term bioassays constitute the major tests, especially in the evaluation of carcinogens—the disease of concern in our society.

Schach von Wittenau (1987) has examined the strengths and limitations of long-term animal bioassays for carcinogens. He raises several important questions, such as: Is the dose given in animal bioassays within a pharmacokinetic range that is relevant to man? He points out that compounds given at low doses go through metabolic pathways that may be different from pathways followed after giving high doses. Indeed, at high doses, the administration of the MTD, the Maximum Tolerated Dose (which is routinely utilized in cancer research), may overwhelm normal metabolic pathways and detoxication mechanisms. Such findings from high-dose testing are then compared to use of the test compound in humans. In the case of foods, food components, or food additives, lower doses are given for a longer time—perhaps for the entire life of the person so exposed.

Schach von Wittenau asks: Does the dose under study provide a stimulus not likely to be exerted in humans under the foreseeable conditions of use? I believe that the answer to that question is "yes, routinely" and almost always the case in toxicity studies of materials common to food. In trying to compress the time scale because of the cost of testing and the shorter life-span of animals to produce an effect in test animals, we sometimes overload the model system thereby rendering the model invalid according Schach von Wittenau.

Others on this program will discuss risk assessment techniques and herein lies another limitation in the system. Schach von Wittenau points out that the statisticians and their computer capabilities transform cancer research into a mathematical exercise. Orientation moves from the animal house into the computer center. Schach von Wittenau points out that cancer evaluation requires the skills of persons other than mathematicians. Cancer evaluation requires qualified pathologists—those scientists and artisans who look at the microscopic and macroscopic changes observed in animals being bioassayed, observing the morphologic and anatomic changes—many of which are subtle—which separate a benign change from one that might indicate the potential for morbidity and mortality.

Schach von Wittenau reminds us that the cause of the change from which the cancer is defined must be considered. He cites Riley's 1975 paper in *Science*. Riley reported that mice housed in a noisy environment developed mammary tumors much earlier than siblings kept in a quiet environment. No carcinogen was under evaluation. Apparently it was the stress that was carcinogenic. Riley's work clearly demonstrates the dependence of tumor emergence upon distortion of the test system's homeostasis and the generation of what Schach von Wittenau calls "pseudocarcinogens." "In other words," he says " . . . for a model to be useful, we must be sure that the stimulus that we provide reflects human reality, and we must also understand to what extent the reaction of the biological system we use mimics the response of man." The validity of the model is often only a wishful guess, he writes, constituting another major limitation in toxicologic testing procedures.

Ames and coworkers (1987) have also examined the limitations of relying on animal tests as predictors for cancer in people. They point to species variation in response to 392 chemicals in their database. They report that 226 were carcinogens in at least one test, but 96, about one-fourth of the compounds, were positive in the mouse and negative in the rat, or the other way around. Ames et al. point out that "qualitative extrapolation of cancer risks from rats or mice to humans . . . is unlikely to be as reliable." They note also that tobacco smoke and alcohol, which they identify as "the two largest identified cause of neoplastic death in the United States," are not easily detected in standard rodent carcinogenicity tests. Their findings provided part of the impetus in their developing the Human Exposure Rodent Potency, or HERP, index, frequently discussed in cancer evaluation.

Equally disconcerting for the food toxicologist is Ames's observation that "quantitative extrapolation from rodents to humans, particularly at low doses, is guesswork that we have no way of validating." Ames says that it is guesswork because of the lack of knowledge in at least six major areas:

The basic mechanisms of carcinogenicity.

The relation of cancer, aging, and life-span

Order and timing of events in the carcinogenic process.

Species differences in metabolism and pharmacokinetics.

Differences in natural defences against cancer—one species vs another.

Human heterogenity in resistance to cancer.

LIMITATIONS IN TOXICOLOGY STUDIES—THE DECREASING ZERO

Unfortunately, toxicologic evaluation of discrete, defined chemical entities present in food at high levels is only one aspect of the toxicologist's responsibilities. Because of markedly improved capabilities in analytical chemical techniques, the presence of exquisitely low levels of materials can be detected with a specificity and sensitivity unheard of as little as a decade ago. At this point in time, toxicology testing begins to interact with societal decisions. Food, its availability, its value, its safety has at one time or another crossed the minds of probably everyone in our society. It is now that the limitations in toxicologic testing become more apparent. From my standpoint as a toxicologist, I believe we face a minimum of three basic limitations in that phase of our work. These are:

1. An inherent lack of sensitivity in the biological responses we measure versus a high degree of sensitivity and specificity in analytical chemical technology.
2. The misuse and overextrapolation of toxicologic data in search of the never-achievable goal of absolute safety.
3. Failure to provide assurance and comfort to a troubled general population. "They" who feel that "we" in food technology, or technology in general, arc poisoning them.

Thanks to the sensitivity and specificity of new analytical chemical techniques, it is routinely possible to measure the presence of a xenobiotic in a biological system at the parts per million level and, often, at the parts per billion level. In order to better appreciate this sensitivity, let's consider it from the standpoint of some common descriptors that might be useful in your interaction as a food scientist with the general public whom you seek to serve, as well as other nontoxicologists within your organization.

I know of at least three common analogies which are used. First, there is the population analogy. One part per billion is the ability to seek out and identify one citizen of the People's Republic of China out of its entire population of one billion people. Second, there is the time analogy. One part per billion is one minute in all of the time since Christ was born until the present. Third, is the martini analogy. A part per billion is roughly two teaspoons (10mL) of vermouth in thirty/100,000 gallon tank cars of gin or vodka. A dry martini, indeed.

Compare that with the fact that in biology we are currently dealing with systems that are sensitive only to the equivalent of a part per thousand basis, by definition, a million times less sensitive than the technology available to the analytical chemist. Siu et al. (1977) describe this limitation as follows.

> Given a set of experimental conditions with n number of control and treated animals, respectively, what increase in untoward responses in the latter group over those in the controls should be taken as evidence of toxicity?
>
> If n equals 1,000, an upper limit of 2.3 affected animals would give a 90% confidence of the absence of toxicity. Such a degree of assurance, however, would hardly be comforting to the average person as far as cancer is concerned.

That person would prefer a much higher confidence together with an associated incidence of, let's say, less than one tumor per 500,000 test animals. I would parenthetically point out that that's not good enough. Regulatory authorities nowadays consider an insignificant risk to be one in a million. Siu et al. note that to obtain such a projection (2.3 affected animals over controls) with 0.999 confidence would require study of over three million test animals.

The tools and testing methods available to the toxicologist just do not have the sensitivity and specificity of the methodologies available to the analytical chemist. As a result, the chemist is able to measure potential toxicants in our environment with great precision and accuracy. The ability of the toxicologist to comment with any degree of accuracy as to the toxicologic significance of these low-levels materials, if any, is severely limited.

The second limitation mentioned is our search for absolute safety. As absolute safety is unattainable, we do the next best thing and attempt to use safety factors as a guide. Note I said "guide" and not "rule." Toxicologists like to use safety factors. They provide some degree of comfort by linking the amount of material that induces toxicity in a test organism and then compare that amount to the amount that a human might reasonably be exposed to. Such a rationale calls for the toxicologic evaluation of a compound and the construction of a dose-response curve. That is, giving a dose, or doses, sufficiently high in experimental animals to induce a toxic effect and lower doses where little or no effect is seen. Then, by extrapolation, conclude that a lower dose is safe for man. The toxicologic guidelines have been codified (21CFR § 170.22) and state "Except where evidence is submitted which justifies use of a different safety factor in applying animal experimentation to man, 100 to 1 will be used; that is: a food additive for use by man will not be granted a tolerance (for use) that will exceed 1/100th of the maximum amount demonstrated to be without harm to experimental animals." The 100-fold safety factor is derived from an anticipated 10-fold variation between animals and humans and another 10-fold span between different humans.

Along with that guideline comes another toxicologic limitation. Let's assume a food technologist discovers a potential nutrient that is to be used in food at greater than 1% of the diet. By definition, you cannot feed greater than 100% of the substance in a toxicologic evaluation. Moreover, unless the material invented provided all of the nutrient components of a control diet, the toxicologic effects of a nutritionally insufficient diet could ensue. Regulatory authorities take this into account and they also recognize that a number of food constituents, such as vitamins A and D, have less than 100-fold safety factors in comparing the toxic levels that may be demonstrated in animals and the nutrient use of these two vitamins in man. The Redbook guideline advocates a general maximum of 5% of the test substance in the diet.

Another weakness in toxicologic testing is the interpretation of carcinogenicity studies. Toxicologists may be interested in a wide variety of toxic manifestations. However, the suggestion that our environment, food included, may be a factor in cancer has been widely embraced by our society. Frightened by cancer statistics, cancer and its control have major social interest.

IARC/NTP AND EXPERT COMMITTEES

For decades, the International Agency for Research on Cancer (IARC), among other groups, has been evaluating the toxicologic data in the literature on a wide variety of materials and processes. Animal data from chronic studies, short-term tests believed to be predictors of carcinogenicity, and epidemiological evidence in humans are all taken into consideration in IARC's evaluations. Monographs are published in which the data are summarized. Quality of the data are considered as descriptors are attached to the conclusions. Evidence for carcinogenicity is separated as to data in humans vs. animals vs. short-term tests. Agreed-upon descriptive words are used to characterize the studies, specifically "sufficient," "limited," "inadequate," "no data."

But then, as a result of the deliberations, IARC makes lists based on the descriptors in the monographs and categorizes the compound or process. IARC establishes a decreasing order of numerical ranking depending on the evidence of carcinogenicity. IARC category 1—the strongest—is assigned to those compounds where there is human epidemiology indicating carcinogencity. Category 2 has two subcategories, A and B. Category 2A is assigned to those materials where there is "limited evidence" of carcinogenicity in humans but where the data are not so clear-cut—bias, confounding effects, etc. cannot be excluded. When sufficient evidence is available from animal studies, but not humans in IARC's opinion, a category of 2B is assigned.

Compounds evaluated, but in which the data are insufficient to draw a sound conclusion, are placed in category 3, and category 4 is assigned to those substances evaluated in which there was no evidence of carcinogenicity.

Herein lies another limitation in toxicologic testing and one that engenders particularly strong feelings. Many persons influential in cancer policy, like Shubik, Hutt, and others, vociferously argue against "pigeonholing" carcinogens by placing them on a list. For example, Shubik, at this year's winter meeting of the Toxicology Forum (1988), inquired as to what use these lists of categories are in terms of human health. Shubik worried aloud that the whole exercise is "a big joke," a waste of resources. If any list of cancer-causing substances were to be promulgated, it should be by cancer mechanisms, Shubik advocated. He accurately observed that the force or reason for creating these lists in the first place is in response to legislative bodies like the U.S. Congress.

All that effort does little to advance knowledge on cancer and its prevention according to Shubik—clearly a limitation in toxicology.

Ex-FDA General Counsel Peter Barton Hutt, also speaking at the winter Toxicology Forum (1988), commented from the standpoint of Food and Drug Law on the merits of lists of carcinogens and how lawyers use the lists which toxicology developed and the role of toxicologists in general. Hutt said " . . . the field of toxicology has failed to convince the American public of two things: either, one, that you know what you are doing, or two, that if left to you own devices that you will succeed in adquately protecting the public from a safety standpoint." Hutt goes on to say that toxicology has contributed to its own problems. Discussing *lists* of toxicants, Hutt asked the toxicologists, "Who makes up these rules? Who makes up these lists? It is all of you people. It isn't me. I never made up a rule or a list in my entire four years at FDA. I talked to a lot of people who advised me how to do it and followed their advice. So, we have met the enemy, and they are you."

LISTS FROM LISTS

This semi-quantification of toxic effect, in this case cancer, now is further simplified and a quantal "all-or-none" format is embraced to satisfy a legal requirement. Let's take a further look at that interaction. Section 262 of Public Law 95-622, published November 9, 1978, for example, states that the Secretary of Health and Human Services shall publish an annual report which contains a list of all substances which have two characteristics: (1) which either are known to be carcinogens or may reasonably be anticipated to be carcinogens; and (2) which a significant number of persons residing in the United States are exposed. Key definitions, such as "known to be carcinogens," "reasonably be anticipated," and "significant numbers" are not defined. It is at this point in time that the toxicologist must turn to risk assessment techniques to achieve some predictable reality and satisfy the law. Like you, I wait in vain for lawmakers to write laws and regulations based on sound science.

Nowhere has the limited success of toxicologic interaction with politics become more evident than in California. Food scientists had better know the basics of California's Proposition 65—the so-called "Safe Drinking Water and Toxic Enforcement Act of 1986." Although subject to further action, perhaps in the courts, the toxicologic impact of this law (which was passed by referendum) calls for the governor to publish annually a list of carcinogens and reproductive toxicants to which California citizens are "exposed" and, presumably, not protected by the myriad of federal and state laws already pertaining to public health.

To assist the governor, a blue ribbon advisory group of toxicologists has been created to assist in the promulgation of the list of carcinogens and reproductive toxicants. I believe that virtually all of the state's Scientific Advisory Panel meetings, and the numerous hearings completed by the state, on Proposition 65 have been attended by one or more of the participants of this program. My observation is that the toxicologists on the Scientific Advisory Panel who develop their list of carcinogens from the IARC and NTP lists, among others, very well know of, and have gone out of their way to point to, the limitations of the studies as described in the NTP or IARC monographs.

Many of the SAP members have participated in the NTP and IARC programs themselves. Investigators like Ames, whose work is widely quoted and whose papers strongly influenced this talk, are leaders in carcinogenicity research and know from their own experience the strengths and limitations of laboratories, investigators, protocols, results, and the numerous other factors impacting upon the soundness of toxicologic tests.

My concern is that many of the factors which must be taken into consideration are not. I would submit that when it comes to satisfying the political requirements of a list of toxicants, a compound is listed or it is not. And that, by definition, is a major limitation in toxicologic testing. Simply put, a compound having evidence of carcinogenicity in animals, no matter how limited the data, is often listed. It is presumed—no, it is even reported in the press—that a compound, by virtue of its being placed on the governor's list, is a carcinogen—to man. Who else does the justifiably suspicious public worry about? The B6C3F1 mouse? The Fischer 344 rat? Of course not.

One simple comparison I recently made was to examine the list of carcinogens published by the State of California as of January, 1988, and ask "How did IARC classify this compound? How did NTP classify this compound?" It may come as little surprise that the number of carcinogens listed, that is, assumed to be and reported to be carcinogens in man, well exceeded those human carcinogens listed by the IARC and NTP.

Chemical & Engineering News summarized the status of over 175 carcinogens listed under Proposition 65 (Baum, 1988). It is interesting to note that of 162 compounds recommended for placement on the governor's list—sure to be interpreted as representing a cancer hazard to humans—only 25, or 15%, have been categorized as category 1 by IARC or NTP.

Ebert

Most (110) had been classified in category 2A or 2B, and 26 of the 162 had not been listed by IARC or NTP at all—other data being presumably used with these 26.

One might sarcastically inquire—"Why worry about human data?" For in California, it appears that positive responses in any animals species, and under almost any conditions of response, will get the compound listed.

There will be those who argue that such an attitude is callous—that toxicologists who insist on having human and animal evidence indicating toxicity do so to the detriment of people. The lack of acceptability on the part of the public to separate human from animal data represents, to my thinking, another great limitation in toxicologic testing.

Hutt (1988) pointed out that the public wants more than a "vague general assurance from a group of toxicologists." Toxicologic testing is not providing that assurance. Our firm is interested in consumer attitudes and the public's perception of the products sold by member companies in associations which our firm manages. One such study was, in our view, quite troublesome and should create concern for food scientiests and toxicologists (Ebert, 1987). *Self* magazine published in its "Trends in Nutrition" series the results of a survey of attitudes in women, aged 30 to 65, toward a selected group of poorly perceived food ingredients. Table 14.1 lists seven materials which, to my recollection, have been the subject of IFT Scientific Status Summaries or have been otherwise reviewed from a toxicologic standpoint and the results of toxicologic testing summarized. They are ranked from the standpoint of safety concern. Perhaps we should take some comfort that cholesterol was rated the item of greatest concern, with 86% of those surveyed saying that they were "very concerned" or "slightly concerned." in good agreement with clinical and toxicologic evidence. The percentages do not add up to 100 because not every material was recognized by every person surveyed. Consider the percentages of concern of those surveyed for food additives that have been studied—studied by the protocols described in this paper, reviewed by toxicologists in the GRAS Review, or having received other national and international review—and which have been allowed for use by national and international governments. The table ranked salt third in terms of concern, with 83% of those surveyed expressing worry. Saccharin was ranked fifth, with 75% of those surveyed expressing concern.

At the recently completed American Cancer Society Writers' Forum for Medical Writers, Dr. John Ashby of ICI was asked if he knew of any compound that got a "bum rap" in receiving a carcinogenic rating. He replied, "Yes. Saccharin." Dr. Vincent DiVita of the National Cancer Institute agreed with him (Gentry, 1988).

TABLE 14.1 Attitudes Toward A Selected Group of Poorly Perceived Ingredients (Women, 35–65 Years of Age)

Ranking	Material	Percent of subjects surveyed who are:			
		Very concerned	Slightly concerned	Unconcerned	Neither
1	Cholesterol	50	36	1	11
3	NaCl	46	37	2	12
5	Saccharin	40	35	2	17
6	MSG	40	28	1	17
7	NO_3	38	28	1	18
10	Caffeine	28	43	3	23
11	Vitamin-fortified foods	20	35	4	32

Source: Adapted from data compiled by Mark Clements Research, Inc., National Family Opinion, Inc., SRI-VAL, Inc., and published in *Self* Magazine and Ebert (1987).

MSG was rated sixth, with 68% of those surveyed expressing concern. This in spite of the fact that in 1987 FAO/WHO markedly liberalized its views toward MSG (WHO, 1987) by removing the numerical ADI from glutamates and allocating an ADI of "not specified." FAO/WHO also removed the previous specific prohibition of MSG used in foods specifically designed for infants.

I wonder how many persons in the general public or in food science, for that matter, know that? The safety base for MSG is extensive, but until that information is assimilated by the general public, the information gathered from toxicologic tests will have its value severely diminished. A great limitation of toxicologic testing, as I see it, is that the results are poorly disseminated when the findings indicate little or no toxicity and extensively disseminated when the opposite occurs. We had better get going.

The *Self* magazine data, illustrated in Table 14.2 does not indicate much improvement with time. The percentage of those expressing an opinion of being "very concerned" over the safety of food additives is basically unchanged from 1981 to 1986—42% and 43%, respectively, claiming that they are "very concerned." Saccharin's reputation has even slipped in that time, 35% being "very concerned" in 1981 increasing to 40% being "very concerned" in 1986. MSG's rating of "very concerned" increased from 31 to 40% during a time interval when any number of papers reaffirming its safety to man appeared in the literature.

TABLE 14.2 Trends in Attitudes Toward Poorly Perceived Ingredients

Material	Percent very concerned		
	1986	1983	1981
Food additives and chemical perservatives	43	44	42
Cholesterol	50	46	41
NaCl	46	50	36
Saccharin	40	38	35
MSG	40	40	31
NO_3	38	39	35
Caffeine	28	32	26
Vitamin-fortified foods	20	23	25

Source: Adapted from data compiled by Mark Clements Research, Inc., National Family Opinion, Inc., SRI-VAL, Inc., and published in *Self* Magazine and Ebert (1987).

Thus, the concerns continue and the limitations of toxicologic testing continue to be discussed. Many scientists at the American Cancer Society briefing that I mentioned have discussed toxicologic testing. They accurately note that toxicologic testing is costly. I have not even begun to consider economics in this talk. Cheaper, quicker, more reliable tests are needed. Michael Shelby warned that we are spreading our toxicologic efforts so thin that "we are not focusing enough effort on those chemicals that present the greatest hazard."

Like you, I anxiously await the deliberations of the experts in risk analysis. Perhaps, unlike the toxicologists' tests, our mathematically oriented colleagues utilizing the statistical approach in risk analysis can put this entire matter in better perspective.

REFERENCES

Ames, B. N., Magaw, R., and Gold, L. 1987. Ranking possible carcinogenic hazards. *Science* 236: 271.

Baum, R. M. 1988. Businesses feel first impact of California's toxic law. *Chem. Eng. News* 66: 19.

Gentry, C. 1988. Cancer researchers declare saccharin got a bum rap. *St. Petersburg (Florida) Times,* March 22, p. 1-A.

Ebert, A. G. 1987. Interaction of the food industry with the academic community. *Am. J. Clin. Nutr.* 46: 216.

Food & Drug Administration. 1982. Toxicologic principles for the safety assessment of direct food additives and color additives used in food. Bureau of Foods, U.S. Food & Drug Administration, Washington, DC, pp. 14–19, Appendix III, Fig. 1.

Hayes, J. R. and Campbell, T. C. 1986. Food additives and contaminants. Ch. 24. In *Casarett and Doull's Toxicology: The Basic Science of Poisons,* (Ed.) Klaasen, C. D., Amdur, M. O., and Doull, J., p. 785. MacMillan Co., New York.

Hutt, P. B. 1988. Discussion remarks at the Toxicology Forum 1988 Annual Winter Meeting, Bethesda, MD, pp. 97–105.

Newsome, R. L. 1988. The risk benefit concept as applied to food. *Food Technol.* 42(3): 119.

Riley, 1975.

Rulis, A. M. and Hattan, D. G. 1985. FDA's priority-based assessment of food additives II general toxicity parameters. *Reg. Tox. Pharmacol.* 5: 152.

Schach von Wittenau, M. 1987. Strengths and weaknesses of long-term bioassays. *Reg. Tox Pharmacol.* 7: 113.

Shubik, P. 1988. Discussion remarks at the Toxicology Forum 1988 Annual Winter Meeting, Bethesda, MD, p. 40.

Siu, R. G. H., Borzelleca, J. F., Carr, C. J., Day, H. G., Fomon, S. J., Irving, G. W., Jr., LaDu, B. N., Jr., McCoy, J. R., Miller, S. A., Plaa, G. J., Shimkin, M. B., and Wood, J. L. 1977. Evaluation of health aspects of GRAS food ingredients: Lessons learned and questions unanswered. *Fed. Proc.* 36: 2522.

World Health Organization, Geneva. 1987. Evaluation of Certain Food Additives and Contaminants. Thirty-first Report of the Joint FAO/ WHO Expert Committee on Food Additives. *Technical Report Series No. 759,* p. 29.

15

Pros and Cons of Quantitative Risk Analysis

W. Gary Flamm

Food and Drug Administration
Reston, Virginia

INTRODUCTION AND BACKGROUND

For our purposes, "quantitative risk assessment" (QRA) is defined, consistent with the National Academy of Sciences' report on *Risk Assessment in the Federal Government* (1983), as the application of cancer incidence data obtained from properly conducted studies by which laboratory animals are administered a carcinogen to assess the risk of cancer posed to humans from exposure to that carcinogen. The process of QRA has four discrete steps.

First, a decision must be made about the animal study following a thorough review and evaluation of the pathology, toxicology, and statistics. The questions are: (1) Is the tested chemical a carcinogen? (2) At which organ, tissue, and cellular site(s) was cancer induced? (3) What was the combined incidence of cancer? The next step in the process involves establishing the relationship between the doses of carcinogen administered and the degree of response observed (incidence of cancer induced), and, by using some mathematical model, to extrapolate this dose-response curve down to dosage levels equivalent to levels of human exposure. The third step is the assessment of the level of human exposure to the chemical in question. While this step may sound simple, it actually is not, often requiring exposure distribution data on a variety of sub-populations that may be especially at risk and a maze of complex food consumption considerations. Suffice it to say this is often an area of great debate and dispute. The fourth and final step, referred to as "risk characterization" by the NAS report, involves merging the animal data and its extrapolation to low dose as facilitated by some type of mathematical model with human exposure data toward the assessment—or more correctly an estimation—of the risk of cancer posed to exposed human populations.

The entire field of QRA is young, barely a decade and a half old. How does QRA differ from the rest of toxicology and safety assessment? Why does QRA differ? What caused QRA to come into being? How were carcinogens regulated before QRA? To what extent is there scientific consensus over the appropriateness of QRA for use in regulatory decisions? These are the critical questions demanding answers, if an understanding of QRA's pros and cons is to be gleaned. The term "pros and cons" is selected over "strengths and weaknesses" because the latter would imply scientific merit versus a lack thereof. Scientific merit is only one of the issues which QRA encompasses. Its chief purpose and function is to resolve disputes. Disputes over how carcinogens should be regulated regardless of whether they are environmental contaminants, pesticides, drug residues in food-producing animals, or food and color additives—disputes that develop between government and industry. The ultimate issue to be resolved is at what, if any, level is the carcinogen to be allowed or regulated.

To understand how profoundly vexing resolution of the cancer issue is, we need to address the above questions about what makes the toxicology of cancer induction so special and the unique history of food regulation preceding the birth of QRA. It is important to understand that the fundamental underlying principles used in setting tolerances (maximum acceptable levels) for chemicals in food has been that the dose, not the substance, is the poison and at some low enough dose there is no toxic effect whatsoever (Kokoski and Flamm, 1984). In other words, the concept is that there are threshold dose levels for toxicants, and unless the dose is high enough to overcome the threshold, no toxic effects will occur. For toxic substances that produce acute effects such as death, which are observable soon after administration, the existence of thresholds is intuitively obvious to all of us. Common table salt is lethal to humans when taken as a single dose of 30 g or more. But no one dies, as we all know, when a hundredth of that dose is consumed. Obviously, thousands of everyday examples involving food, drugs, household items, and other common exposure can be used to make the point that thresholds as a practical matter do exist for toxicants.

But, what about cancer—do thresholds exist for it or not? The real answer, unfortunately, is no one knows, but there is every reason to believe that cancer induction, like other forms of toxicity, is dose dependent. It is important to stress that clear dose dependency depends upon everything else in the experiment being held constant except for the administered test compound. While this may sound simple, it often is anything but simple. The test compound can, for instance, make the food unpalatable, leading to undernutrition, or the reverse can occur. Or the test compound can cause secondary effects which are known or suspected to produce cancer in their own right, thereby confusing the interpretation of the outcome of the experiment.

One thing is for certain, cancer does not occur immediately following exposure. In both humans and animals, it is well established that the development of cancer does not occur until many months and, in some cases, decades after the exposure which induced it. So, unlike the situation described for acute toxicity, establishing the relationship between exposure and the event that caused it is not so simple for cancer. In fact, it is enormously complex.

Another factor we can count on is that, for certain carcinogens at least, exposure to the carcinogen(s) add up and count toward the overall risk of cancer being induced, even when the exposures are separated by years. For example, the cancer risk from smoking a pack of cigarettes a day for 20 years is essentially the same whether it was accomplished over a 20-year period (without interruption) or over 30 or more years repleat with starts and stops (Lawrence and Paulson, 1981). So, the two incontrovertible statements that can be made about the induction of cancer by chemicals is that the disease occurs long after exposure and that the effects registered from individual, separate exposures are recorded or remembered by the cells affected which later develop cancer. This is clearly a different concept than that described for common table salt, but does it mean *a priori* there is no dose, no matter how low, that is beneath the threshold for cancer induction? Again, the answer is, no one knows.

QRA has been embraced as a solution to the dilemma that our peculiar brand of ignorance and knowledge has caused. QRA rests on the principle that cancer induction is dose dependent and so, its advocates say, it should be possible to estimate effects at low dose without having to address the threshold question, which they argue, correctly, cannot be answered, at least for certain types of carcinogens. These same QRA advocates tell the affected industry they should welcome QRA as the best hope of averting the rigid application of the Delaney no-risk concept (FD&C Act, 1981), while at the same time they will argue that consumer activists and environmentalists should be delighted with the large number of conservatisms built into QRA which ostensibly serve to protect fully the public health. In other words, QRA is, in their words, a compromise in which everyone is left happy. But are they? The answer, of course, is no, as industry is more often than not dismayed over the burden imposed by the conservatisms of QRA and consumerists are upset over the departure, which they think is entirely unnecessary, from the Delaney principle that carcinogens should not be added to food under any circumstance or for any reason whatsoever.

Perhaps it would be naive to expect both industry and consumer activists to be pleased by any single solution to so vexing a public health problem, but what about the experts in carcinogenesis—they are happy, right? Well, no, they are not happy either, for reasons that will be discussed later. How, then, without the industry's, consumerists', or experts' support, can QRA exist as a functional tool used by every regulatory agency in the United States charged with regulating chemical carcinogens? Perhaps the answer lies not in the virtues of QRA, but in the difficulties which beset regulatory agencies before QRA came into existence.

Prior to QRA, the name of the game was stalemate. Even when the Delaney anticancer clause did not legally apply (as it does with food and color additives and residues of carcinogenic animal drugs), if a substance was found to be carcinogenic, the only tenable regulatory policy was to insist upon zero levels, zero exposure, and zero risk.

As the tools and capability of analytical chemistry grew, insisting upon zero became more and more unrealistic. Soon it became apparent that given the extraordinarily low level at which analytical chemists could measure chemical contaminants in food or anything else, all substances, no matter how pure, could be shown to be contaminated with one carcinogen or another. So, as a practical matter, the idea that we humans could be absolutely protected from chemical carcinogens died as a viable scientific concept. In its place, U.S. regulatory agencies have adopted QRA, for, despite all its faults, it is a process on which policy decisions have been and will be based. Use of QRA avoids the stalemate of the past and offers a means of settling disputes while avoiding or appearing to avoid the use of post hoc reasoning.

Most other nations of the world are still not employing QRA (Flamm, 1986). You could argue they have not caught up with us yet or that we have gone off on some crazy tangent. For the most part, these nations are using case-by-case, post hoc decision making in coming to terms with their carcinogen problems. Sometimes they are very tough, invoking a total ban against the offending carcinogen, while, on other occasions, they appear extremely tolerant. Consequently, both industry and consumerists in the United States have been prompted to hold up the regulatory actions of specific nations as examples of what we in the United States should follow while forgetting those other decisions they despise in principle. But the question lingers in the wake of California's Proposition 65, is QRA what America wants? U.S. regulatory agencies think so and have thought so for the past 10 years. The purpose of this article is to let you decide for yourself by proving some insights and what is hoped are useful entries to the literature.

BASIC ASSUMPTIONS OF QRA

QRA depends entirely upon scientific assumptions, many of which are not subject to proof or even investigation and others which can at least be better defined by additional study or investigation. Many of the scientific assumptions are identical to those inherent in the use of animal toxicity data in general for assessing safe conditions of use or exposure to humans. The common assumption which ties the entire field together is that the experimental animal used in the study provides a reliable model for predicting what would occur in humans if humans were exposed to comparable levels or doses of the toxic substance. Since humans are much larger than the rats or mice used in toxicity studies, a correction for the size difference needs to be made in calculating what constitutes comparable dosage between humans and the experimental animal. There are a variety of ways by which this scaling up for larger size can be accomplished. However, the scaling is generally based either on body weight or body surface area differences. The quantitative outcome of picking one scaling factor over the other can amount to differences in risk (or allowable levels) of as much as 12-fold.

Often, there are no data to support one approach over the other, and selection depends entirely on policy options. Such options are likely to generate controversy, particularly when different regulatory agencies choose different options. Closely related to the issue of which scaling factor is most appropriate is the whole question of interspecies comparative pharmacokinetics (PK) and metabolism between humans and the animal model. Is the chemical in question absorbed at the same rate in the animal model as it is in humans? Is the chemical distributed throughout the body of both organisms in identical ways and metabolized to the same metabolites, in the same relative amounts, and eliminated by the same mechanisms and at the same rates? The answer to these questions is "probably not," and though it may be possible in some instances to shed light on the differences that may exist between the animal model and humans, the usual situation is that very little metabolic or PK information is available.

Assumptions, not scientific facts, are used to support and arrive at a final numerical value of risk to humans. This helps explain why regulatory agencies appear to act so conservatively in terms of the assumptions they adopt in any given risk assessment exercise. It also helps to explain why any additional data that are relevant to the above questions concerning human-animal model comparisons are more likely to result in a lowering of the estimated risk than in the increase in risk. Many other factors apart from metabolic and pharmacokinetic ones are known to influence the outcome of an animal carcinogenicity study. These factors include time, age, and duration of exposure, dietary or nutritional status, immunological, endocrinological status, and, perhaps most importantly, inherent sensitivity to cancer at the cellular level.

Examples abound of controversies on the subject of differences in intrinsic sensitivity to cancer between the animal models and humans, but the best example is probably liver cancer in the mouse. In the United States, human liver cancer (hepatocellular carcinoma) is relatively rare, having an incidence of less than one in a thousand individuals. However, in the mouse strain most extensively used for carcinogenicity studies (the $F_1B_6C_3$ hybrid), spontaneous liver cancer is extraordinarily common; in the male the lifetime incidence is 30–50% and in the female, it is 10–20%. The obvious question that arises and has become the central focus of much controversy is, should the mouse liver be considered an appropriate model for human cancer, given the observation that the incidence of spontaneously occurring liver cancer in the mouse is hundreds of times higher than it is in humans. Coupled to this problem and further exacerbating the controversy is the debate over MTD (maximum tolerated dose), which is the highest dose fed to the experimental animal. The argument made by the federal government (National Toxicology Program, regulatory agencies) is that the highest possible doses consistent with long-time survival of the animal must be administered in carcinogenicity studies for the studies to have adequate sensitivity and usefulness in protecting the public health. The argument made often by industry and occasionally by other groups as well is that such high doses cause a variety of physiological changes which may be immunological, hormonal, or result in persistent cellular injury and repair that predisposed the organism toward a higher incidence of cancer at one organ site or another. They argue that such agents might not be carcinogenic at all, but are simply substances that are acting indirectly and only at high dose to cause a physiological disturbance resulting in a higher incidence of cancer at some specific organ site.

Returning to mouse liver, the argument is that the mouse, unlike humans, has a liver that has already been initiated or triggered to develop cancer, and all that is needed for cancer to occur is for injury, followed by cellular proliferation, to take place. Once injured, the cells within the liver begin to divide and replicate to repair the injury, but as this proliferative response also involves the triggered cells, it leads ultimately to the development of neoplasms and finally to frank cancer (Berenblum, 1974). Whether this scenario is accurate or not cannot be stated scientifically, but the scenario serves to illustrate that assumptions, not facts, fill the voids that constitute QRA and that regulatory agencies use these assumptions to fulfill their view of their responsibilities (a) to resolve issues/disputes and (b) to protect the public health (Flamm and Lorentzen, 1988). You can hear them ask, if not QRA, what tools would you have us use for performing functions (a) and (b)? The following section of this article includes a discussion of some alternatives to QRA set in, to the extent possible, a historical perspective.

In addition to concerns over mouse liver being overly sensitive, similar concerns have been raised for mouse lymphoma, rat mammary, adrenal, and thyroid cancer, to name a few. Oddly, few scientists mention the fact that carcinoma of the colon/rectum or prostate are rarely seen in either the mouse or the rat, while they are among the most common cancers in males in the United States. To suggest that cancer is a rare disease within the United States would be idiotic, rather it's very common. Of course, we don't know what its causes are. The problem is the cancers common in the rat and mouse models are not necessarily the cancers that are most common in U.S. populations. So, are rats and mice a good model or not? The way regulatory agencies in the United States have dealt with this question has been by taking the position that while the model and QRA itself may not be perfect, nothing in the field of toxicology and safety evaluation is and unless there are demonstrably better models and approaches, animal models and QRA will continue to be used to meet the objectives under their responsibility.

In addition to the controversy over whether the animal models used are overly sensitive and the effects of maximum tolerated dose on the animal model, there is the much debated question of the shape of the dose-response curve and whether there is a threshold or not. Once again, regulatory agencies have taken the position that in the absence of data and scientific knowledge to the contrary, the most conservative assumptions must be applied. Failing this, the regulatory agencies argue they are left defenseless when brought before the courts on charges of failing to fulfill their responsibilities as given to them by the Congress. The agencies argue that unless you can prove there is a threshold, you shouldn't regulate as if there is one. Health-related conservatism in the scientific assumptions used is the consistent tread which ties together the entire structure of QRA as used by U.S. regulatory agencies. Since the entire process of QRA commonly involves dozens of scientific assumptions that must be made, there are many bones of contention that can be chewed on by anyone made unhappy by the outcome of the final decision which was ostensibly based on QRA. It is small wonder QRA has become a big target of criticism by industry, consumerists, and scientists in general, but given the lack of available scientific facts, perhaps it should be subjected to close public review and scrutiny. Indeed, the agencies seem to think so and often subject their QRAs to public peer reviews. To some extent, this has helped to get the issues out in the open and subject to the kind of open and frank deliberations they deserve. Whatever the problems or deficiencies of peer review, QRA is worse by far when peer review is not conducted.

The final bone of contention is the estimation of human exposure. In certain cases, human exposure can be very accurately calculated, in other cases, it can be confidently estimated, but in still other situations, it is virtually impossible to calculate, estimate, or predict human exposure. Here again, regulatory agencies have tended to act with utmost conservatism by making worst-case estimates in situations where accurate estimates are not possible. Since exposure estimates or overestimates are far removed from "high science" and consist of common everyday concepts, the regulatory agencies are particularly vulnerable to criticism, particularly from industry which often knows far more about human exposure to the chemical in question than the agency.

The picture of QRA that emerges is one of a process, rather than a discipline of science—a process consisting of many steps whose stepping stones are built of assumptions, not scientific facts. A range of uncertainty bounds each stepping stone, the truth presumably lies somewhere within the bounds, and the range may be as much as two or three orders of magnitude. Since the range of uncertainties describing each assumption is likely to be independent of other assumptions, the ranges become multiplicative. When only the most conservative assumptions are made throughout the process, the likelihood is that many of the assumptions will represent overestimates of human risk by 10- or 100-fold leading to a combined overestimate of perhaps a millionfold or more. This is why, in recent years, there has been such a cry for research to define better the assumptions which underlie QRA. Unfortunately, so many of the tractable assumptions are case-specific. Not only are they case-specific, but they are also highly resource-intensive. The nation could not begin to afford extensive research on each case, but nor could the cause of public health as perceived by our society allow such issues to be ignored. So in steps the regulatory agencies to do what it and everyone else knows is not scientifically sound or supportable. What a wonderful target they make and oh, so vulnerable.

ALTERNATIVES TO QRA

The question is, before the birth of QRA, how did scientists determine safe levels for carcinogens in the human environment? The answer is, they did not. Consequently, regulatory/policy decisions were either stalemated, postponed, ignored, or a total ban was invoked. It has often been argued that the entire process of carcinogen regulation (if it can be called a process) was at best haphazard, sometimes giving the perception that safe substances are being banned and dangerous ones are being left on the market or in the environment.

The absolute need for some kind of quantitative assessment arose in the late 1960s and early 1970s. Ironically, it was the Delaney anticancer clause itself which forced, for the first time, the Food and Drug Administration to undertake the development of QRA for coping with residues of carcinogenic drugs (or feed additives) used in animals intended for human food. The Delaney clause contains a specific exemption for carcinogenic additives to the feed of food-producing animals, provided the addition does not result in injury to the animal or its offspring and leaves no residue at the time the animals are marketed as food. The problem was how to define or establish that there was "no residue" within the meaning of the Act. After much pondering, the Agency concluded that if the residue(s) could not be detected by an approved analytic method and if that method was sensitive enough to protect the public health from cancer, the terms of the Delaney clause would be satisfied. But the question remained how to determine what levels of residue are low enough to be considered consistent with public health protection. One answer emerged: use animal data which are the only data available and extrapolate these data to low doses for assessing human risk. Thus, QRA was born, though it has gone through many changes since those early days and will undoubtedly go through many more (Flamm and Lorentzen, 1988).

But surely there must be other ways to regulate carcinogens besides using QRA. And there are. As mentioned earlier, most other nations do not use QRA for decision making. They use instead a great variety of techniques, methods, and framewords for accomplishing what we in the United States try to accomplish through QRA. To some extent, these governments are able to make their decisions far from the glare of publicity and are less often called upon to document and defend every nuance of their decision making to all interested parties. In the United States, there are many interested parties and, in general, these parties have a much stronger egalitarian mindset than exists elsewhere. Americans insist that government, particularly government in Washington, be open to public scrutiny and that government policies be fair. Fairness among egalitarian Americans means equal treatment. To assure equal treatment, government types believe rules and procedures must be developed and used with strict adherence (Rayner and Cantor, 1987). Post hoc judgments that are untethered by rules and procedures and perceived as imposing health risks upon the American people are totally unacceptable to most Americans (Rayner and Cantor, 1987). Consumer groups are quick to point a finger and demand public hearings if they sense government is guilty of post hoc judgments or departures from standard rules and procedures. The courts, which exist to resolve disputes, can be expected to rule against the Agency whenever their actions are judged as having departed from set procedures or to lack consistency.

Does this mean that in the United States there is no alternative to QRA? Of course not. It does mean that in the United States the options or alternatives to QRA are limited. The following appears viable within the confines of our society: 1) a Delaney-type no-risk approach, (2) a safety factor approach, (3) a nonparametric approach, and (4) an approach which combines QRA with other "science" to arrive at a more scientific, less assumption-dependent risk assessment.

The no-risk approach has the advantage of pure simplicity and of being clearly on the side of the angels. Indeed, at first blush, we would all vote for this approach to avoid cancer. Unfortunately, but not surprisingly, now that we have such supersensitive ways of detecting carcinogens, we know that carcinogens can be found everywhere and in all products. To implement a no-risk cancer policy given this fact is clearly impossible if the concept that there are no thresholds for carcinogens is accepted as operational. The only way such a no-risk policy could be implemented would be by trickery and deception. Or government could declare that there are thresholds and regulate accordingly. However, since there is no scientific consensus that threshold exists, such a policy would be doomed to failure.

The safety factor approach is used for many other forms of toxicity such as reproductive toxicity and target organ toxicity. This approach could also be used for carcinogens, even though it would have to be acknowledged that there are no known or ascertainable thresholds for carcinogens. For the approach to work, all that would be required is a safety factor large enough to satisfy most interested parties. The factor would have to be extremely large to do this. Consumerists would undoubtedly want the safety factor to be large enough to assure that the resulting risks do not exceed an "acceptable risk" as determined by QRA. Acceptable risk is generally an upper limit estimate of one cancer in one million human lifetimes. To achieve this low level of risk with a safety factor approach, a factor of at least 10,000 would have to be divided into the highest dose level at which no induction of cancer was observed in the animal experiment. While industry might object initially, it would ultimately learn to work within these boundaries, as well as the present boundaries. The problem is such an approach would ignore differences in dose response slopes and be viewed as nonscientific, possibly antiscientific. Such an approach might well cut short efforts to introduce additional scientific advances into the overall QRA process. On these grounds, it seems unlikely that the safety factor approach for regulating carcinogens has much chance of success or would, at this time, allow or be able to incorporate scientific advances.

The nonparametric approach (Flamm and Winbush, 1984) is somewhat similar to the safety factor approach, except it can take advantage of the experimentally determined dose-response curve. However, instead of using a mathematically sophisticated model for extrapolation to low dose, it simply assumes strict linearity in dose response at doses below the experimental range. This approach stands halfway between the safety factor approach and the types of QRA which employ complex mathematical models such as the computer-driven multistage model. It often produces risk values which are virtually identical to those generated by one-hit, multistage, multihit or any other model which possesses or can be made to possess a strong linear component. It has the advantage of making full use of the shape and slope of the experimentally generated dose-reponse curve without the pretentions that the shape and slope of the dose-response curve at doses far below observable ones are ascertainable by the model. It could properly be argued that this approach is not an alternative to QRA, but just a variant of QRA. It is actually the approach used and favored by FDA in the food area, though generally FDA scientists will look at a variety of methods, but in almost all cases, each method will possess a strong linear component. In reality, linearity is the dominant feature in virtually all the QRA conducted by FDA and EPA (Flamm and Winbush, 1984). The reasons for this are often questioned, but the best answer seems to be that the linearized extrapolation provides a considerable degree of assurance that the estimated risk is not being understated. Indeed, the unashamed objective of QRA in regulatory agencies is to avoid unstating the risk and to assure the policy objective of protecting the public health is met (Flamm, 1987).

In the past 2 or 3 years, we have seen a new and unprecedented effort to introduce new or additional science into QRA. Originally, QRA was, or at least seemed to be, closed to any scientific information or considerations beyond simple cancer incidence data from either humans or experimental animals. Now, however, in large part because potentially relevant data are being developed by industry and submitted to regulatory agencies, the use of data which may or may not help to replace scientific assumptions with scientific data is becoming commonplace. No scientist worthy of the title could lament this advent, but it is clear that these changes will challenge and strain regulatory scientists to the limit. To pretend that this is gradual evolution rather than abrupt change is unhelpful. Denial of truth only postpones sought-after goals and objectives. It should be recognized we are entering a new area where patience and perseverance is essential. Again, this approach is not so much an alternative to QRA as it is a modification to reduce dependency upon scientific assumptions and to shift that burden to scientific data. The burning question which will arise again and again is, when is the scientific evidence sufficient to be dispositive? There is likely to be great frustration over this question and many threats from the industry to cease and desist in their efforts to generate credible scientific information unless a means can be found by regulatory agencies to introduce such information and allow it to impact on QRA. While they should not be blamed for that attitude, patience nevertheless is an essential ingredient to success. Let us all hope that success will come in reasonable time.

THE PROS

The advantages of QRA are fivefold:

1. provides an appearance of consistency
2. an appearance of scientific sophistication
3. recognizes that risk is related to dose or exposure
4. eliminates post hoc judgments
5. highly useful in settling issues and disputes

Providing the appearance of consistency is highly regarded by the courts, those in government responsible for setting priorities (i.e., agency heads, appropriation committees of Congress, and the Office of Management and Budget), and American society in general. Consistency is, to some extent, the handmaiden to equal treatment, all of which plays very well in our egalitarian society. Should you think it not important, suppose, for instance, the EPA had two disparate methods for determining miles per gallon estimates on new cars, but kept secret which method they used when reporting mpgs. None of us would be pleased. Consistency in the way government reports its findings is viewed as essential (Huber, 1987). QRA appears to meet this test. In reality, this consistency is only illusionary, as will be pointed out in the next section, but this section is reserved to support QRA.

The appearance of scientific sophistication through use of computer-driven mathematical models that are understood by only the cognoscente helps in some cases to deflect criticism of the models and the approach. This has not stopped certain notable pioneers in the field of experimental carcinogenesis from being highly critical of QRA. However, since the criticism has not been matched by proposals for alternative approaches, these critics have had little impact to date. The apparent sophistication of QRA has partially succeeded in stilling criticism, and its only viable challenger is the nonparametric approach, which does not differ significantly from most QRA, either in concept or numerical outcome. The guts of both approaches is a strong linear component which is trusted to prevent an understatement of actual risk.

Recognition that risk of cancer is related to dose is the great triumph of QRA. But, here again, cancer experimentalists will argue for caution. The factors affecting the probability of cancer development are complex and dependent on a host of exogenous and endogenous factors. Nevertheless, the dose-dependency concept is fundamental to safety evaluation and QRA makes possible its use for carcinogens. A progressive step to be sure, but with progress goes problems and new responsibility. The tendency in traditional QRA is to ignore these problems, since seldom are there data to do otherwise. Filling the vacuum of ignorance are scientific assumptions. In the minds of many, the biggest and most critical assumption is that the dose-response curve is linear beneath the lowest observable effect. This assumption results in the calculation of relatively high risks, even at doses that are hundreds and thousands of times less than the lowest dose producing cancer in the experimental animal. There have been many arguments raised to refute and criticize linear extrapolation. The most cogent of these is, why should risk of cancer be linearly related to dose below the observable range when it is clearly nonlinear (in certain cases) in the observable range? Arguments to account for this seeming inconsistency have been advanced (Flamm and Lorentzen, 1988), but they are, and are likely to stay, theoretical.

A fourth heralded virtue of QRA is it avoids post hoc judgments. Its proponents are quick to say that QRA assures science, not politics, will prevail in the final scientific evaluation proclaimed by the regulatory agency. The less scientific the judgment allowed to enter the QRA process, the truer is the statement. Unfortunately, keeping out scientific judgments does not always serve the best interest of society. As will be discussed later, additional science can help improve the "accuracy" of risk assessment and can relieve some of the burden placed on industry. But determining when the scientific evidence suffices for inclusion into QRA is presently a matter of considerable dispute. There is a great need to have open and public discussion as to how scientific consensus can be treated in a timely and effective manner to support the inclusion of additional science into risk assessment. Such discussion should involve all interested parties and include a mechanism to assure recognition of real-world practicalities.

The fifth and final pro is undoubtedly the quintessential reason for using risk assessment—it settles disputes and the courts have even upheld their use for this purpose. Indeed, the Supreme Court overturned and admonished OSHA in the early 1980s for its regulatory policy on benzene (1980) because it failed to consider or explain its regulation in terms of risk assessment. Other courts (Court of Appeals, 1984) have upheld FDA's use of QRA, which was applied to a carcinogenic contaminant in a color additive in order to avoid invoking the Delaney clause when the Agency believed it possible to establish safe conditions of use despite the presence of the carcinogenic contaminant. Many consumer advocate groups are now proponents of QRA, believing that it offers a constructive way of assuring equal treatment. So, regulatory agencies, consumerist groups, the courts, and even the Congress are evidencing support for QRA. It seems to be the American thing to do, or is it?

THE CONS

The greatest weakness of QRA is it depends entirely on unproven—and some say—unlikely assumptions. These assumptions can be placed in the following three categories and arranged in order of their descending weakness. The linearized mathematical extrapolation from high to low dose is the most criticized since, in many instances, such extrapolations span several orders of magnitude in dose. To assume knowledge of the dose-response relationship at doses so many orders of magnitude below the observable range has only little to do with science, but a great deal to do with belief, doctrine, and policy objective. When a previously trusted and relied-upon substance such as formaldehyde is found to induce cancer and is deemed a serious risk to humans at levels of exposure common to humans, the debate becomes quite heated. The dose-response relationship for formaldehyde is extremely steep; halving the dose that induces a high incidence in nasal cancer results in a precipitous drop in cancer response, perhaps by as much as 50-fold (Gaylor, 1983). Is it fair, appropriate, or scientific to act as if the dose-response curve for formaldehyde suddenly becomes linear just barely below the lowest observable dose? While it is unlikely to become immediately linear and hence unlikely to be true, science has failed, to date, to provide clear evidence of when formaldehyde's plunging dose-response curve levels off to become linear. Again, the tendency on the part of regulatory agencies is to use a cautious approach which avoids criticism from powerful groups who pursue the "health agenda." When assumptions that can reasonably be considered as "highly unlikely" are adopted, insisted upon, and adhered to in policy decisions, QRA loses credibility as an effective process.

Next in the order of descending weakness is the reliability of the animal model for predicting human cancer. Critics argue that since the mouse does not predict well for rat cancer, why should it be expected to predict better for human cancer? How can cancer incidence data in the animal model be relied upon to predict quantitatively for humans when it is known that changes in diet, routes of administration, and subtle changes in dosage regimen can result in very substantial differences in response? The answer is, they can't. But proponents of risk assessment assert that this is why the assumptions used must be sufficiently conservative so that any error in estimating risk is on the side of the public health. Others argue that judgments which are based on such inaccurate measures will not and cannot in the end serve the public's best interests. Some of these parties argue that differences in metabolism and pharmacokinetics between humans and the animal model are so great much of the time that unless additional information is developed, QRA, as currently defined, is useless.

Third, and last, assumptions about human exposure are often highly contentious. Even regulatory agencies disagree sometimes by surprising amounts. FDA, over the past decade, has made great progress in improving its databases, which make possible more accurate estimates of human exposure. Sometimes the contentious issue is over how much dirt a child eats in a day. Again, the regulatory agency tends to take a position that cannot be criticized for underestimating exposure, but may be subject to scorn from those who believe the estimates to be ridiculous.

Another often heard criticism of QRA is it provides only the illusion of scientific sophistication and is in the minds of such people a shell game instead with complicated rules masquerading as science. To take limited experimental cancer incidence data obtained at only one or two doses and to plug these data into a highly sophisticated mathematical model for extrapolation down to doses that are thousands of times below the lowest effect level for assessing human risk requires a great leap of faith. But more unsettling than this realization is the criticism that QRA shuts out scientific judgment to the detriment of better decision making. While good examples of this having happened are not commonplace, they do exist. The reason for this is to avoid post hoc judgments where "political and socioeconomic" considerations are feared will deny Americans their rights by subjecting them to unfair health risks. Such fears can lead to a "no loss at any cost" philosophy which can be paralyzing. Without some degree of trust in those entrusted to carrying out the laws of the land, science and reason fall before fear, mistrust, and doctrine. Society must decide whether to trust in a limited way public officials and to risk being disappointed occasionally or to insist upon processes which exclude judgment and do not require trust but incur the high costs of being overly fearful.

HOPE FOR THE FUTURE

Some of my colleagues will say the best hope for the future is to put QRA in the trash can or worse. But they are less clear about what will replace QRA. Are we to return to stalemate, etc., or do we adopt a more "European approach." To do this, we might have to change the social consciousness temperament of Americans, hardly a proper task for scientists or government officials.

It would seem that proceeding forward into the future with QRA is inevitable. But can it be improved, and how might that be accomplished? Hope for improvement rests with research directed and focused on both generic as well as specific compound-related questions. The generic questions can be divided into two large groups: (a) molecular and cellular mechanisms of carcinogenesis, and (b) ways of determining target dose and relating target dose in the animal to target dose in the human. Mechanism studies will help to determine whether cancer findings in the animal are relevant to humans. The artificial sweetener saccharin produces bladder cancer in rats, but not in mice. To definitively assess the relevance of the rat studies to humans, an understanding of the mechanism by which saccharin acts to induce bladder cancer is probably necessary. Industry in general is sensitive to this need, and the Chemical Industry Institute of Toxicology (CIIT) in particular is making impressive progress in delineating the mechanism by which certain substances may be inducing cancer. The question of target dose is being addressed in several ways. Pharmacokinetics, DNA adducts, and sensitive biomarkers are being studied for their usefulness in reducing the uncertainties associated with the scientific assumptions that are an integral part of QRA. Studies that focus on a specific carcinogen and seek to develop a better understanding of how results in an animal model can be related to humans are expected to provide valuable anecdotal information, which should provide an eventual matrix of knowledge. In short, research offers hope rather than despair. Let's hope that hope prevails.

REFERENCES

Benzene decsion, 1980. Industrial Union Dept. *AFL-CIO* v. *American Petroleum Institute*, 448 U.S. 607.

Berenblum, I. 1974. *Carcinogenesis as a Biological Problem*, p. 36–50. North Holland Publishing Co., Amsterdam.

Court of Appeals 6th Circuit Constituent Policy. 1984. *Scott* vs. *FDA*, 728 F. 2d 322.

Federal Food, Drug and Cosmetic Act, as amended, Sec. 409, 512, 706 1981.

Flamm, W. G., 1986. *Risk Assessment Policy in the U.S. Risk and Reason: Risk Assessment in Relation to Environmental Mutagens and Carcinogens*, p. 141. Alan R. Liss, New York.

Flamm, W. G., 1987. Editorial, *Regulatory Tox. and Pharm.* 7: 343.

Flamm, W. G. and Lorentzen, R. J. 1988. Quantitative risk assessment (QRA): A special problem in the approval of new products. In *Risk Assessment and Risk Management of Industrial and Environmental Chemicals*. Scientific Publishing Co., Inc., Princeton, NJ.

Flamm, W. G. and Winbush, J. S. 1984. Role of mathematical models in assessment of risk and in attempts to define management strategy. *Fund. Appl. Toxicol.* 4: 5395–5401.

Gaylor, D. W. 1983. Mathematical approaches to risk assessment: squamous cell nasal carcinoma in rats exposed to formaldehyde vapor.

In *Formaldehyde Toxicity,* (Ed.) Gibson, E. Hemisphere Publishing Corp. 24: 279–283.

Huber, P. W. 1987. Little risks and big fears. In *Regulatory Toxicology and Pharmacology.* Academic Press, Inc. 7(2)

Kokoski, C. J. and Flamm, W. G. 1984. Establishment of acceptable limits of intake. In *Proceedings of the Second National Conference for Food Protection.* DHHS, Washington, DC.

Lawrence, C. E. and Paulson, A. S. 1981. *Cigarette Smoke: Camcer Risk at Low Dose, The Analysis of Actual Versus Perceived Risks,* (Ed.) Covello, V., Flamm, G., Rodricks, J., and Tardiff, R., p. 169. Plenum, London, New York.

National Academy of Sciences, National Research Council. 1983. *Risk Assessment in the Federal Government: Managing the Process.* National Academy Press, Washington, DC.

Rayner, S. and Cantor, R. 1987. How fair is safe enought? The cultural approach to societal technology choice. *Risk Analysis.* 7(1): 3–9.

Index

Abnormalities, behavorial:
  associated with vitamin deficiencies, 227
Acesulfame K, sweetness, 152
Activity, physical:
  as protective factor for cancer, 8
Additives, food, 2
  categories of, 400
  concerns about, 426
  Delaney Clause, and regulation of, 400, 401
  excretion through kidneys, 373
  as a factor in cancer deaths, 206
  and hyperactivity, 225
Adulteration, definition of, 401
Aflatoxin:
  carcinogenicity, 13
    epidemiological evidence of, 17, 18
    evidence against, 20, 21
  in corn as added poisonous or deleterious substance, 400
  in corn and peanuts, as environmental contaminant, 401
  detoxification of, 17
  dose-response relationship for, 17, 18
  exemption from Proposition 65, 403
  human susceptibility to, 16, 17
  as initiator of DNA damage, 23
  and interaction with hepatitis B virus, 12, 21–24
  mutagenicity of, 16, 24
  seasonal variation in levels of, 18
  species differences in metabolism of, 16
  structures of, 12
  as a tumor promoter, 18
  withdrawal of exposure to, 19
Aflatoxin B_1, 104, 122, 126, 127
  carcinogenic potency of, 13, 16
  effect of indoles on, 133, 134
  formation of DNA adducts with, 129

Aflatoxin B_1 (*cont'd.*)
  mutagenicity of, 39
  structure of, 12
  TD_{50}, 15
Agents:
  food coloring, and hyperkinesis,
    257, 278, 279
  nitrosating, 59, 61
    reactions and equilibria, 61
Alcohol (*see also* Ethanol):
  and cancer deaths, 206
  as cancer risk factor, 31
  as hepatotoxic agent and promoter
    of liver cancer, 23
  inhibition of xenobiotic metabolism
    by, 366
Alitame, sweetness, 152
Allergens, food,
  in codfish, 264, 265
  in cottonseed, 265, 267
  in cows' milk, 264, 265
  in eggs, 265, 266
  in green peas, 265, 267
  as naturally occurring food pro-
    teins, 263–267
  nature and chemistry of, 263–267
  in peanuts, 265, 267
  in rice, 265, 267
  in sesame seeds, 267
  in soybeans, 265, 267
  in tomatoes, 265, 267
  traces of, and adverse reactions,
    268, 269
Allergies, food,
  diagnosis of, 261, 262
  as explanation of nutrition-
    behavior connection, 236
  IgE-mediated, 256, 257
    symptoms of, 260
  non-IgE-mediated, 256
  persistence of, 262, 263
  prevalence of, 262
  treatment of, 267–269
  true, 258–260
    as caused by naturally occurring
      substances, 258

    immunologically-mediated, 258
    role of IgG4, 260, 261
    role of IgE, 259, 260
    tolerance levels in, 268
Allergy, fish, 257
Allergy, food,
  exercise-induced, 261
  incidence of, 255
  involvement of the immune system
    in, 256, 257
Allyl isothiocyanate, 211
  dose-response assessment, 216, 217
  exposure assessment, 217
  hazard identification, 216
  risk characterization, 217
  risk estimate of, 220
Alternariol methyl ester, 11
Amides, 61
  nitrosation of, 59
  substituted, 60
Amines:
  heterocyclic,
    abbreviations for, 35
    adducts with guanine bases, 38,
      40
    carcinogenicity of, 36, 37
      in primates, 43
    chemical names of, 35
    chemistry of, 33–36
    in cooked foods, 32
    IQ-type, 32–35
      mutagenicity of, 35, 39
      structures of, 33
    metabolism of, 38
    mutagenicity of,
      in Chinese hamster lung cells,
        41
      inhibitors of, 43, 44
      in *Salmonella typhimurium*, 38,
        39
    non-IQ-type, 32–35
      mutagenicity of, 35, 39
      structures of, 34
    other effects of, 46
      atherosclerotic, 46
      atrophy of salivary glands, 46

promotion of carcinogenicity of, by phorbol ester, 43
quantitation of, in foods, 44, 45
relationship between carcinogenicity and mutagenicity of, 40–42
nitrosation of, 59
secondary, 59, 60
Amino acids, pyrolysates of, as source of heterocyclic amines, 32
Anaphylaxis, systemic, 260
Anticarcinogen, from fried ground beef, 5
Anticarcinogens:
beta-carotene as potential, 4
as blocking agents, 125–127
in cellular protection, 185–188
in food, 3
in inhibiting carcinogen-DNA adduct formation, 128–132
as precursor conversion inhibitors, 124, 125
as suppressing agents, 125, 127, 128
Anticarcinogenesis:
by food components and additives, 103–117
mechanisms of, 123–134
quantitative, 128–132
Antioxidants:
as anticarcinogens, 103–112
in cellular protection, 185–188
as modifiers of carcinogenesis, 106, 120
Apigenin, 112
Apples, as source of Folpet, 211, 212
Ascorbic acid (see also vitamin C), 61
as inhibitor of nitrosamine formation, 125
as modifier of carcinogenesis, 106, 110, 124, 125
in protection against free radicals, 173, 191
in protection from nitrate, 78
reaction with dinitrogen trioxide, 63
reaction with nitrite, 89

structure of, 109
Aspartame, 151
acceptable daily intake of, 231
as cause of migraine headaches, 272
as cause of urticaria, 272, 278
effects of,
appetite-stimulating, 236
appetite-suppressing, 236
on behavior, 233–236
on changes in eating behavior, 235, 236
on childhood hyperactivity, 234, 235
on mood states, 236
elevations in plasma phenylalanine from, 234
FDA-approved uses of, 233
intake of, 232
metabolism of, 234
as a nutritive sweetener, 231
sweetness of, 152
Aspergillus, 13
Assessment:
behavioral, 242, 243
dose-response,
of allyl isothiocyanate, 216, 217
of ethylene dibromide, 214
of Folpet, 212
of polycyclic aromatic hydrocarbons, 215
exposure,
of allyl isothiocyanate, 217
of ethylene dibromide, 214
of Folpet, 212
of polycyclic aromatic hydrocarbons, 215
nutritional, 241, 242
quantitative risk, 207, 209–211, 219
alternatives to, 437–440
basic assumptions of, 433–437
the cons of, 442–444
definition of, 429
history predating, 432
principle of, 431
process of, 429

Assessment (*cont'd.*)
  the pros of, 440–442
  strengths, limitations and uncer-
    tainties of, 219
  risk,
    advantages of, 220, 221
    definition of, 209
    steps in regulatory process of, 209
Atherosclerosis:
  initiation of, 298
  lipid hypothesis of, 300–307, 310
  lipoproteins and, 315–320
  myocardial infarction in, 298
  pathologic process of, 308, 309
  plaque accumulation in, 298
  response-to-injury hypothesis of,
    308–310

Bacon, fried,
  as source of N-nitrosothiazolidine
    carboxylic acid, 72
  as source of non-volatile nitro-
    samines, 86
  as source of volatile nitrosamines,
    71
Barley, as cause of celiac disease, 270
Beef:
  broiled,
    cholesterol oxidation products in,
      311, 312
    heterocyclic amines in, 45
  dehydrated, cholesterol oxidation
    products in, 314
  extract, heterocyclic amines in, 45
  ground, fried,
    as anticarcinogen, 5
    heterocyclic amines in, 44, 45
  precooked, cholesterol oxidation
    products in, 311, 312
  as source of mutagens, 32, 35
Beer:
  decreased nitrosamine content of, 74
  nonvolatile nitrosamines in, 73
  volatile nitrosamines in, 71, 75, 86

Behavior:
  antisocial,
    and abnormalities in carbohy-
      drate metabolism, 239
    and dietary manipulations, 226
    and sucrose, 237, 239, 240
  aspartame and, 230–236
  influence of diet on, 225
  influence of nutritional status on,
    226–230
  juvenile delinquent, interaction
    with sugar, 240
  nutritive sweeteners and, 230–234
Benzo [a]pyrene, 4, 104, 127
  absorption of, 341
  7, 8-epoxide of, 175
  mutagenicity of, 39
  mutagenic metabolites of, 185
Benzoates, as cause of urticaria, 272,
  278, 283
Bilirubin, in protection against free
  radicals, 173
Bioassays:
  carcinogenicity, 14
  in experimental animals, 14
Bread, as a source of nitrate, 65
Broccoli, as a source of allyl isothiocyanate, 216
Brussel sprouts:
  as a source of indoles, 114
  as a source of isothiocyanates, 116,
    211
Butter, cholesterol oxidation products
  in, 314
2-(3)-*tert*-Butyl-4-hydroxyanisole
  (BHA), 3
  absorption and excretion of, 345
  carcinogenic status of, 106
  as cause of hives, 257, 272, 278,
    279, 283
  effects on nitrosamine carcino-
    genesis, 120
  as epigenetic tumor promoter, 107
  excretion of, 373

as inducer of glutathione-S-transferase, 185
as inducer of NADPH (quinone acceptor) oxidoreductase, 186
as inducer of phase II enzymes, 186
as inhibitor of tumor formation,
107
as modulator of carcinogenesis, 104,
106, 107, 122, 124–127
structure of, 105
3, 5-di-*tert*-Butyl-4-hydroxytoluene
(BHT):
carcinogenic status of, 106
as cause of hives, 257, 272, 278,
279, 283
cytochrome P-450-catalyzed conversion of, 183
effect on glutathione, glutathione
reductase, and glutathione peroxidase, 186
as epigenetic tumor promoter, 107
as inhibitor of tumor formation,
107
in inhibition of LDL modification,
317
as modulator of carcinogenesis, 104,
106, 107, 124, 125, 126
structure of, 105
in termination of free radical reactions, 191

Cabbage:
as source of indoles, 114
as source of isothiocyanates, 116,
211, 216
Caffeic acid, 112
as an anticarcinogen, 124
Caffeine:
attitude toward, 425
trends in, 426
concern about, 424
effect on behavior, 226
as naturally occurring toxicant in
coffee, 398

as suppressing agent for carcinogenesis, 127
Cancer:
bladder, 153–161
breast, 102
causes of, 205, 206
chemoprevention of, 101
colon, 4, 102
death from, 2
dietary recommendations and, 102
epidemiological associations with
dietary components, 102
esophageal, 80, 102
liver,
and aflatoxin, 19
etiology of human, 19
lung, 2, 102, 205
pancreas, 102
prostate, 102
risk of human, from cyclamate
and saccharin, 161
stomach, 2, 77, 78, 80, 89, 102
Cancers, risk of developing, 1
Carbohydrate:
consumption of,
and changes in plasma tryptophan, 228
effect of behavior, 230
dietary, effect on xenobiotic metabolism, 364, 365
to protein ratio and activity patterns, 229
Carcinogen, nitrosamide as direct acting, 63
Carcinogenesis:
dietary modifiers of, 101
enhancement of,
by diet, 6
by fat, 6
initiation of, by oxidative damage,
103
modulation, ambivalent, 133, 134
modulation of,
effect of animal species, 120, 122

Carcinogens (*cont'd.*)
  effect of exposure protocol, 121–123
  target organ variability, 120, 122
substances that modulate, 3
Carcinogenicity, animal, factors influencing, 434
Carcinogens:
  cellular defense against, 170
  comparison of IARC, NTP, and Proposition 65 lists of, 423, 424
  concentrations of, in diet, 3
  in cooked foods, 31
  estimates of human exposure to, in quantitative risk assessment, 431
  in food, 3
  latency of effects of, 431
  listed, and Proposition 65, 403
  lists of,
    created by IARC, 421
    known, 421–423
    limitations of, 421, 422
  naturally occurring, 3
  FDA regulation of, 399
  and Proposition 65, 404
  strengths and limitations of animal bioassays for, 416–418
  TD_{50} as potency measurement of, 208
Carnosine, in protection against free radicals, 173
β-Carotene, 170
  as an anticarcinogen, 104, 110, 111
  epidemiological studies of intake of, 110
  in protection against free radicals, 173–191
  structure of, 109
Carotenoids, as inhibitors of tumor progression, 122, 127
Catalase, 104, 170, 173, 174, 190
Catecholamines, as neurotransmitters, 228
Cauliflower:
  as source of indoles, 114

as source of isothiocyanates, 116, 211, 216
Celery, in exercise-induced food allergy, 261
Characterization, risk, 210, 212
  of allyl isothiocyanate, 217
  of ethylene dibromide, 214
  of Folpet, 212
  of polycyclic aromatic hydrocarbons, 215, 216
  of safrole, 218
Cheese:
  cheddar, cholesterol oxidation products in, 314
  cottage, cholesterol oxidation products in, 314
Cheeses:
  powdered, cholesterol oxidation products in, 314
  volatile nitrosamines in, 71, 75
Chicken:
  broiled, heterocyclic amines in, 45
  dehydrated, cholesterol oxidation products in, 314
Chlorogenic acid, 112
Chocolate:
  lack of involvement in true food allergies, 263, 272
  and migraine headaches, 257
Cholesterol:
  attitudes toward, 425
    trends in, 426
  concern about, 424
  dietary, 318–320
  role in atherosclerosis, 300, 301, 306
  serum, and dietary fats, 318
Cinnamon, as a source of safrole, 217
Citrinin, 11
  as a tumor promoter, 23
CLA, 5, 6
  as anticarcinogen, 5, 6
  formation of, 5
  in heat-processed foods, 5
Clams, as common allergenic food, 263

Coffee:
  caffeine in, 398
  polycyclic aromatic hydrocarbons
    in, 211
Colors, artificial food,
  and behavioral disorders, 272
  and childhood hyperactivity, 237,
    278
Communication, risk, 211
Comparison, risk, 211
  of natural versus pesticide carcino-
    gens, 220
Conjugates, glutathione, formation of,
  177
Contaminants:
  chlorinated hydrocarbon, as tumor
    promoters, 118
  environmental, as category of
    added food constituents, 401
Contamination, microbiological, 1, 2
Cosmetics, N-nitroso compounds in,
  70, 73, 74, 75
Cottonseed, allergens in, 265, 267
Crab:
  allergens in, 265, 266
  as a common allergenic food, 263
Criminality, adult, and sucrose, 237,
  239, 240
Cyclamate, 151
  carcinogenicity of, 152, 153
  as promoter of bladder tumors,
    155–157, 160, 161
  sweetness of, 152
Cyclohexylamine:
  carcinogenicity of, 153
  as metabolite of cyclamate, 152, 153
Cysteine, as an electophile scavenger,
  171, 172
Cytochrome P-450 monooxygenases
  (*see also* oxidase, mixed function):
  in cellular protection, 183
  in conversion of BHT, 183
  effect of mineral depletion on, 369,
    370

effect of protein-energy malnutri-
    tion on, 363
  effect of vitamin status on, 367–369
  in metabolism, 169, 355–357
  of heterocyclic amines, 38

Deficiencies:
  nutritional, 1
  vitamin, and behavioral abnormali-
    ties, 227
  vitamin/mineral,
    effect on absorption of toxicants,
      344, 345
    as explanation of nutrition-
      behavior connection, 236
    and hyperactivity, 225
Delaney Clause:
  in regulation of food and color
    additives, 400–402, 404
  as stimulus of quantitative risk as-
    sessment, 437
Deoxynivalenol, 11
  structure of, 12
Deprivation, acute protein-energy, ef-
    fect on behavior, 226, 227
Diet:
  as a factor in cancer deaths, 206
  specific avoidance, in treatment of
    food allergies, 267–269
Diethylnitrosamine (*see also* N-nitro-
    sodiethylamine), 104, 106, 127
  TD_{50}, 15
Diethylstilbesterol:
  as a co-carcinogen and tumor pro-
    moter, 117, 118
  TD_{50}, 15
Diets, high-fat, as tumor promoters,
  117
7, 12-Dimethylbenz[a]anthracene
    (DMBA), 104, 106, 122
Dimethylhydrazine, 106
Dimethylnitrosamine (*see also* N-ni-
    trosodimethylamine), TD_{50}, 15
Dinitrogen tetroxide, 61

Dinitrogen trioxide, reaction with ascorbic acid, 63
Disease, celiac,
  as form of food allergy, 269–271
  as an idiosyncratic reaction, 278
Disorders, metabolic food, 257, 271, 273–277
  causative substances of, 272
DNA, covalent binding to, 183, 184
DT-diaphorase, 104

Eggs:
  allergens in, 265, 266
  as a common allergenic food, 263
  fresh, cholesterol oxidation products in, 313
  powdered, cholesterol oxidation products in, 311
  spray-dried, cholesterol oxidation products in, 312
Electrophiles, protection against, 170–172
Ellagic acid, 112
  as a blocking agent for carcinogenesis, 125, 126
Environment, occupational, N-nitroso compounds in, 70, 71, 75
Enzymes:
  conjugation, 357, 358
  phase II, induction of, 186
  protective, induction of, 185–188
Epoxide hydrolase, 108, 170, 357, 362
  role in cellular protection, 175, 176
Epoxides, as ultimate carcinogens, 175, 176
Equivalence, nitrosáting, 61, 62
Erythorbate, as inhibitor of nitrosamine formation, 125
β-Estradiol, as a co-carcinogen and tumor promoter, 117, 118
Estragole, as a carcinogen, 218
Ethanol (see also alcohol):
  and esophageal cancer, 102
  induction of mixed function oxidase, 359, 360

inhibition of glucuronidation by, 366
TD_{50}, 15
Ethoxyquin:
  as inducer of glutathione-S-transferase, 185
  as inhibitor of aflatoxin B_1-induced hepatocarcinogenesis, 107
  as modulator of carcinogenesis, 104, 106–108
  structure of, 105
Ethylene dibromide (EDB), 211
  dose-response assessment, 214
  EPA ban of, 24
  exposure assessment, 214
  hazard identification, 214
  mutagenic effects of, 214
  as nematocide and pesticide, 213, 214
  risk characterization, 214
  risk estimate, 220
  TD_{50}, 15

Factor, safety, in toxicologic extrapolations, 420
Fat, dietary, in enhancement of carcinogenesis, 6–8
Fats:
  dietary, and serum cholesterol, 318
  processed, 2
Fatty acid hydroperoxides:
  in atherosclerosis, 304, 305, 311, 315, 321–323
  in serum lipoproteins, 315
Fatty acids:
  omega-3:
    antiatheromatous effects of, 320–322
    as inhibitors of tumor formation, 117
    properties of, 320, 321
  unsaturated, as inhibitors of mutagenesis of heterocyclic amines, 43

Favism, 257
  as metabolic food disorder, 272,
    273, 276, 277
Ferulic acid, 112
  as anticarcinogen, 124
Fish:
  broiled:
    low content of heterocyclic
      amines in, 46
    as risk factor in stomach cancer,
      43
  broiling, as source of mutagens, 32
  charred, as potential carcinogen, 46
  cod:
    as common allergenic food in
      Scandinavia, 264
    as source of allergen M, 264, 265
  as a common allergenic food, 263
  gastric formation of N-nitroso
    compounds with, 46
  mercury in, 400, 401
  oils, as inhibitors of tumor forma-
    tion, 117
  smoked:
    nonvolatile nitroso compounds
      in, 86
    and stomach cancer, 102
  tolerance for PCBs in, 401
  volatile nitrosamines in, 71, 75
Folpet:
  dose-response assessment, 212
  EPA classification as probable hu-
    man carcinogen, 212
  exposure assessment, 212
  hazard identification, 212
  mutagenicity of, 212
  risk characterization, 212, 213
  risk estimate, 220
  use as a fungicide, 211
Food and Drug Administration, 1, 2,
    397–405
Food, Drug, and Cosmetic Act, 398
Foods:
  common allergenic, 263, 264
  fried in tallow, cholesterol oxida-

tion products in, 311
  smoked, polynuclear aromatic hy-
    drocarbons in, 211
Free radicals:
  in bioactivation of mutagens and
    carcinogens, 172, 173
  protection against, 172, 173
Fruits:
  citrus,
    lack of involvement in true food
      allergies, 263
    as source of Folpet, 211, 212
  source of nitrate, 65
Fungi:
  climatic conditions for growth of,
    22
  toxigenic, 13
Fusarium, 13

Gallic acid, as an anticarcinogen, 124
Garlic, as a source of organosulfur
    compounds, 116
Glucocorticoids, in retarding tumor
    development, 8
Glucuronyl transferase, 108, 355, 357,
    362, 370
Glu-P-1:
  carcinogenicity of, 36, 37
  mutagenicity of,
    in Chinese hamster lung cells, 40,
      41
    in *Salmonella typhimurium,* 39
  structure of, 34
Glu-P-2:
  carcinogenicity of, 36, 37
  mutagenicity of,
    in Chinese hamster lung cells,
      40, 41
    in *Salmonella typhimurium,* 39
  structure of, 34
Glutathione, 170
  in cellular nonprotein thiols, 183
  effect of BHA administration on,
    186

Glutathione (*cont'd.*)
  as an electrophile scavenger, 170,
    171, 177, 178
  intracellular content of, 176
  liver content of, 177, 185
  maintenance of, 177
  as a metabolic cofactor, 358–360
  mitochondrial pool of, 183
  in protection against oxidative
    damage, 188–191
  as substrate for glutathione peroxi-
    dase/reductase, 173, 174
Glutathione peroxidase, 104, 112, 170,
  173, 174, 186–189
Glutathione reductase, 108, 170, 173,
  174, 186
Glutathione-S-transferase, 104, 107,
  108, 116, 127, 170, 178, 179, 189
  355, 357, 358, 360
  enhanced activity by BHA feeding,
    185
  specificity for glutathione, 178
Goods, baked, as source of nitrite, 66

Heme, as inhibitor of mutagenicity of
  heterocyclic amines, 43
Hemin, as inhibitor of mutagenicity
  of heterocyclic amines, 43
HERP (human exposure dose/rodent
  potency dose), 208, 417
Histamine:
  as mediator of allergic reactions,
    259, 260
  role in histamine poisoning, 271,
    273
Honey, 230
  per capita consumption, 231
Horseradish, as source of allyl isothiocyanate, 211, 216
Hydrogen peroxide, 103, 170, 173
  role in microsomal lipid peroxi-
    dation, 191
Hydroperoxides, organic, metabolism
  of, 189, 191
Hydroxyl radical, 103, 128, 173, 191

Hyperactivity:
  and artificial food colors, 237, 257,
    278, 279
  in children, 225
  effects of aspartame, 234, 235
  effects of sucrose, 237, 238
  and salicylates, 237
Hypercholesterolemia, 317–320
Hypoglycemia, reactive,
  and diet, 236
  prevalence in criminal populations,
    239, 240

Ice cream, cholesterol oxidation products in, 314
Identification, hazard:
  of allyl isothiocyanate, 216
  of ethylene dibromide, 214
  of Folpet, 212
  of polycyclic aromatic hydrocar-
    bons, 215
  of safrole, 217, 218
Imbalance, nutritional, 1
Indoles:
  as anticarcinogens, 114, 115
  effect on aflatoxin B1-DNA adduct
    formation, 129–132
  induction of glutathione-S-transfer-
    ase, 360
  as inhibitors and promoters of car-
    cinogenesis, 133, 134
  structures of, 115
Infarction, myocardial, in atherosclerosis, 298, 320
Infection:
  and cancer deaths, 206
  chronic hepatitis B virus, and car-
    cinogenicity of aflatoxin, 16,
    21–23
  incidence of, 21
Intake:
  estimated dietary aflatoxin, 17
  excessive caloric, as risk factor for
    cancer, 8

total caloric, in enhancement of
carcinogenesis, 6–8
total energy, in enhancement of
carcinogenesis, 6–8
total fat, in enhancement of carcinogenesis, 8
Intermediates, reactive, covalent binding of, 183, 184
Intolerance, lactose, 257
diagnosis of, 274
effect of age on, 274
metabolic defect in, 274
as metabolic food disorder, 272, 273
prevalence of, 274
symptoms of, 274
tolerance for lactose in, 275
treatment of, 275
Intoxications, allergy-like, 256
Iodine, maternal, deficiency of and
brain development, 227
IQ, 32
atherosclerotic effect of, 46
carcinogenicity of, 36, 37
mutagenicity of,
in Chinese hamster lung cells, 40,
41
in *Salmonella typhimurium,* 35, 39
structure of, 33
suppression of carcinogenicity by
quercitin, 43
Iron, deficiency of:
and diminished neuropsychological
function, 227
effect on metabolism of xenobiotics, 369
Isothiocyanates, as anticarcinogens,
116, 122, 127

Juices, fruit, as source of nitrate, 65

Kale, as source of allyl isothiocyanate,
216

Lead:
effects on neuropsychological function, 227, 228
in pottery, as an environmental
contaminant, 401
Lettuce, as a source of Folpet, 211,
212
Level, concern, in FDA's Redbook,
410–416
Linoleic acid, derivatives of, as anticarcinogens, 5
Linoleic acid hydroperoxides, as inducer of atherosclerosis, 304
Lipids, oxidized,
dietary, effect on xenobiotic metabolism, 365, 366
role of, in atherosclerosis, 310–316
Lipoproteins:
low-density,
and diet, 317
oxidized and modified, 315, 316
role in atherogenesis, 315–317
high-density, and atherosclerosis,
317
Lobster:
allergens in, 265, 266
as a common allergenic food, 263

Magnesium, dietary, effects on xenobiotic metabolism, 369, 370
Malnutrition:
chronic protein-energy, effect on
brain development and cognitive functioning, 226
effect on drug uptake and distribution, 352, 353
effect of excretion of xenobiotics,
373
forms of, 241, 242
protein-energy,
effect on absorption of toxicants,
344
effect on xenobiotic metabolism,
363, 364
Management, risk, definition of, 209

Margins, safety, as estimated by 1/R values, 414–416
Meat:
  broiled, polynuclear aromatic hydrocarbons in, 211
  charred surfaces of, as mutagenic, 32
  and colon cancer, 4
  creatinine in, 32
  cured,
    nitrate in, 65–67
    nitrite in, 66, 67, 90
    nonvolatile nitrosamines in, 86
    occurrence of nitrosamines in, 57
    as source of urinary N-nitrosoproline, 80–82
    volatile nitrosamines in, 71
  fresh, as source of nitrite, 66
  fried, and pancreatic cancer, 102
  smoked,
    nonvolatile nitrosamines in, 86
    as source of mutagens, 32
Mercury:
  effects on neuropsychological function, 227, 228
  in swordfish, as an added substance, 400
Metabolism:
  comparative, in quantitative risk assessment, 433
  hepatic toxicant-drug, 355–370
  xenobiotic, regulation by dietary factors, 359
Microorganisms:
  dangerous, 2
  oral, role in nitrite formation, 64
Milk:
  acidophilus, in treatment of lactose intolerance, 276
  cows':
    as a common allergenic food, 263
    as source of allergens, 264, 265
    dried, volatile nitrosamines in, 71
    evaporated, cholesterol oxidation products in, 314
    lactose-hydrolyzed, in treatment of lactose intolerance, 275
    tolerance for PCBs in, 401
    whole, cholesterol oxidation products in, 314
Minerals, trace,
  depletion of, effects on xenobiotic metabolism, 369, 370
  essentiality for development and function of brain, 227
Models, mathematical, of dose-response, 210
Modulators, of carcinogenesis, 3, 104, 120–123, 135
Monosodium glutamate:
  and asthma, 272, 278
  attitudes toward, 425
    trends in, 426
  and Chinese restaurant syndrome, 257, 272, 278, 279
  concern about, 426
Mortality:
  annual summaries of cancer, 2
  trends in cancer, 2
MTD (maximum tolerated dose):
  in quantitative risk assessment, 434
  in toxicological testing, 416
Mushrooms, poisonous, 399
Mustard, as source of allyl isothiocyanate, 211, 216
Mutagens:
  cellular defense against, 170
  in cooked foods, 31, 44
Mutton, broiled, heterocyclic amines in, 45
Mycophenolic acid, 11
Mycotoxins:
  carcinogenic, 13, 14, 23–25
  chemical structure vs. biological activity, 14
  control of, in prevention of human liver cancer, 24, 25
  in foods, 11–14
  role in esophageal cancer, 24

NADPH:
  effect of ethanol intake on, 366
  as a metabolic cofactor, 358, 360
NADPH-cytochrome P-450 reductase,
    191, 355, 356
NADPH (quinone acceptor) oxido-
    reductase, 186
Neurotransmitters, precursor control
    of, 228–230
Nitrate, 57, 58
  absorption of, 67
  attitudes toward, 425
    trends in, 426
  content of, in saliva, 78
  de novo synthesis of, 64, 68, 85
    from ammonia, 70
    from arginine, 70
  endogenous formation of, 58, 64,
    67–70
  in the immune system, 92
  human exposure to, from food and
    water, 64–67, 85, 91
  intake and increased risk of gastric
    cancer, 77, 78
  metabolism of, 67–70
  as reservoir of nitrite, 61
Nitric oxide, 60, 61
Nitrite, 57, 58
  endogenous formation of, 64, 67–70
  human exposure to, from food, 64
  level in saliva, 68, 78
  metabolism of, 67
  rate of loss from stomach, 88, 89
  reaction with ascorbic acid, 89
  from reduction of nitrate,
    by oral microorganisms, 61, 64,
      68, 85, 90
    by the immune system, 85, 92
  synthesis from arginine, 70
Nitrogen:
  chemistry of, 60
  oxidation states of, 60, 61
  oxides of, 60
Nitrogen dioxide, 60
N-Nitrosamide, 58, 62, 63

direct-acting carcinogens, 63, 64
endogenous formation of, 64, 82
general structure of, 59
Nitrosamine, 124
  activation to carcinogens of, 63
  carcinogenic, 73
  exposure to exogenous, 74, 75
  exposure of smokers, 71
  formation of, in bacon and beer, 71
  general structures of, 59
  in initiation of chemical carcino-
    genesis, 206
  metabolism of, 78, 79
  nonvolatile, 58, 62
  in smokeless tobacco, 72
  volatile, 58, 73, 74, 76, 86, 90, 91
    in foods, 71
Nitrosation, 59
  of amines and amides, 60
  chemistry of, in the stomach, 76
  endogenous, 78–92
    effect of ascorbic acid on, 83, 84
    factors affecting, 82–85
    influence of gastric pH on, 83
    thiocyanate as catalyst for, 85
  of fava beans, 77
  gastric,
    kinetic model for, 88
    simulated, 76
  inhibition of, ascorbate-mediated,
    61
N-Nitroso compounds, 57
  biological activity of, 62
  biological markers of exposure to,
    86, 87
  carcinogenic, 59, 71, 87–89, 91, 124
  carcinogenicity of, 62, 70
  endogenous formation of, 58, 76, 77,
    84, 86–90
  exposure to,
    from endogenous vs. exogenous
      sources, 85–91
    from exogenous sources, 70–76,
      86
  in food and drink, 71

N-Nitroso compounds (*cont'd.*)
  formation of, 58, 61
  interspecies differences in organ
    sites of carcinogenicity of, 64
  involvement in human cancer, 64
  link to oral cancer from tobacco
    snuff, 64
  nonvolatile, 71–74
  precursors to, 62
    and risk of cancer, 76, 77
  structure-activity relationships for,
    64
  in tobacco products, 71
  volatile, 71, 72
N-Nitrosoamino acids:
  gastric formation of, 76
  noncarcinogenic, 58
  precursors of, 80
  in urine, 79–81
N-Nitrosodiethylamine (*see also*
    diethylnitrosamine), 63
  in cigarette smoke, 75
  gastric formation of, 76
  mutagenicity of, 39
  in smokeless tobacco, 72
N-Nitrosodimethylamine (*see also* di-
    methylnitrosamine), 120, 124,
    127
  in beer, 75
  in cheese, 75
  in cigarette smoke, 75
  in dried foods, 75
  endogenous formation of, 79, 80
  in fish, 75
  in fried bacon, 75
  gastric formation of, 76
  as a liver carcinogen, 64
  metabolic activation of, 87
  metabolic products of, 78, 79
  mutagenicity of, 39
  in occupational environments, 71,
    75
  in smokeless tobacco, 72
  uptake of, by hepatocytes, 374

N-Nitrosoproline:
  endogenous formation of, 88, 89
  in smokeless tobacco, 73
  urinary excretion of, 79–82, 84, 90
N-Nitrosopyrrolidine, 120, 124
  in cigarette smoke, 75
  in fried bacon, 75
  in smokeless tobacco, 72
N-Nitrosothiazolidine carboxylic
    acid:
  in bacon, 72
  in urine, 79
Nitrous acid, 61
Nitrous anhydride, 61
Nivalenol, 11
  structure of, 12
Nutmeg, as a source of safrole, 217
Nutrition, role of, in health and dis-
    ease prevention, 331, 332
Nuts, tree, as common allergenic
    foods, 263

Oats, as a cause of celiac disease, 270
Ochratoxin, 11
Ochratoxin A, 11
  carcinogenicity of, 16
  as initiator and promoter of tumors,
    23
  structure of, 12
Oils:
  fish:
    as inhibitors of tumor formation,
      117
    in reducing platelet aggregation
      and arterial spasm, 320
  peanut, soybean, and sunflower, as
    non-allergenic, 269
  processed, 2
Oncogenes, role of, 207
Onions, as a source of organosulfur
    compounds, 116
Oranges, as a source of Folpet, 211,
    212

Organosulfur compounds, as anticarcinogens, 116
Oxidase, mixed function (*see also*
cytochromee P-450 monooxygenases), 355–357
effect of dietary protein on, 362, 363
effect of starvation on, 360, 361
induction by naturally occurring
plant constituents, 359, 360
Oxides, of nitrogen, reactions and
equilibria, 62
Oxygen:
bioactivation of, 173
free radical oxidant species of, 170
as contributors to cellular injury,
170
Oysters, as a common allergenic food,
263

Papain, as a cause of true food allergy, 258
Parabens, as a cause of urticaria, 283
Patulin, 11
structure of, 12
as a tumor promoter, 23
Peach, in exercise-induced food al-
lergy, 261
Peanuts:
allergenicity of products made
from, 269
allergens in, 265, 266
as a common allergenic food, 263
Peas, green, allergens in, 265, 267
Pellagra, and psychosis, 227
Penicillic acid, 11
structure of, 12
Penicillin, as food contaminant caus-
ing true food allergies, 258
Penicillium, 13
Penitrem A, 11
Pepper, black, as a source of safrole,
217
Perception, public, 1

Peroxidation, lipid, 104
microsomal, 191
NADPH-dependent, 191
thiol-dependent, 181
Pesticides, 2
chlorinated hydrocarbon, as tumor
promoters, co-carcinogens, and
weak carcinogens, 117
as source on N-nitroso compounds,
70, 73
Phenolics, plant,
as anticarcinogens, 112–114
structures of, 113
Phenylalanine:
plasma, elevation after aspartame
intake, 234
as precursor of catecholamines,
233
Polychlorinated biphenyls (PCBs):
established tolerances for, in milk
and fish, 401
as tumor promoters, co-carcinogens, and weak carcinogens,
117
uptake by hepatocytes, 374
Polynuclear aromatic hydrocarbons,
211
carcinogenic, 214
dose-response assessment, 215
exposure assessment, 215
hazard identification, 215
human exposure to, 214, 215
risk characterization, 215, 216
risk estimate, 220
Products, cholesterol oxidation:
absorption of, 302
in atherosclerosis, 305–307, 309–311,
315, 316, 320–323
in foods, 311–315
in ghee, 304
inhibition of HMG CoA reductase
by, 301
mutagenicity of, 301
in serum lipoproteins, 315

Products, lipid oxidation:
    in the initiation and promotion of
        atherosclerosis, 297–308, 310,
        311, 315, 316
Products, spray-dried dairy, choles-
    terol oxidation products in, 313
Prolactin, in promotion of mammary
    cancer, 8
Promoters, tumor, 3
    in foods, 117–120
Promotion, tumor:
    by cyclamate, 155–157, 160, 161
    by saccharin, 155, 157–161
Prooxidants, endogenously produced,
    103
Proposition 65, California, 402–405,
    422–424, 433
Propyl gallate:
    as modulator of carcinogenesis, 104
    structure of, 105
Protease inhibitors, as antitumor
    agents, 116, 122, 127
Protection:
    afforded by cytochrome P-450
        monooxygenases, 183
    cellular aspects of, 184–191
    against electrophiles, 170–172
    against free radicals, 172, 173
    against oxygen-mediated toxicity,
        173, 174
    against quinones, 189, 190
    types of, 173–184
    water and cellular, 173
PR toxin, 11

Quercitin, 112
    as inhibitor of carcinogenicity of
        IQ, 43
Quinones, protection against, 189, 190

Reaction, nitrosation, 59
Reactions:
    anaphylactoid, 256, 257, 271
        causative substances of, 272
        histamine poisoning as an ex-
            ample of, 271

idiosyncratic, 257, 271
    categories of, 278
    causative substances of, 272
    list of food-associated, 278
    role of specific foods in, 279
    metabolic, 256
Regulation:
    of naturally occurring substances in
        food, 398–400
    under Proposition 65, 402–405
    of substances added to food, 400–
        402
Research:
    diet-behavior, criteria for evalu-
        ation, 244
    nutrient-behavior, guidelines for,
        243–245
Residues, pesticide, 2
Rhubarb, oxalic acid in, 398
Riboflavin, deficiency of, effect on
    xenobiotic metabolism, 367
Rice, allergens in, 265, 267
Risk:
    definition of, 409
    de minimis, 401
    estimates, upper-bound, 220
    Q1* as statement of, 212, 213
Rugulosin, as initiator and promoter
    of tumors, 23
Rye, as a cause of celiac disease, 270

Saccharin, 151, 444, 445
    attitudes toward, 425
        trends in, 426
    carcinogenicity of, 153, 154
    mechanism of tumor promotion by,
        159, 160
    as promoter of bladder tumors, 155,
        157–161
    sweetness of, 152
    TD_{50}, 15
Safety, absolute, as limitation in toxi-
    cology testing, 420
Safrole, 211
    dose-response assessment, 218

epoxidation of, 356
exposure assessment, 218
hazard identification, 217, 218
induction of cytochrome P-450, 360
risk characterization, 218
risk estimate, 220
TD_{50}, 15
Salicylates, and childhood hyperactivity, 237
Salicylic acid, absorption of, 341
Sardines, broiled, as a source of mutagens, 32, 35
Sassafras, oil of, as source of safrole, 217
Scallops, as a common allergenic food, 263
Selenium:
   as an anticarcinogen, 104, 106, 111, 112, 127
   as prosthetic group of glutathione peroxidase, 112, 187, 188
Sensitivities, food,
   definition of, 256
   as explanation of nutrition-behavior connection, 236
   immunological, 256, 257
   nonimmunological, 257, 271
   causative substances of, 272
Sensitivity, food:
   incidence of, 255
   primary, 256
   secondary, 256
Serotonin:
   effects on behavior of animals, 229
   as a neurotransmitter, 228, 229
Sesame seeds, allergens in, 267
Shellfish:
   as cause of anaphylactoid reactions, 272
   in exercise-induced food allergy, 261
Shrimp:
   allergens in, 265, 266
   as a common allergenic food, 263
Smoking, 335
   as cancer risk factor, 31

cigarette, as cause of lung cancer, 205, 206
Snuff, tobacco,
   link to oral cancer, 64, 71
   N-nitroso compounds in, 71
Sour cream, cholesterol oxidation products in, 314
Soybeans:
   allergens in, 265, 267
   as a common allergenic food, 263
   in Japan, 264
Sterigmatocystin, 11, 15
   as an animal carcinogen, 16
   as initiator and promoter of tumors, 23
Steroids, as co-carcinogens and promoters, 117
trans-Stilbene oxide, as enzyme inducing agent, 187
Strategy, anticancer, 8
Strawberries:
   as cause of anaphylactoid reactions, 272, 273
   lack of involvement in true food allergies, 263
Sucralose, sweetness of, 152
Sucrose (see also sugar):
   in fruits, cereals, and vegetables, 230
   and hyperactivity, 225, 238
   ingestion of, and antisocial behavior, 239
Sugar (see also sucrose):
   and behavior, 236–240, 272, 278
   and breast cancer, 102
   date, as a nutritive sweetener, 230
   and hyperkinesis, 257
   intake of, and hyperactivity, 238
   interaction of, with juvenile delinquent behavior, 240
   per capita consumption of, in developed countries, 232
   refined, per capita consumption of, in U.S., 231
Sulfites, and asthma, 257, 272, 280, 281

Sulfotransferase, 355, 357, 358
Sunset yellow, as a cause of chronic
urticaria, 283
Superoxide anion radical, 103, 128,
173, 188–191
in modification of LDL, 316
quinone-stimulated formation of,
189
Superoxide dismutase, 104, 170, 173,
174, 189, 317
Sweeteners:
artificial, 151
corn, per capita consumption of,
231
nutritive, and behavior, 230–234
total caloric, per capita consumption of, 231

Tallow, heated, cholesterol oxidation
products in, 311
Tannic acid, 112
Tartrazine, as cause of asthma and
urticaria, 272, 278, 279, 282, 283
TD$_{50}$, measure of carcinogenic potency, 208
Testing, toxicology,
amount required, 411–416
Decision Tree as a system for, 408,
409
failure to provide assurance of
safety by, 424
FDA's Redbook and, 409–416
of food and color additives, 409–
416
limitations of, 413–420
lists as, 423
Theory, selective clonal expansion, 23
Thiamin, deficiency of, effect on
xenobiotic metabolism, 367
Thiocyanate, as catalyst of endogenous nitrosation, 85
Thiols:
as electrophile scavengers, 171
nonprotein, 184
in prevention of lipid peroxide formation, 181

in promotion of lipid peroxidation,
181
in protection against free radicals,
179
role in cellular protection, 176–181
Thrombosis, in atherosclerosis, 298,
320, 321
Tobacco:
smokeless, nitrosamine content of,
72, 74, 75
as source of N-nitroso compounds,
70, 71
α-Tocopherol (see also vitamin E):
as anticarcinogen, 108, 110, 124, 125
as chain-breaking antioxidant, 182
in protection against free radicals,
173, 191
Tomatoes, allergens in, 265, 267
Toxicant, reproductive, and Proposition 65, 403, 404, 423
Toxicants, naturally occurring,
concept of threshold dose levels for,
430
as posing acceptable risk, 398
and Proposition 65, 403
ordinarily injurious safety standard
for, 398–400
Toxicology, interactions with politics,
422–424
Toxins, microbial, 2
Trichothecenes, 11
Trp-P-1:
carcinogenicity of, 36, 37
as monoamine oxidase inhibitor, 46
as mutagen, 32
mutagenicity of,
in Chinese hamster lung cells, 40,
41
in Salmonella typhimurium, 39
structure of, 34
Trp-P-2:
carcinogenicity of, 36, 37
as monoamine oxidase inhibitor,
46
as mutagen, 32
mutagenicity of,

in Chinese hamster lung cells, 40, 41
in *Salmonella typhimurium,* 39
structure of, 34
Tryptophan:
and behavior in rats, 229
plasma, changes with carbohydrate consumption, 228
as precursor of serotonin, 228
sedative-like effects of, 230
Turkey:
dehydrated, cholesterol oxidation products in, 314
precooked, cholesterol oxidation products in, 311, 312
Tyrosine:
influence on brain catecholamine levels, 229
and improved performance, 230
plasma, effect of aspartame intake, 233

Urethane, 104, 123, 127
TD_{50}, 15
Uric acid, in protection against free radicals, 173

Vegetables:
green and yellow, and colon cancer, 4
nitrate in, 65–67, 90
nitrite in, 66, 67
Vitamin A:
as anticarcinogen, 110, 111
depletion of, effect on mixed function oxidase activities, 368
Vitamin C (*see also* ascorbic acid), 170
deficiency of, effect on drug metabolism, 367, 368
as inhibitor of nitrosation, 82, 110
as modifier of carcinogenesis, 104, 110
protection from nitrate by, 78
structure of, 109

Vitamin E (*see also* α-tocopherol), 170
as anticarcinogen, 104, 106, 108, 110
deficiency of, decrease in mixed function oxidase activities, 368, 369
as inhibitor of lipid peroxidation, 181, 182
as inhibitor of tumor promotion, 108
RDA of, 110
structure of, 109, 181
Vitamins, effect on the mixed function oxidase system, 367–369

Water:
contaminated, nitrate in, 65–67
drinking, carcinogenic nitrosamines in, 73, 75
participation in cellular protection, 173, 175
as substrate for epoxide hydrolases, 175
Wheat:
as cause of celiac disease, 270
as a common allergenic food, 263
in exercise-induced food allergy, 261
Whiskies, as source of polynuclear aromatic hydrocarbons, 211

Xenobiotics:
absorption of, 333–345
effects of food on, 344, 345
analysis of, 419
distribution of, 345–353
elimination of, 353–376
excretion of, 370–376
exposure to, 331
metabolism of, 353–370
effect of starvation, 360, 361

Yogurt:
cholesterol oxidation products in, 314
in treatment of lactose intolerance, 276

Zearalenol, 11
Zearalenone, 11
  structure of, 12

Zinc, inadequate, and changes in
  neurotransmitter levels, 227